Getting Your ADL Groove in Gear with PAPS: Preparing for Surgery

Getting Your ADL Groove in Gear with PAPS: Preparing for Surgery

Living Your Life after Surgery

LARRY CIPOLLA

Getting Your ADL Grove in Gear With PAPS: Preparing for Surgery
Living Your Life After Surgery

Larry Cipolla
Life-long Learner, Life-long Gardener

© 2020 Cipolla Companies, Inc.,
CCi Gardening Connections. All rights reserved.

No part of this book may be used or reproduced in any manner whatsoever without the prior written permission of the author except in the case of brief quotations embodied in critical articles or reviews. While we are not vengeful, we are provokable.

This book may be purchased in quantity for educational, business and sales promotion use. Contact *okikumapress@gmail.com*

ISBN: 978-1-6600-9919-1

Publisher: OkiKumaPress, Minnesota, United States of America
Cover: Ralph Hagen and Cartoon Stock.com
Front and back covers and internal graphic layout: Wordzworth, UK
Grammar resources: Chicago Manual of Style, 16th edition.
BISAC: Health & Fitness and Medical General
First Printing: 2020
Font Style: Effra

I dedicate this book to anyone who has had or is thinking about having elective surgery.

To anyone who is feeling apprehensive about whether to have elective surgery.

To those who have wondered why they waited so long to have that elective procedure.

To those who have enduring pain, discomfort and the daily aggravation of having to live with a lower quality of life and being less active than they would like to be.

To those who have put off surgery because of their concerns regarding post-surgical rehabilitation protocols due to their current physical condition.

To those who have finally made the decision to have surgery.

And to anyone who has a passion for gardening, sports or other active daily living activities (ADLs) and perhaps agonized a bit about how the surgery and rehabilitation process would affect when and how they could return to their passion as quickly as possible.

PERSEVERANCE: THE FORTUNATE ONE

On a different road I travelled
With lessons many unraveled.
On that road came fame
As worldwide clients came.
Through perseverance and striving,
By doing and not just trying,
With beads of perspiration,
Without doubts or hesitation,
With ups and downs,
With smiles and frowns,
With mistakes enough,
I kept hanging tough.
By doing the work I got it done
And could say I had won,
All the while having fun.
I took the path less traveled by,
And never once had a regret or sigh,
And kept my head held high.
Nor not by sitting on a fence,
But moving way ahead hence
And that made the difference.
And I became the fortunate one,
I, the fortunate second son.

CONTENTS

Perseverance: The Fortunate One	vi
Disclaimer	x
Acknowledgements	xi
Why This Book Now	xii
What You Will Learn	xiii
Structure	xv

MODULE 1 PREPARING YOUR MIND AND BODY	**1**
Overview	1
Elective Surgery	2
Arthritis	4
Pain Management	9
Non-Surgical Options	11
Behavior Change and You	26
Module Summary	34
Your Notes	36

MODULE 2 PREPARING YOUR INSIDE WORLD	**37**
Overview	37
Sports Envy Have I	38
Organizing Your Indoor Space	44
Navigating after Surgery	53
Module Summary	63
Your Notes	65

MODULE 3 PREPARING YOUR OUTSIDE WORLD	**67**
Overview	68
Planning for after Surgery before Surgery	68
Extending Your Season	77
Container Options	82
Ergonomic Toys and Tools	100
pH and Plant Care	104

Module Summary	107
Your Notes	110

MODULE 4   PREPARING YOUR WATER WORLD   111

Overview	111
Hydroponic Gardening	112
DWC: The Passive Hydroponic System	120
Plant Options	142
Module Summary	148
Your Notes	152

MODULE 5   COLLABORATING WITH YOUR MEDICAL CARE-TEAM   153

Overview	153
Butts, Binging, Boozing and You	154
Whom to Trust	160
Communication and You	166
Surgery: Go or No Go	170
Module Summary	177
Self-Directed Action Plans (SDAPS)	178
Your Notes	179
My Self-Directed Action Plan	180

MODULE 6   EXERCISING FOR YOUR PRE- POST-CONDITIONING   183

Overview	184
Terms of Movement: Range of Motion	185
Exercises for Body Parts	189
Module Summary	224
Your Notes	226

APPENDICES   227

MODULE A1   PREPARING MIND AND BODY   229

Arthritis: Natural Remedies	229
C and A Words	231

MODULE A2   PREPARING YOUR INSIDE WORLD   235

Mobility Devices and Aids	235
Re-Organizing Where You Live	235
Preventing Falls	236

MODULE A3 PREPARING YOUR OUTSIDE WORLD	**239**
Yard and Gardening Benefits	240
Beware: Botanicals and Allergies	241
Critter Control and You	246
MODULE A4 PREPARING YOUR WATER WORLD	**253**
Foodies for Food	253
Food and Ailments	256
Hydroponics	260
MODULE A5 COLLABORATING WITH YOUR CARE-TEAM	**273**
Your Guide to Elective Surgery	273
Post-Surgery Protocol	274
Force Field Analysis: Making Decisions	277
MODULE A6 PROTOCOL EXERCISES	**279**
Do Not Make Resolutions	279
Low-No Sweat Exercises	280
Stretch Exercises: Sitting or Standing	285
Exercises to Avoid	290
Non-Food Diet for Weight Loss and Conditioning	291
Exercise Machines	295
Bibliography	**299**
General References	299
Gardening References	300
Arthritis References	303
Collaborating with Your Care-Team	303
Long and Ridiculously Long Urls	305
Index	**307**
A Last Word or Two	**309**
Biography of Author	**311**
Other books by the author	311

DISCLAIMER

I am not a surgeon or physician. I am not a medical person. I am a quasi-bionic person having had multiple (five and counting) orthopedic surgeries and some soft-tissue procedures (four and counting). I am a master gardener, a life-long gardener and a life-long learner. All information included in this book is provided as a courtesy service to you. All recommendations should not be substituted for direct professional advice from your personal physician and medical team. Contact your medical-care team about any of the recommendations and exercises identified in this book. I do not know your specific situation. Your medical team will be more familiar with your condition and the procedure they have (or will have) identified for you and your post-surgery protocol. Establishing a collaborative dialog with your team would be wise thing to do.

ACKNOWLEDGEMENTS

Thank you Allina Health Systems, Twin City Orthopedics and Sports Orthopedics with their superb surgeons, physicians, fantastic nurses, nurses' aides and physical therapists who endured my requests to push my exercise routine and encouraged me during my rehabilitation process. A special thank you to my orthopedic surgeon who encouraged me to write this book.

CREDITS

All poems and photos are from the author unless otherwise noted and credited. Other photographs, illustrations, cartoons and quotations are from the public domain and free online sources and are noted within the text or in the extensive bibliography. A special thank you and gratitude to cartoonists Bill Abbott, Tim Dolighan, Joseph Farris, Ed Fischer, Randy Glasbergen, Christophe 'Hagen' Granet, Dave Granlund, Seppo Leinonen, Astkhik Rakimova, Jeff Stahler and John Wagner.

WHY THIS BOOK NOW

This is your guide to helping you prepare for and recover from an elective surgical procedure. There are different types of elective surgeries. The focus in this book is on joint-related procedures brought on by arthritis, sports injuries, long-suffering pain or other issues. Pro-active preparations (PAPS) ahead of your scheduled procedure can help you cope with surgery and for completing your post-surgical rehabilitation protocol and get back to your daily living activities (ADLs).

This book is about thinking through, planning and implementing some important and practical tasks *before* surgery so you can return to and enjoy your ADLs *after* surgery with less stress and frustration. All the exercises described and illustrated in this book are low-impact and could be easily integrated into your pre-surgery preparations and your post-surgery protocols. Implementing these recommendations and those you receive from your care-team could help you become better prepared, mentally and physically, for your surgical procedure.

You cannot control or do the actual surgery. Surgeons tend to prefer to do that for you. What you can control is what you do before and after surgery. And that is what this book is all about. Whether you are having elective orthopedic surgery or any other type of surgical procedure that requires rest and rehabilitation for a period of time, planning ahead, prioritizing and implementing what you could be doing before that surgery can relieve almost any anxiety level you may be having about when and how you will be able to return to your ADLs.

This book is about accessibility and your active daily living activities, your ADLs. Your ADLs make up your lifestyle, whether it is gardening, playing cards or board games, sports activities or fitness classes. The PAPS (Pro-Active Preparations) in this book can help you better prepare for an upcoming procedure by providing you with practical tips and best-practices, so you can get your life-style in gear sooner and as comfy as possible. G*etting Your ADL Groove in Gear with PAPS: Preparing for Surgery,* will help you prepare for what you could be doing inside and outside your living space before entering the operating room.

WHAT YOU WILL LEARN

This is a comprehensive practical guide and reference book. Through six easy-to-read modules and hundreds of photos, diagrams, charts and illustrations, the author clearly identifies how you can get your ADL groove back safely and how to maintain positive behavior changes after surgery to keep you in better condition to do whatever it is that you want to do.

Would you like to learn how to have less pain from an arthritic condition? Are you interested in non-surgical options that you can use while waiting for your surgery? (re: **Module One)**?

Are you looking for simple, practical ways to organize your home and make it safer and more accessible while you recover from surgery? Will you need to learn how to navigate with crutches or a wheel-chair or other assistive aids during your rehab period (re: **Module Two)**?

Are you interested in ideas for making your outdoor world safer and more accessible while reducing the time and energy you spend maintaining that world after surgery (re: **Module Three)**?

Would you like to return to gardening within days (yes, days) of your release from your medical-care facility using a proven, low-cost alternative to soil-based practices (re: **Module Four)**?

Have you tried to lose weight, quit smoking or cut back on your alcohol consumption with fad-diets or other programs without much long-term success? Would you like to cut through the *fog factor* while communicating with your care-team by asking specific questions and understanding what types of questions they typically ask you (re: **Module Five)**?

Would you like to learn which low-impact exercises you can easily do while sitting, lying down or standing, regardless of your weight or age or physical condition and whether you are at home, at work or at your club? Would you like to learn how a wide range of strength and flexibility exercises targeted to specific body parts could help your running or swimming or softball or golf or tennis game and keep you in better shape for whatever sport or non-sport activity you are involved in (re: **Module Six)**?

Would you like to learn how some botanicals may not be as safe as advertised? Or, discover which veggies and fruit contain the most residual pesticides? Or, learn how you can reduce your potential exposure to E-coli? Or how Tai Chi and yoga can provide you with greater flexibility and balance? Or go more in depth about what you have read in each module (re: **Appendices** and the **Bibliography)**?

STRUCTURE

There are six modules, each flowing from one to the other. Each can stand on its own. Read the entire book. Read the modules that appeal to you the most. Each module includes a summary of selected key points and provides a quick reference for that module. There are dozens of pictures, illustrations, cartoons, quotations and poems to reinforce key points throughout the book.

Each module focuses on accessibility and flexibility and what you can do prior to and after your elective surgical procedure. We start with preparing your body and mind for your upcoming elective procedure. Next, we discuss very practical ways that you can do to organize the inside of your home and how they can help you reduce your pre-surgical stress level. From inside we move outside into your yard and garden and identify how you can achieve greater accessibility and mobility, especially if you require the use of assistive devices such as wheel-chairs, walkers, knee-walkers, crutches or canes.

We move on to an alternative to soil-based gardening that can allow you to return to your ADLs within days after discharge from your medical facility. You will learn how to garden the year-round without having to use hand tools or expensive equipment, materials and supplies.

Lastly, we provide you with a simple **Five-Ws Plus Three** questioning process for communicating with your care-team and a series of illustrated low-impact exercises that you can do at anytime, anywhere. We include specific exercises for your neck and shoulders, elbows, hands and wrists, upper and lower back, lower spine area, hips, knees, ankles and feet. These exercises can help you whether you are a gardener, a dedicated or not so dedicated sports-person, a Tai Chi or yoga or Pilates-person or someone who just prefers to bob up and down in a pool or soak in a hot-tub. And these exercises are for folks who have been a bit adverse to exercising in the past. We make it easy and comfy for you.

Appendices: The six appendices provide you with more information about selected topics covered in each corresponding module, coupled with photographs, tables and charts.

Bibliography: The extensive bibliography can expand your knowledge on a wide range of topics covered in this book.

Index. Cross-references can facilitate your search for a specific topic.

Author Biography. There is a short biography along with a brief description of other books by this author. You are invited to contact the author at *okikumapress@gmail.com* or *larryc7021@gmail.com* with your questions, concerns and feedback.

Thank you for buying my book. I appreciate it very much. Please know that you have done your part to stamp out hunger and poverty. I trust you will find this book informative and very worthwhile and, in the process, learn a lot and read something that will put a smile on your face or maybe even bring out a giggle or two.

MODULE 1

PREPARING YOUR MIND AND BODY

The Focus and Outcomes of this Module are ...

- Osteoarthritis and Elective Surgery
- Non-surgical options and treatments
- Exercises for pain management
- Changing Attitudes and Behaviors

Overview

Many surgical procedures require that you modify your behavior. Everyday activities such as bending, squatting, kneeling, reaching, lifting, turning, squeezing, pulling, pushing and even walking may be a problem for you, depending on what body part gives you the gift of pain that day. And if you do those activities repetitively throughout the day you may find yourself in greater pain and more continuous discomfort. This module can help you prepare yourself mentally and physically for your procedure. The changes to your behavior may be short-term, at least until you have completed your protocol as prescribed by your physician. They could also be long-term and affect how you go about your daily living activities log after your surgery.

You don't realize how much you depend on a body part until the function of that body part is lost or diminished.

Elective Surgery

Elective surgery is a planned affair. You planned for it in advance, certainly weeks and probably months in advance, whether it is for joint repair or replacement for a body part in your neck, shoulders, elbows, wrists, hands, hips, knees, ankles or feet or an internal *soft-tissue* part. You may have scheduled surgery for those body parts because of an arthritic condition which has limited your ability to engage in your ADLs. Perhaps your level of pain has increased beyond the point of tolerance. The procedure you agreed to, whether you were dragged kicking and screaming or not, was a collaborative or quasi-collaborative effort between yourself, your surgeon and perhaps others on your care-team based upon test results, X-rays and conversations with your family and friends and others.

Elective surgery is not a medical or life-threatening emergency. You may have been putting it off. Yet, upon completion of your procedure you certainly should realize a better quality of life with less pain and more mobility.

There are at least three different classifications of elective surgery. *Semi-elective surgery* may need to be done to preserve your life, but it does not need to be performed immediately. That sounds odd, but ... *Urgent surgery* is surgery that can wait until you are medically-stable or a pre-condition has been resolved. By contrast, *non-elective surgery* does involve an urgent medical procedure. It is essential to your survival. Acute appendicitis is an urgent and life-threatening issue. Immediate surgery is critical. A surgery to repair a hernia could be elective if your surgeon recommends that it be done, say, within the month or so. An ulcerated hernia, where a part of the

Surgical Classifications

Diagnostic	Curative	Elective/Therapeutic	Palliative
Goal to identify the nature or cause of disease	Aim to cure potentially life threatening condition, prolong life	Aim to cure non life threatening condition, may relieve pain or distress if underlying condition is not life threatening	Goal to relieve pain or distress with no attempt to cure the underlying condition
Examples	**Examples**	**Examples**	**Examples**
▪ Cystoscopy ▪ Hysteroscopy ▪ Biopsy ▪ Cervical Mediastinoscopy ▪ Colonoscopy	▪ Resection/Excision of mass/cancer/tumor ▪ Coronary Artery Bypass Graft surgery ▪ Valve repair/replacement ▪ Transplant	▪ Joint Replacement ▪ Reconstruction ▪ Uterine Fibroid surgery ▪ Gastric bypass	▪ Pleurex catheter placement ▪ Esophageal dilation ▪ Ureteral stent placement ▪ Suprapubic tube placement

intestine bulges from that herniated area would probably not be considered elective, but a condition that should be treated immediately.

These types of surgeries can extend your life or improve your physical or psychological well-being. Some examples of elective surgery include, but are not limited to, cosmetic and reconstructive procedures. While not life-threatening they can improve your self-esteem and confidence. Cataract surgery, liposuction, a face-lift or tummy-tuck or breast reduction or enhancement are other examples of optional, elective procedures.

Are you coping with pain
With no energy drain?
If so, your head may say no,
But if yes, your head says go.
Your quality of life
Is better without strife.
And your body will thank you.
That I surely do know.

So why bother with elective surgery? It is simple: one or more of your body parts is not functioning properly. Your body is telling you that it needs to be fixed. You find it difficult or at least a bit bothersome to do what you like to do when you want to do it. Your situation is causing you pain. You want the pain to go away. You want to enjoy a better lifestyle or at least have the option of being as active as you want without being hostage to the pain and malfunctioning body part(s). You may also want to be able to socialize and engage with your family and friends more actively than you are able to do now.

No doubt, your first hope will be to have a pill or an injection that will cure what ails you and make everything all nice and better. No surgery. No hospital stays. No rehab. No big hospital bills. Nice thoughts, but not always realistic. Pills and injections are short-term remedies at best. They can mask your pain, but the problem will still be there. Rather than putting off the inevitable, it may be wise to sign up for the surgery your doctor has recommended. Go for the long-term solution. And, of course, you may have already decided to do just that.

Procrastination makes easy things hard,
hard things harder.

—MASON COOLEY

Orthopedic Surgery: a brief history. Generally, elective orthopedic surgery and arthritis go together. Orthopedic surgery or orthopedics is a type of surgery associated with the musculoskeletal system in your body. Surgeons can choose to use surgical and nonsurgical procedures for different diseases, infections, tumors, injuries to joints and bones and congenital issues.

Wartime and war related injuries influenced the treatment of certain injuries. During the Middle Ages injured warriors were said to be treated with cloth or bandages soaked in *horses' blood* which then dried to form a stiff, but unsanitary splint. I understand they do not do that anymore, which is very nice to know. Maybe even the horse thought that was nice to know.

The word orthopedic comes from the Greek words *correct* and *child* – correcting musculoskeletal deformities in children. Nichols Andry, a professor at the University of Paris, coined the word in French, in 1741.

The use of arthroscopic techniques was developed in the early 1950s by Dr. Masaki Watanabe of Japan. The goal was to perform minimally invasive cartilage surgery and reconstruction of torn ligaments (soft tissue repair). Arthroplasty is a more involved elective process where a musculoskeletal joint is replaced, remodeled or realigned. This surgery can help relieve pain and restore joint function caused by arthritis or other types of joint trauma. Joint replacements are typically used with knees, hips, shoulders, elbows, wrists, ankles, spine, and finger joints.

Total hip replacement was pioneered by Sir John Charnley in the 1960s, who designed a stainless-steel one-piece femoral stem and head and a polyethylene component secured to the bone with bone cement. His invention formed the basis for all modern hip replacements.

Arthritis

Arthritis is Non-Discriminatory. When you wake in the morning do you feel a bit stiff and experience some pain? Does it take your knees a while to get started? Chances are that one of the primary reasons is because the pain and stiffness you experience is caused by arthritis. There are different types of arthritic conditions. All are equal-opportunity afflictions. They can affect anyone at almost any age.

Millions of Americans (and a whole bunch more around the world) need some type of orthopedic procedure. Severe arthritis could have adversely affected your joints to the point where now surgery is a given. The CDC (Center for Disease Control) estimates that fifty-two million people are diagnosed with arthritis every year. Thirty-percent are between the ages of 45 and 64; forty-nine-percent are over age 65. *Osteoarthritis (OA)* is the most common form of arthritis. OA is also known as degenerative joint disease. According to the *Centers for Disease Control and Prevention (CDC)*, about 30 million adults in the United States have OA. That makes OA one of the leading causes of disability in adults. Yet, arthritis is not necessarily an adult or senior affliction.

Always remember that you are absolutely unique,
Just like everyone else.

—MARGARET MEAD

Arthritis can affect any joint in your body. Joints form the connections between your bones. Joints support you and help you move around. Damage to your joints, whether from disease or an injury, can impede that movement and affect your lifestyle. Joint pain is very common. Knee pain seems to be the most common in folks, regardless of age. Joint pain can range from being an irritant to debilitating. Joint pain can include different types of arthritis, bursitis, gout, strains, sprains and a whole host of injuries, sports related and otherwise.

Arthritis is an all-encompassing label used to describe different diseases or processes. Wear and tear of the joints can cause damage to the cartilage. When your cartilage wears down to the point where your physician says your joints are basically

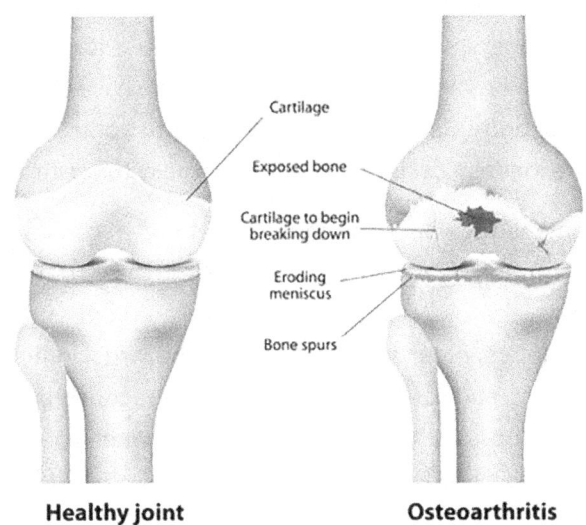

bone-on-bone, perhaps it is time for joint replacement. There are at least three basic common types of arthritis

- **Osteoarthritis (OA).** This is a degenerative form that involves the breakdown of cartilage in your joints. Your bones rub against each other. Bone-on-bone. You experience pain and stiffness. Swelling can occur.
- **Rheumatoid Arthritis (RA).** This is a chronic joint disease where your body's immune system attacks the cartilage. Your fingers can become deformed. Swelling, stiffness, tenderness and redness are common symptoms. It can potentially affect your internal organs and lead to disability.
- **Post-traumatic Arthritis.** This type of arthritis can develop after an injury to the joint. The cartilage has been damaged.

Connections: Arthritis, Cartilage and You. What does cartilage have to do with arthritis and you? As it turns out, a lot. A membrane called the *synovium* produces a thick fluid that helps keep the cartilage healthy. The synovium can become inflamed and thickened as wear and tear on the cartilage occurs. This may lead to inflammation, which produces extra fluid within the joint, resulting in swelling—and possibly the development of OA.

Cartilage is a resilient, smooth and elastic tissue. It serves as a shock absorber. It is a rubber-like padding that covers and protects the ends of long bones at the joints. Cartilage is a bit like the *goldilocks* of tissue in your body. It is not as rigid as bone, nor is it as flexible as muscle. Cartilage has several functions in our body. It reduces friction and acts as a cushion between joints and helps support our weight when we run, bend, and stretch. It holds bones together, such as the bones of our ribcage. Some body parts are made almost entirely of cartilage: the external parts of our ears, our nose, our bronchial tubes and other body parts that we have become accustomed to having as part of our body. Cartilage is the precursor to bone. In children, the ends of the long bones are made of cartilage, which eventually turns into bone.

When cartilage is damaged or worn away, the affected joint becomes painful, stiff, and limited in its range of motion. When there is a decrease in the volume and thickness of cartilage, you have cartilage loss. Damage to your cartilage can be caused by different factors—obesity, genetics, older age, occupational hazards, infections or injuries from high-impact sports, such as football or running or racquet-ball. It can occur as a result of repetitive actions, such as swinging your arms when you play tennis or golf or do hammering actions if you are a carpenter.

Previous damage to a joint can cause problems in the normal smooth joint surface and be a significant cause in the development of arthritis. A *tibial plateau fracture*, where a broken area of the bone enters the cartilage of the knee joint, can cause arthritis. A significant loss or damage to cartilage can contribute to the progression of osteoarthritis. The greater the progression, the greater the pain, creating a lower quality of life.

When the cartilage cannot cushion the joint because of prolonged wearing and tearing, your hip or knee (and other affected joints) are not able to glide or move smoothly as you move. This causes a dilemma. When you experience joint-pain you tend to avoid using that joint. You favor the other hip or the other knee, which then further weakens the surrounding muscles of your *bad* knee and makes moving that joint more difficult and more painful for you. In the case of those lower body joints, you will tend to rock a bit as you walk. Maybe you have become bow-legged or maybe your knees turn in a bit. Your normal gait is gone and the greater the pain, the more you will rock or sway. You may even walk bent over. When you choose to delay surgery, you may find that you will need both joints replaced. Nice thought. And I am not sure that many health-care facilities are offering you a two-for-one BOGO-free sale.

According to the folks at the Mayo Clinic, "Osteoarthritis causes cartilage — the hard, slippery tissue that covers the ends of bones where they form a joint — to break down. Rheumatoid arthritis is an autoimmune disorder that first targets the lining of joints (*synovium*). The most common type of arthritis, osteoarthritis involves wear-and-tear damage to your joint's cartilage — the hard, slick coating on the ends

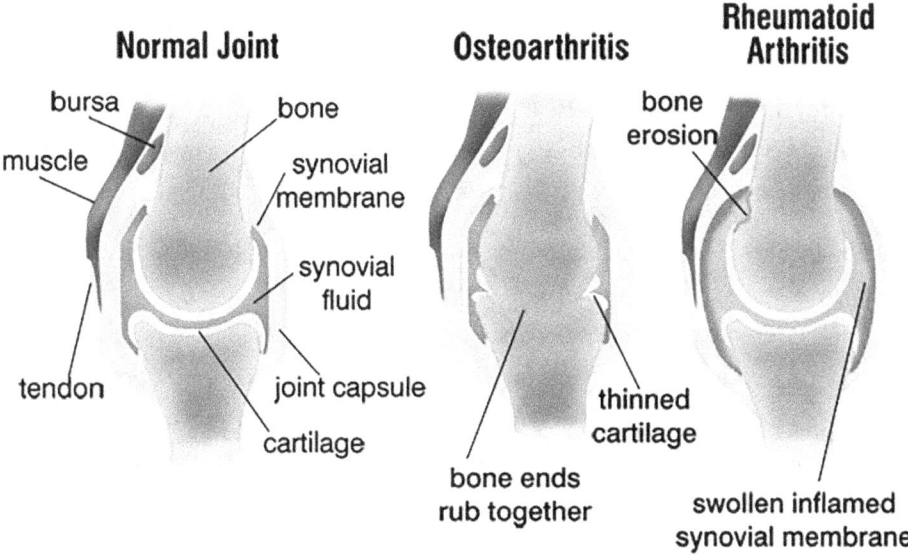

of bones. Enough damage can result in bone grinding directly on bone, which causes pain and restricted movement. This wear and tear can occur over many years, or it can be hastened by a joint injury or infection (Mayo Clinic, 20350772)."

While cartilage is very beneficial to the body, it does have a drawback: it doesn't heal itself as well as most other tissues. The cartilage cells known as *chondrocytes* do not often replicate or repair themselves, which means damaged or injured cartilage will not likely heal well without medical intervention. Unlike other types of tissue, cartilage does not have a blood supply. Because of this, damaged cartilage takes much longer to heal, compared with other tissues.

Osteoarthritis and Heart Disease. The bad news: If you have OA you could have an increased risk of death from cardiovascular disease. The really bad news: If you have knee or hip OA your chances to die of chronic heart disease or heart failure are twenty-percent higher than folks without that condition. See your physician-surgeon, please.

According to Martin Englund, a professor at Lund University in Sweden and lead author of an extensive scientific study of 469,177 Swedes ages 45 to 84, the risk increased with the duration of the disease. He indicates that "because when you have pain, you're inactive, and this inactivity, along with obesity, increases the risk for cardiovascular disease."

Walk, don't run. If you have OA, running is probably not high on your ADL wish-list. You may not be a big fan of pain. Walking may not be much better for you, depending on your physical condition and the extent of your OA. So, you sit. Martin suggests that you "learn how to move and keep moving without injury." Walking is one option that most people can (and should) do.

As painful as it may be initially, include walking as an integral part of your ADL-things-to-do-today. Power-walking? No. Marathon-walking? No. Stroll around a mall or grocery store or garden center or big-box building supply company. Do you live in a high-rise or apartment complex? Walk the halls. Walk around the parking lot.

Start slowly. Start with just five, ten or fifteen minutes a day, every day, and build up your pace and extend your time over time. Get up and move. Get in the habit of walking. Of course, you will experience some pain and that should go away as you move and work your joints. By the way, if you experience pain the first time you start walking, do not give up. One time anything doesn't count for much (actually, it just counts as one-time). As you continue to walk you will find yourself walking with less pain and discomfort. There is no wonder drug for OA. Your OA is giving you pain now just by sitting and being less active than you could be. Walk. What do you have to lose?

Pain Management

At some point, arthritis did not bother you as you went about your daily activities and routine. At some later point, it did. Maybe a lot. It did interfere with your daily activities. Have you had to alter how you play sports or how you exercise or walk or work in your yard and garden? Can you still do yoga or Tai Chi? Are high-impact exercises no longer on your to-do list? Got joint pain? As your condition became more bothersome, you probably experienced pain in your fingers, hips, knees, or other joints. Grinding or clicking in the joint is a common sign. Symptoms can range from mild to severe and change over time. There is no cure for arthritis but there are options you can do prior to walking through the surgical-door.

Pain is a not so subtle message from your body that something is amiss, something is not right. As we age and we wake up in the morning we may find that another part of our body has decided to inflict pain on us. Or, the pain we had yesterday seems worse today. Osteoarthritis, poor blood circulation, nerve damage, disease, an injury, being over-weight, take your pick.

There is no question that it is easier to grab your bottle of happy pills and make that part of your world go away. You may find that is your best remedy or at least a temporary solution. Sometimes your pain is not a big deal and goes away. Sometimes you just decide to cope with it. Sometimes it is chronic or severe and diminishes your way of life. We, you, me may have had to modify our daily living activities because of that pain or discomfort. We have had to change.

We need to change our behavior and attitude about what we do and who we do it with. Maybe you are sitting more now and doing less walking than you did. Maybe you find yourself avoiding certain active social or family events because of your pain. Maybe standing is a problem or just getting up out of a chair or getting in and out of your car is a bit more difficult for you. Or maybe lifting something, almost anything, over your head brings another exciting level of pain. Twisting a door-knob? Pain.

Pain Meds and You. There is a problem with taking drugs, whether prescribed or over-the-counter. Drugs are drugs. Yes, they can alleviate your pain. Many are designed to do just that, which is a nice feature. Yes, they can help you cope or have a pain-free hour or day. But sometimes, at some point, you really don't need to take anything, period. Yet, you continue to rely on them to help you start your day or to help you get through the day or to help you sleep at night. After a while they become a habit that psychologically may help you cope, but medically they are not doing anything positive for you.

Continuing to take whatever it is that you think you should be taking is a bit like painting over a rusty chair. It looks good and it makes you feel good to not have to put up with seeing the rust any longer, but the rust is still there. The problem may be hidden, but it is still there. Have a chat with your physician. What do you think (s)he will say?

We develop a routine and before it becomes a habit, we believe that it is helping us and hopefully it is doing just that. Then the ritual of the habit takes over. Ask yourself, why do you continue to take the meds that you do? Are they really helping you and how do you know? Test this out. Every day or two either reduce the number of meds you normally take each day or extend the time period between dosages, whether they are prescribed or over the counter. Has your pain level increased? Has it stayed the same? If your pain level has not increased, then extend the time or reduce the number of meds you take each day. At some point soon, you will realize that you do not need them. Have another chat with your physician. What will (s)he say?

Research has shown that opioid pain medications can help you cope with pain within the first week or so of your procedure. After that, not so much. According to Christopher J. Centeno, M.D., who is an international expert and specialist in regenerative medicine, research has shown that replacing an opioid with, say Tylenol, is just as helpful (or more so, because it is not addictive). There are ways you can manage your pain or at least manage how you go about your ADLs without being dependent on prescription or over-the-counter drugs.

Check with your primary physician about some of the non-addictive options currently available. Some could provide temporary relief, but they will not cure your damaged joint so be prepared that at some point you may need that surgical procedure.

There are all types of pain. Some are caused by an injury. Obesity can also cause pain because it puts a lot of stress on your hips, back, and knees. Losing some weight, even if you are only moderately overweight, will benefit you. Regardless, ask your primary physician what (s)he recommends. You may be able to treat your pain-level yourself. At the very least you could protect your injury from further injury. Sounds simple enough, right? Do you need a physician to tell you that? Rest, elevate, and ice your injury for about fifteen-minutes or so throughout the day. A physical therapist may offer some more specific time intervals and icing procedures.

> *I had an Achilles Tendon and Posterior Tibial Tendon repair in 2001. I was in a soft cast for about ten-days, had forty-five staples removed, then placed in a hard cast for about three months. I was on pain-meds for ten days, then switched to Tylenol, three-times a day for about two years. Habit. My primary physician*

wanted to know why I was still taking Tylenol. Pain? No. Then why? Because. My doctor was not impressed with my response. I got into that habit and when I stopped, I still had no pain. I couldn't believe that I was taking them just for whatever reason. Easy to develop a habit. Changed my behavior. Changed my attitude. Or, changed my attitude, then changed my behavior.

Non-Surgical Options

Surgery could work for you. Consuming or applying prescribed or over-the-counter medications could work for you. There are different activities you could stop and start doing to alleviate your pain level. One activity to stop is to avoid any high-impact sports or exercise classes or other activities that aggravate a joint or cause you more pain. There are non-surgical options that could help relieve your pain level. Some could work for you. Others, maybe not so much.

- **Braces and Straps.** You could enjoy some daily relief by using a brace or wrap around your affected joint, especially if you have joint pain in your arms, knees or feet. Compression or elastic bandages are two options. There are over-the-counter braces and straps for thumbs and wrists and other body parts. Your physician could prescribe a customized brace. Some braces include stiff plastic or metal to provide you with support.

- **Chiropractic therapy.** Chiropractic adjustment is a procedure where specialists use their hands or a small instrument to apply a controlled, sudden force to a spinal joint. The goal, also known as spinal manipulation, is to improve spinal motion and improve your body's physical function. If you have spinal pain, this may help.

- **Pills and Smells.** Aroma therapy is relatively new, at least for traditional Western treatments. These inhalers include different herbal scents and fragrances, such as lavender, chamomile, rose, hyssop, frankincense and others. They may not alleviate your pain directly but could help you relax and chill for a bit. You could take a pill. Glucosamine and chondroitin supplements are available and could work for you if you still have enough cartilage left in the joint. If you have bone-on-bone, forget it. Herbal supplements are popular with some folks, but their side effects are not known and there is very little rigorous research to document their benefits, if any. And they may cause you additional problems if you take herbals with, say a prescribed or over-the-counter medication. Usually, you will be required to stop using herbals prior to your surgery. Check with your favorite physician.

- **Pins and Needles.** Cortisone is the old name. Steroid injections are the new name. Injections of rooster-comb and other goodies could be recommended. Folks with arthritis, joint diseases or tendinitis often receive these shots. The results are temporary. They take about a week to kick in and for some people relief is measured in months. For others, relief is a couple of weeks at best. The one downside to these injections, and any of the options listed here, is that while they may provide some relief, they can hide a more serious condition and cause further damage to the joint. You may get relief from the symptom, but the problem is still there. Your pain will still be with you. In Asia, acupuncture is a normal treatment for a variety of ailments. Acupuncture stimulates points on or under the skin. The practitioner sticks lots of tiny needles in various parts of your body to alleviate pain levels. It is catching on in the USA and other countries. Many advocates say it works for them. Will it work for you? You will know.

- **Physical Therapy.** You can strengthen the muscles around a joint with physical therapy, which can stabilize the joint, improve your range of motion, and reduce your level of pain. Therapists can use ultrasound, ice, heat, manual manipulation, and electrical nerve stimulations. Heat tends to bring more blood to the affected area and may not be wise if your joint is swollen. Ice is better for reducing that swelling.

- **RICE it.** Rest, Ice, Compression and Elevation. Ice works. Ice reduces the swelling and, as a result, usually reduces the pain associated with swelling. Remove your brace or wrap and apply ice packs for about fifteen minutes at a time, several times a day. Elevate the joint, knee or foot above the level of your heart.

- **Topical Creams (Agents).** Hot peppers have a substance called *capsaicin* which is known to relieve joint pain associated with arthritis. Capsaicin blocks pain signals to the brain and triggers the release of endorphins, which block pain. One side effect includes a burning sensation in the area where you applied the cream. That sensation is temporary. Its intensity varies from person to person. A product called Ben Gay contains capsaicin. There are others. Wash your hands with soap after using these creams. If you do not wash your hands and then rub your eyes, you may experience another level of pain on another body part.

Wraps and creams and shots and pills are easy. No energy required. Someone sticks you with a needle or you spread a cream on your area of pain or enclose it with a wrap or brace. There is a temporary relief from your pain. You could go about your ADLs. No one, generally, will know that you are wearing a brace or had an injection or ingested whatever it was that you ingested. Privacy. At some point, you may want to take a more pro-active and physical approach to managing your pain. The **E-word** may not be high on your wish list.

Exercise and you. Exercise is any movement that makes your muscles work and requires your favorite body to burn some calories. How many calories you burn is contingent on the amount of effort you expend. Exercise can include, but is not limited to, swimming, running, jogging, dancing and walking. Exercise can make you feel happier. It can help you lose weight and increase your energy levels. It can increase your flexibility and mobility. It can help you relax. It can help your brain and tends to allow you to live a bit longer. And it can reduce your pain level. Low-impact exercises are a great starting point.

You can exercise by yourself or in a group. You can exercise at home, at work or at the local YMCA and senior center. You can exercise with or without weights. You can do it without wearing any special clothes. If you are home alone, you can even do it buck-naked. Whether you are relatively mobile or use a wheel-chair, you can exercise standing, sitting, bending, kneeling or lying on your bed or floor. Exercising while you are having pain may sound a bit counter-intuitive, illogical. Exercise causes you pain, right? So why bother engaging in more pain?

You can engage in exercises that range from low-impact to high-intensity. A physical therapist or a personal trainer can provide you with suggestions. You can register for small or larger classes, classes for flexibility and balance, aerobic swimming classes and much more. Check out what is available where you live. What do you want to do? What are you willing to do? What is your physical situation? How should you start?

Tai Chi is one option. Yoga is an option. Pilates yet another option. Choose one or engage in them all. Engaging in HIIT (high-intensity interval training) may not be a smart option, given your physical condition. Practice putting on a golf green could be a possibility but playing eighteen holes may not. Playing pickle-ball could be a way to exercise without creating excessive stress but playing tennis or racquet ball or hand-ball may not. Stretch exercise classes and swing dancing lessons may be better for you, but a heart-pounding cycle class may not.

Yard and garden activities can help. It helps, in part, because while you are gardening you are exercising. You are moving, pushing, pulling, standing, kneeling, crouching, lifting, walking back and forth from your garden to your house or shed and walking within your yard and garden. And depending how extensive your garden is or how strenuously you garden, you are probably exercising your lungs and doing a little cardio as you garden.

And just to clarify a bit: your pre- and post-surgical exercise programs should not be designed for you to compete in the Olympics. They should be designed to get you moving safely and at a comfy-level that works for you. For any exercise, start slowly. Depending on the exercise, initially you may want to exercise for five, ten, fifteen or thirty minutes. What can you do now? Don't worry about how long or how much you could do later? Work on the *now*. Get into the habit of exercising a little each day, every week. Build up to other exercises. Build up to exercising longer. Build up to exercising more aggressively as you gain confidence in what you are doing and the progress you are making. You are not going to get a prize for rushing through an exercise routine. Go slow. Go easy. Go safely. But go.

That all may sound fine, but here you are in your comfy home sitting in your comfy chair. So why should you venture outside to go to your local YMCA or club to exercise? Besides, it is winter. It is cold outside. It is icy and snowy. It is cloudy. It is sunny. It is rainy. It is windy. It is humid. Or maybe it is stifling hot and humid or just plain sticky hot and humid. You believe it is more comfy-dandy to sit inside fussing with your remote and gazing outside rather than go outside and dabble in dirt or drive all the way to the Y. Right?

Barriers and You. Going out in public to, say, a health and fitness club, the YMCA or even to the exercise room or pool in your building may create tension for you. Are you embarrassed about how you look and how people may respond to you? Are you concerned that you will not be able to do the exercises as well as others in the room? Depending on where you go you may be in a sea of strangers. You haven't seen them before. Decision time. What would you rather do: sit in your comfy cozy chair watching television, chatting on the phone, texting to whomever and taking a nice low-impact nap? Or, would you rather go to your local YMCA or gym and exercise where you will see skinny folks who wear a size zero and folks who sport six-pack Abs and bulging muscles that are larger than your legs and watch folks in exercise classes doing things you thought impossible to do? Decision time.

Why are you leaving your comfy chair? You are going to exercise. You want to get in better shape for your upcoming procedure and to stay in shape after your procedure. You are not going to invite folks over for a cup of coffee and make them your best friends forever. Don't get yourself all worked up thinking about what they may be thinking. And your friends? They aren't going to say anything about how you look. You have been chumming with them for a long time and whatever it is that they may have said they said it a long time ago. Look on the bright side—maybe your pals will give you kudos for taking positive steps to reduce your weight and become more active, vertically, as you did years earlier (the good old days). And just maybe your efforts will encourage them to get up and out and join you. What's the big deal? Get up and out there. Meet new friends. Live a better life.

Probably the easiest low-impact exercise to start with is to just start walking. A bit pedestrian perhaps, but effective. Getting up from your chair and walking about your house or place of work for just five minutes every hour or so is exercise. That may not sound like you are doing much but sitting in your chair isn't doing much for you either. Getting up and about to grab a nice sweet or fatty treat may not exactly qualify, however. And when you go to your senior center or YMCA or club you can not only walk but talk and chew gum at the same time. Maybe even scratch your nose or something. Multi-task.

Stop the talk.
Get up and walk.
Stop the stall
And walk the mall
Whether slim or stout,
Get out and about.
Start short and slow
Then aim to go
Longer and more.
Just get out the door.

Exercise by Walking. Simple. Effective. Low-impact. There are different ways to walk. You can walk in water. You can walk on a machine. You can walk on flat surfaces or up and down low hills or take a hike in the park. Consider these low-impact suggestions to get you started.

- **Walk and eye-shop.** Do you live near a mall? Grocery store? A big-box home improvement center? Grab a cart for support and motor up and down the aisles. People will think you are looking for something to buy. No need to buy anything. Just walk and look around. No one will kick you out.

- **Take a Hike.** Maybe someone has told you to take a hike. So, do it. Walking can improve your circulation and strengthen the muscles that support your joints. You do not need any special equipment or clothing except a good comfy pair of shoes. You can walk almost anywhere. Walk around your house. Go up and down stairs. Walk in the hallways in your building. Do not walk on uneven surfaces or sidewalks that need repair. Use that mall or enclosed space to extend your walking program. If your mall is circular in design, find out how long each level is and hike it. How long did it take you to make one complete circuit? And if you cannot walk the entire level, how far did you get? Use that as your bench-mark and strive to reduce the time it takes you to go past that point. Use that as a goal to walk beyond that place the next time. Start easy. Did you reduce the time by ten-seconds? Thirty-seconds? More? Fantastic. Did you manage to walk past that first stopping-point? How much further? Did you walk all the way around?

> **NOTE:** Just an FYI and for comparison sake, there are four levels in the Mall of America (MOA, Bloomington, Minnesota). Each outer ring or the exterior wall of the MOA is over one-mile (1.5 miles actually) or over four-miles total if you walk all four levels or walk four-times around one level. You could burn 80-100 calories walking around in just twenty-minutes. You can entertain yourself by window-shopping while you walk. No stopping to shop. Keep walking.

- **Treadmills**. I find them safer to use than, say, walking along a street without a sidewalk or busy highway. If your local YMCA or club has them, use them. You can control the speed. You can control the duration. You can control the elevation or angle. All (or most) treadmills should have bars on each side to help you keep your balance and steady yourself. You can hang on to them for dear-life or touch them when you feel a need to do so. Most have a panic stop button that will bring the machine to an abrupt stop. Most have a screen where you can track your progress on an oval circuit, or visualize yourself walking along a hiking trail, or select a television or music station to listen to or you could plug in your media-device and listen to snappy tunes.

- **Walk and wander.** You may like to walk or exercise but doing it alone may not be high on your wish-list. No friends? No one to play with? Grab a pal to walk with you. Introduce yourself to a stranger. If they bite, bite them back. Exercise together. Motivate each other. The time will pass by quickly. You will be chatting about whatever throughout the whole time and getting your exercise RDAs in. Form a routine. Form a habit of getting up and out and about. Enroll in a class or two. Meet others. Establish a friendly relationship, even if it is only while you are at the club.

- **Walking and Water Aerobics.** Both exercises can help relieve your pain and lessen further joint damage. Both can help you lose weight. They are easy on your joints, especially if you are overweight or just starting an exercise program or have not been exercising for many years. Both are easy to do. Both are low-impact options to consider.

- **Walk against the tide**. Splashing and bouncing up and down is good but walking in a *lazy river* is better. Does your facility have one of those water therapy units, usually referred to as a *Vortex* unit? It is in the swimming pool where you can walk *against* the current? You don't swim you say. Not to worry. You use the Vortex to walk, not to swim. You get in water up to your waist or chest. The idea is to walk against the current, not with it. Walking against the current helps build strength and stamina. It can help you lose weight. Walking with the current is just a time and space issue—you are only passing the time and taking up someone else's space in the pool. Go against the tide.

- **Walk, Splash and Squirt.** Water aerobics can help alleviate hip or knee arthritis. Get in and up to your chest or shoulders. At that level you are taking a lot of weight off those joints. You may not be too excited about water aerobics but like the idea of getting in the pool. So, get in there and splash around. Splash your neighbor. Chase each other. Play a game of catch-me-catch-me. What if it is cold outside? You will be inside. And, by the way, soaking in a hot tub or having a jet of water slam into parts of your body doesn't get it. That is not exercise.

- **Keep Your Brain Sharp.** There are many ways to exercise your brain. You can do crossword puzzles or Sudoku or play Bridge or chess and other games. Did you know that walking can alter how certain parts of the brain communicate and coordinate with one another while improving your memory function? Are we talking about power-walking? Nope. A relatively recent study suggests that "exercise does not need to be prolonged or intense to benefit the brain and that the effects can begin far more quickly than many of us might expect" (National Academy of Sciences, University of California, Irvine and University of Tsukuba, Japan, reprinted, Gretchen Reynolds, *New York* Times, 2018). Sounds good to me.

Better good news: the article also points out that the exercises you do are not geared towards marathon conditioning. Apparently, people can improve their memories with a short walk or an easy session of something like yoga or Tai Chi. The basic point: get up and out there and just do it.

Walking is man's best medicine.
Hippocrates

- **Watch your gait.** You may need a walker and perhaps a cane or crutches after surgery. The tendency of most people who use a walker right after surgery is to hunch over their shoulders and as a result lean forward on the walker. This can provide balance, especially the first few days after surgery but it can indicate that you are leaning a bit too heavily on the walker and it may not help with your balance. Straighten your back. When using a walker, keep your posture erect, do not lean on it.

- Keep your hands on the walker, but don't tighten your grip as though you were going to toss it at someone. Walk with your heel down first, then your toes—heel toe, heel toe. When you walk heel-to-toe it will be difficult to slouch and hunch over your walker. For those of you who served in the military (hopefully on our side), you know the routine. Your heel hits the ground first before the rest of your foot. Erect posture. No slouching. Practice walking with a walker before your surgical procedure. Create the habit of heel-toe walking with a good, straight-up posture. It will help you while you rehab.

■ **Walking with care.** Avoid walking on ice or snow or uneven surfaces such as stone pathways or areas where there are cracks and uneven sidewalks or pavement areas.

- If you walk on ice or snow, take baby-steps. Walking at your normal stride on a dry surface will not especially work on a wet or slippery surface.
- Wear solid, comfy shoes with good soles for traction and support.
- Trendy shoes with a deep, non-slip sole can cause problems. The sole can *grab* the soil or grass or a rug as you turn. You can lock your foot while your knee or ankle, or both, go off in different directions. You could lose your balance and tear a tendon or two. You could get a *meniscus tear* in your knee(s). Or you could get a crack in your *tibial plateau*.
- When was the last time you had your eyes checked?
- When was the last time you had your hearing checked?
- Walk in well-lighted areas.
- Make multiple trips instead of trying to carry heavy bags all at once.

Increasing Your Balance. Walking can help you increase your balance. Probably nothing will prevent you from falling. You typically do not plan to fall. You fall accidentally. Yet you can take some precautions to reduce your chances of falling and not only breaking something that you did not want broken, but also avoiding the pain that always comes with a fall. You can fall at any age and anywhere under any condition. Falls normally cause more serious issues than if you were a bit younger. If you tend to become dizzy or light-headed, consult your physician first, before you start any exercise program, walking included. Some ways to improve your ability to balance include the following:

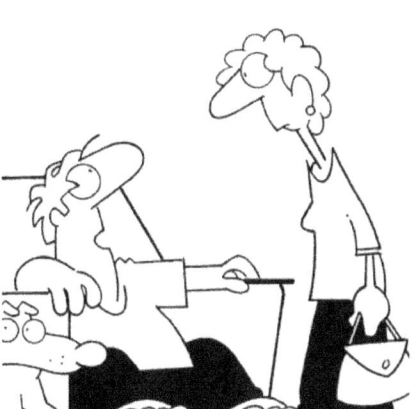

"I did a 30-minute workout today: 15 minutes looking for my sneakers, 10 minutes looking for my sweat pants and 5 minutes on the treadmill."

- **Balance Yourself.** Do you use an assistive-device now? A walker? Cane? Stand on your two feet without your walker or cane and stand by a rail or sturdy chair for support. Let go of your device and stand on your feet. If you feel a tad wobbly, touch or hang on to the rail or chair. Steady yourself. Now, how long can you stand on your two feet without touching anything? Start standing for a few seconds or for as long as you can. Then, gradually build up the time. Can you do that for thirty-seconds? A full minute?

- **Balance Yourself (again).** This could be a toughie. You can increase your ability to prevent falling or stumbling by doing another balancing exercise. Stand next to a table or counter or balance bar. Keep your hands just above them in case you start to wobble a bit. Stand on one foot without holding on to anything. Can you do that for five-seconds? Fifteen-seconds? Keep increasing the time you can stand on one foot to thirty-seconds. Sixty-seconds would be great. Switch your weight to the other foot. Start easy. Doing this on your bare feet is better but a bit more challenging that wearing foot-wear. Start with footwear on a hard, flat surface, then progress to bare feet or incorporate a *Bosu-ball* or balance-board in your program when you feel comfy doing so.

Falling down is easy.
Getting up uneasy.
Not so much fun,
Easier said than done.

Exercise Classes. Take a class in yoga, Tai Chi or Pilates and other classes designed to improve your balance and flexibility. There are classes designed for seniors and other age groups. Check those non-surgical options out. Go to a couple of classes. Are they right for you?

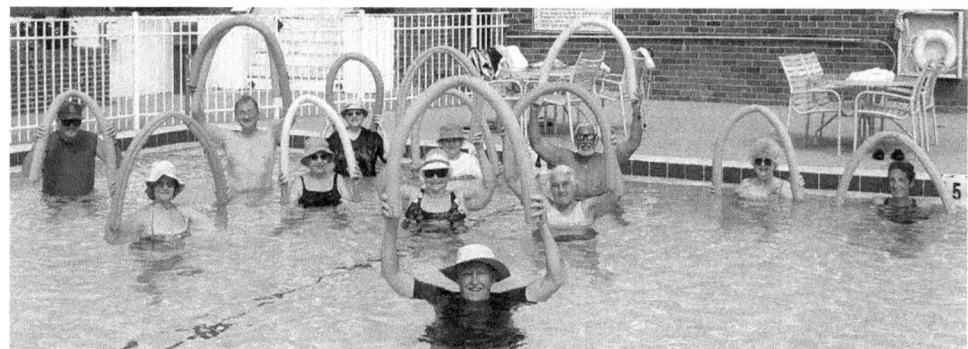

Not too excited about getting all moist and out of breath in a high-impact exercise class? Think water exercises whether you can swim or not. Water helps to keep the weight off your knees and hips. And if you want to lose some weight consider splashing your neighbor, who will no doubt splash you back and chase you around the pool. Great exercise. You can even giggle as you move and motor through the water.

- **Aerobics** can strengthen your heart and lungs and increase your stamina and balance. There should be classes available to you to get your heart started. Walk. Jog. Ride a stationary bike. What else does the facility have to offer you?

- **Endurance**. Work on your endurance when you walk, swim, or bike. Basically, do more and do it longer given what you choose to do when you do it.

- **Stretching** can increase your flexibility and range of motion and help to lubricate your joints. There are many good exercise options to consider (re: **Module Six).**

Taking a class can be a great motivator. There are other options that you can do in an exercise class or on your own.

- **Ride a bike.** Using a regular or stationary bike can work your lower body at even low resistance levels. And if you crank up the resistance level it will give you a good cardio-workout at the same time. Riding a bike or walking on a tread mill could help you lose weight if you keep your heart-rate down. When you exercise at a higher heart-rate you are helping your heart and lungs more than losing weight. *Recumbent bikes.* This type of bike will help you exercise your lower body and reduce the weight and pressure on your joints. It may not help you lose weight, however. *Dual action bikes.* Some bikes will help you exercise your lower body, reduce stress on your knees and hips, while giving you an upper-body workout all at the same time. Depending on how much energy you expend, you could be getting a reasonably good total-body workout on this one machine.

- **Dual action machines.** There are dual action bikes and dual action machines. You sit and push pedals with your feet while using your arms to push and pull handles

PREPARING YOUR MIND AND BODY

on the machine. You can go as fast or as slow as you want. You can create a level of resistance that is comfy for you.

- **Pump Iron**. Consider weight training. If grunting under the weight of barbells or dumbbells are not your thing, then use resistance bands, such as Thera Bands, or very light weights, as in one-or two-pound weights and lots of repetitions. Weights can strengthen the muscles around your joints and help you burn calories and keep burning some calories for a time even after you have completed your lifting for a session. And just to clarify further, you will not be bulking up with a goal of sporting a pair of awesome pipes or six-pack abs. And muscle tissue is not the same as fat tissue. Your muscle tissue, should you bulk up and flex and sport an awesome set of pipes, will not turn to fat if you stop exercising with weights. Cannot happen. Muscle tissue is not fat tissue. Neither can covert to the other. Go for the weights.

- **Do it early**. You get out of bed and probably hit the floor running. Lots of stuff to do early in the morning. Can you get up a couple of minutes earlier? Can you stop or wait a bit doing whatever it is you feel you have to do early in the morning? If you get into your regular routine, you may find that you will not find the time to do it later in the day. Easier said than done, yes; but give exercise an early go if you can. My suggestion is not to do heavy-lifting or heavy-breathing exercises when you first jump out of bed. Stretch. Loosen up those muscles slowly. Do you know any Tai Chi moves? Do those. Later in this book (re: **Module Six)** you will learn about dozens of exercises you can do at home, in your bed or on the floor.

Make sure that you check with your physician or therapist before doing any of these suggestions. Check with them about whether you can do them and whether they have other suggestions for you. Use the ideas in this book as guidelines. Use your medical team to clarify and verify what they recommend you do and when you can do it and how much time and energy you should expend doing it.

Lift Weights. Live Longer. More about pumping iron. Another non-surgical treatment for arthritis and perhaps whatever else ails you, is to lift weights. When you exercise you move, or at least that is one goal. Yet it is not just

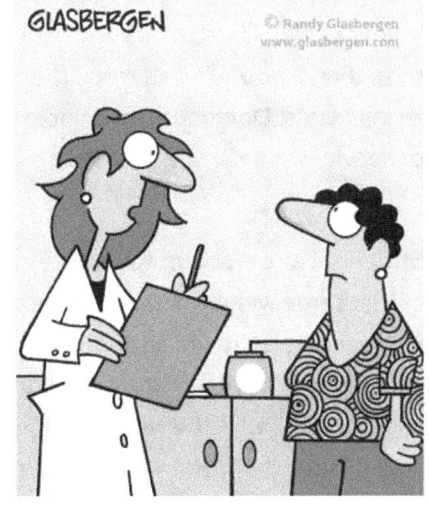

"Sometimes it's good to change your walking routine. Try walking around the block instead of wandering around the kitchen."

getting your body to move that is important to your health. It is getting your muscles toned-up that is more important. Just to reinforce the benefits of using weights, consider some recent research conducted by the University of Michigan indicating that "people with weak muscles don't live as long as their stronger counterparts." The full report, published in the *Journal of Gerontology: Medical Sciences* (Duchowny, 2018) looked at more than 8,000 men and women, whose ages were 65 and older. Strength training with light weights can protect your joints from further injury while strengthening the muscles surrounding those joints.

You could also *lift* with elastic bands or ropes, doing push-ups, sit-ups, and climbing stairs, which allows you to lift your entire body-weight. Other activities include cycling, hiking up hills and walking the golf course rather than riding in a cart. Carry your golf-bag rather than having someone else do it for you and, of course, gardening. In a recent Washington Post article muscle strengthening exercises have been linked to a wide range of health benefits, including but not limited to improved cardiovascular health, better blood sugar control, better bone density, better balance and mobility and improved self-esteem.

For some folks there is a stigma against lifting weights. Consider lifting barbells or just the bar without any weights attached. Barbells weigh about twenty to forty pounds. Start with twenty pounds. Too heavy for you? Then consider dumbbells, which range in weight from one pound to very, very heavy. Start with one pound and as that weight starts to feel too easy for you, grab a heavier weight, say two-pounds or maybe the five-pounder. Lift at home. Lift at your local YMCA. Use weights during your group fitness class. No access or desire to join a club or go to the YMCA? What is in your pantry? Grab a box or can or something. What does it weigh? A few ounces? Less than a pound? Use it to lift and stretch over your head. Use it for biceps and triceps curls. Don't stop and nibble on the contents. Use it as a substitute for metal or heavier weights. Graduate to a one-pound box of salt or a five-pound bag of sugar or flour.

Start light and work up towards ten to fifteen repetitions per set. Do multiple sets at that same weight. You can always use the lighter weights and simply increase the number or repetitions and sets that you do. Use the barbell or dumbbells to increase your range of motion. Stand or sit or lie on your back. With your arms extended down past your waist, lift the weight to your waist. Lift the weights from your waist to above your head. Extend the weights from your waist outward, away from your body. Use the weights and bar on a *universal-type* machine and pull the bar down in front of your body to your chest. Low-impact exercise. Very beneficial.

There are many ways to use weights. Lifting light weights is an easy exercise so long as you do not try to impress folks with how much you can lift, or how fast you can complete a set or how many reps you can do. If someone can lift more than you, so what? If you belong to a club, consider using one of those cute machines that allow you to sit on your butt and pedal with your legs and push and pull bars or levels to give your arms and upper body a workout. One machine for almost all body parts. The more consistently you exercise you will find that, at some point, you will actually be able to exercise, chew gum and carry on a conversation with the person next to you—all at the same time. Amazing. And you can thank the dumbbell (the thing, not the person) for enabling you to do that.

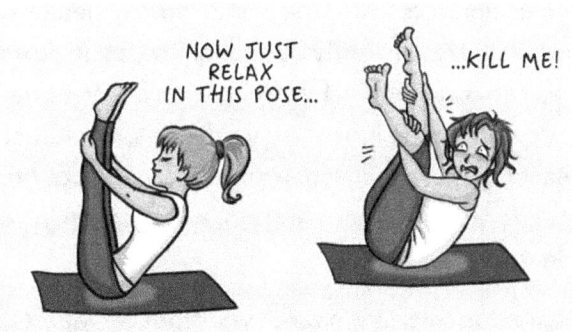

Exercising helps build your overall body tone, strength, flexibility, balance and more. First, you need to learn the correct form for any exercise that you do. A physical therapist can help. A personal trainer can help. You can also learn by watching a personal trainer working with another person (a freebie). Astkhik Rakimova

> When I was younger, I played a variety of sports, including football. If I complained about being sore, my very sympathetic coach, part Neanderthal, part sadist, part village-idiot, would politely suggest that I run up and down the stadium steps with my full football attire strapped to my back and legs. Was I still having pain? Run some more. No pain, no gain was the refrain. A bit off the mark I am now thinking. Maybe that is why I have had multiple orthopedic surgeries. Thanks, but no thanks, Mr. Coach. Of course, genetics could be in play here. But why point fingers?

> **TIP:** When you lift a weight, any weight, do not use rapid, jerky motions. Speed is not the key. Let your muscles do the work. Lift slowly. Pause for a bit at the end of the exercise, then repeat. Yes, you probably want to get that or any exercise done quickly but that is not the point.

Mind and Body Techniques. Another positive non-surgical option for you is meditation. It could help you. Some studies indicate that *meditation* (not medication!) can help relieve pain, ease depression, and often the pain that comes with depression. Usually the pain hits first, then if that pain is on-going and does not seem to subside, depression gets to join the party. You can meditate sitting, standing, and by walking. Do not do this while driving a car or operating power tools. The key is to form a habit. This can be a good habit. Meditation is not a one-time event, but something that you can integrate in your daily activities. Meditation can help you become a bit more peaceful, more focused, less concerned about your pain and more aware of the sounds and fragrances around you. It can help you appreciate your life and life in general.

Meditation certainly may not work for everyone. Give it a go to see if it works for you. Review the following list. Start where you want. Start easy. Get comfy. And build on what works for you. And the best part is that you do not need any special equipment or snazzy fashion-forward or retro-attire. And just for fun and entertainment, you can even do it buck-naked, in the privacy of your home. What the heck. Who's to know? And who would care?

Meditating is easy to do when you are gardening, but maybe not so much if you are playing golf or tennis or basketball or rugby or soccer or jumping up and down in a high-impact (HIIT) exercise class. When you meditate ...

- **Breathe.** Focus on breathing in as deeply as you can, then breathe out, slowly. Breathe through your nose, exhale through your mouth.

- **Commuting to work.** Car pool. Van pool. Take a bus or train. Wear a pair of headsets and listen to some relaxing music. Tune out the noise around you and close your eyes, which should be a clue to the chatter-box sitting next to you to zip it while you meditate.

- **Daydream.** Let your mind wander. Don't focus on your grocery list or what emails you need to send out. Just breathe, relax, get comfy, and maybe even do a mental one-thousand-one count if that helps slow you down a bit. And don't clear your mind, refocus it. Your mind will wander and catch on to something. Focus on that something.

- **Find a quiet place.** Find a quiet spot, a comfy place if possible. You do not need a special room or special pillows or scented candles. Sit where you can be undisturbed, without your cell-phone, television or radio blasting at you. Will soft music help? Get comfy. Shut your eyes. Breathe. You can practice holding your breath for several seconds, then exhale slowly. Are you still working outside your home? Some organizations have quiet or meditation rooms where employees are encouraged to shut it down for a few minutes to relax and chill a bit. Can you find that space and time in your own home? Sitting on a bench by a river or moving body of water can have a soothing effect. Or, just sit and read or think about nothing in particular.

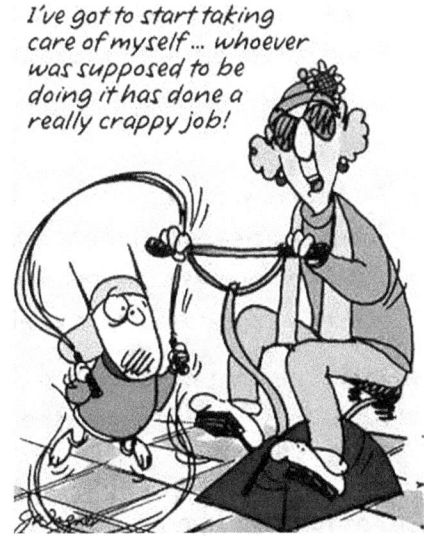

I've got to start taking care of myself... whoever was supposed to be doing it has done a really crappy job!

- **Focus on a body part.** As you get into meditation, let your mind focus on a body part. Where to start? Today, start with your feet and work up towards your head in subsequent days. Or, go from your upper body to your lower body. Breathe. How does your neck feel? What is your foot doing? Move your tootsies. How does that feel? Breathe *up* your body. Don't race to the top. Stop where you want, given the time you have.

- **Focus on your surroundings.** Do you see a light? What is it doing? Where is it coming from, inside or outside the room you are in? Sounds? What are they? Where are they coming from? Do you smell a smell? What is it? Is it a nice smell? Is it a stinky smell? What is it? What makes it pleasant? What makes it stinky? Why is it there?

- **Get an Aquarium.** Dentists, and other pain-masters, often have an aquarium in their waiting area. Watching fish glide through the water. They do not seem to be in a hurry (where would they go anyway?). This can have a calming effect on you. No fighting or quick darting fish. No piranha. Maybe a few goldfish will suffice, especially those with longer pectoral and tail fins, which make their movements appear more graceful, more relaxing.

- **Go with the flow.** Don't fret about where you will meditate or where you will stand or whether you should be on the floor in a sitting lotus position. None of that is important when you first start out. Your biggest hurdle will be to form the habit of meditating. Do it where you are comfy—floor, bed, chair, or leaning against the wall, Remember, we're talking about five minutes or so for your first week. Get comfy. Just be.

- **Got Kiddies Around?** Can you get the little cherubs to go outside and play for a while? Get them out so they can grab some Vitamin D and those rosy-cheeks. Burn off some energy so you can rest and maybe take a short nap. Peace and quiet. Rest. Take some time to just relax. Meditate.

- **Shape a headache.** I am not sure this is a legitimate meditation technique, but when you have a headache focus on that pain and put a shape to it. Consciously make it round. Make it square. Make it elastic. Make it small. Move the shape around. Push it away. Pull it towards you. What happens? Color it. Try different colors. Color it with colors you like and see what happens. Make it go away. It may work for you.

- **Sit for a few.** Sit and meditate for a few minutes each day for a week. Simple enough? Increase the time by another minute or two for the next week. Start with just a few minutes a day for a week. If that goes well, increase by another couple of minutes and do that for a week.

- **Yoga.** There are some positions, such as the Lotus pose, that can help you zone-out. Grab a mat. Sit in a corner or quiet place and chill-out for a while.

Behavior Change and You

Back to change. Like it or not, you will need to change your behavior and attitude if not before surgery, then surely after it. Depending on the type of surgery, you may be restricted from some of your ADLs for just a few weeks or perhaps for several months. You will not be able to do everything you want. You will need to start doing other activities that are linked to your post-surgery protocol as prescribed by your surgeon and physical therapist. That protocol will probably include specific exercises to help you get back in gear and on your road to recovery.

You will need to prepare yourself for surgery by doing some things differently. You may need to exercise more or in a different way. Going out of your home to a facility to exercise, in a public place, could create some stress for you. Some exercises you will not be able to do, initially. Some you will only be able to do with assistive aids, such as a walker or cane or crutches. Some you will only do well after you have had physical therapy by someone (an aide) you do not know. And that someone will recommend changes that will help you rehab quicker so you can get back to your daily living activities in a safer and healthier way.

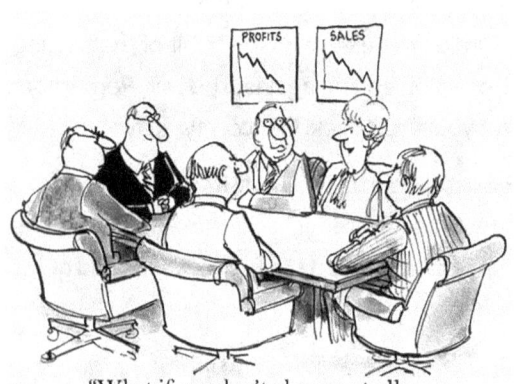
"What if we don't change at all ... and something magical just happens?"

Some folks thrive on change. Others, not so much. In fact, change can create stress and confusion and even despair for some folks and in severe cases lead to depression. Change can be a major stressful event, such as having now to live alone, or to move from a home with a yard to an apartment or condo with limited outdoor recreational space.

Change can be a relatively minor and temporary affair, such as having to drive to work on a different route due to construction. Maybe you have experienced some stress taking that different route. Now you are confronted with a roadblock-a physical and psychological road-block. Where does this new route lead? How long will it take you to get to where you wanted to go? Is it dangerous? Having to change where you shop because your favorite store has closed permanently can cause you to stress out, at least until you find a suitable replacement. A change in your job responsibilities can cause stress. Changes recommended by your medical-team can cause stress, frustration and maybe even make you become defensive.

When you are faced with an event or situation that is not consistent with your core beliefs you will likely feel some level of anxiety. You could become defensive in your response. You can realize stress when your plane is late due to a mechanical or weather-related event. The thought of you missing your connection can cause you to breakout into a sweat or at least create a glow on your skin. In short, change can apply to many things. Regardless, change always requires an adjustment in how you go about your daily activities. There will always be change. And, depending on the issue, you will need to adapt. Changing your attitude and behavior can help make you adapt with less stress.

Change requires that you need to modify your situation or your environment or your physical condition that challenges what you have been doing for as long as you have been doing it. You may need patience. You may need to be a bit calmer and logical, rather than emotional and irrational. Fighting change is a sure way to create additional stress in your life. Procrastinating about changing can cause issues for you. Having to change what you have always done, what you are comfy doing can create a fear about the future, your future. You may know what you need to do to change, but you may not know exactly how that change will affect you. Some fear of that unknown can cause apprehension, whether it is short-lived, transitory, longer-term or permanent. Coping and adapting to change in a positive way requires an adjustment that can be easily managed. For others, rationalization is the key to coping and a way to avoid changing.

On paper, change should be a relatively simple matter. But your brain is not paper. It can make you feel frustrated and resistant. It can also make you feel enthusiastic and pro-active. You have been doing something one way for a long time. Now you need to do it in a different way. So, you adjust and do that something in this new and different way. Simple. But then another part of your brain kicks in. It expects things to be done as usual. Think back to the example about having to change your driving route because of construction or some other issue. When you do something like driving or gardening or working out at your local YMCA or club or other facility in a certain way you tend to do it almost automatically. You have a routine. When driving, you may be day-dreaming or focusing on something while your car automatically seems to take you to where you wanted to go. You may be zoned-out, but somehow your car *knows* the way and brings you to your destination safely. Or perhaps you have gardened in a specific way with the same basic plant varieties. How you prepare your garden and how and what you plant is almost automatic. You have your routine. But perhaps out of the blue someone suggests that you plant other varieties or modify your yard so you can garden in raised beds or containers or that you plant with a specific theme in mind—complementary colors, contrasting colors, textures and so on. Different. Potential stress.

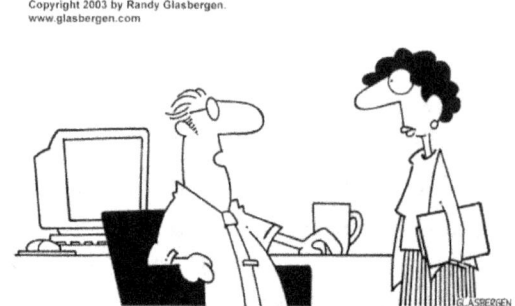

"I'm not procrastinating. I'm proactively delaying the implementation of the energy-intensive phase of the project until the enthusiasm factor is at its maximum effectiveness."

And as we get older our brains become a bit more ridged in that it seems to resist the need to change. Doing something differently is different. Our known behavioral patterns are being broken. We can adjust, of course, or we can resist. When faced with new information we tend to align ourselves with friends or groups that reinforce our earlier beliefs and patterns. We feel comfy and reinforced by people who prefer to do things the way we used to do things. When you find a cadre of folks who tend to agree about something, it is more than easy to disregard the opinions and practices of others in the face of what you believe are undeniable logic and facts. They may be logical. They may be facts and reality, but our brains can easily dismiss that information and allow us to fall back on our preferred habits and opinions. We prefer to live in our comfy-zone. We prefer to believe what we want to believe. We can easily develop an ambiguous relationship with the facts and reality. Group think will be alive and well (*Psychology Today*, Groupthink).

How did you respond when you first learned that you needed surgery? Total acceptance at first? Denial? Anxiety? There was a change. Yesterday you were fine. Today you learned that you need to do something that you may or may not have expected.

David McRaney, in his book about self-delusion, *You Are Not So Smart,* writes*: "The illusion of asymmetric insight makes it seem as though you know everyone else far better than they know you, and not only that, but you know them better than they know themselves. You believe the same thing about groups of which you are a member. As a whole, [you believe] your group understands outsiders better than outsiders understand your group, and you understand the group better than its members know the group to which they belong."* Does this ring any bells for you?

As a result of this self-knowledge you discount conflicting information as bias and false and stick with what you know. In short, you resist change and perhaps even attack it because you think you know better than everyone else and have a group of folks that support your beliefs and, in effect, back up your opinions. Your comfy-zone is alive and well.

Change and Denial. Sometimes folks just don't want to deal with it. Many folks tend not to enjoy discussing disturbing issues—political, religious, climate change, health concerns—that affect them directly or affect someone close to them. Sometimes they fail to take precautions though they sense the danger of not doing so. Change can be a toughie. Denying the need to change is a way some folks cope with that change, regardless of their economic situation or cultural background.

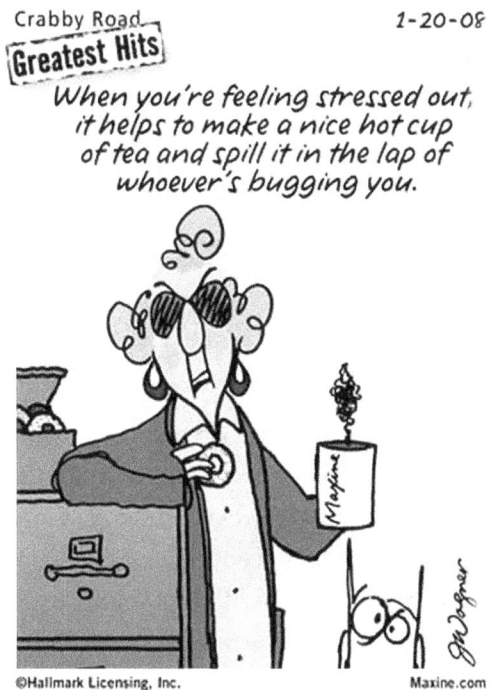

Kari Norgaard talks about denial in her book, *Living in Denial,* and says that "It's not that people don't care [about climate change] and it's not that they don't know, but it has to do with how we manage very disturbing information." She goes on to say that "our species has needed denial to survive." If you know about something, you typically take action in one of two ways. You either take a pro-active approach and do what you can to resolve or remedy the situation. Or, you decide that that *something* is not something that really needs remedial action, so you deny its significance or relevancy (or existence) to what you want to believe.

Those who believe being overweight or who continue to smoke or drink more than what is generally recommended or do not exercise and choose to be more sedentary and though they may fully understand that their situation is more dangerous to their health and well-being, are not likely to take positive action, in spite of what their physician or others recommend. Denial is a handy coping mechanism. And over time can lead to some serious mental and physical concerns.

Resisting Change. Think of a time when you had to make some changes in the past. Did it cause you any stress? Review this checklist of common reasons and note which applied to you then and do you think they will apply again as you move ever closer to your surgical procedure.

- **Loss of control**. Your sense of self-determination made you believe that you had no other options or choices when faced with change.
- **Uncertainty**. Did your brain make you feel like a lemming, that you are sure you would fall off a cliff if you accepted this change?
- **Immediacy**. The change came upon you suddenly with little time for you to think it through.
- **Too Radical**. The change broke your normal habits and routines. No more automatic *stimulus-response.* You had to stop and think a bit about this new change.
- **Lack of competence**. Could you do it? Did the thought of making a change make you feel that you could not do it as well as you believe you had been doing it in the past? What if you fail?

Change may be great for Ye
But not so much I think for Me.
Better for He and She,
To that I agree,
So just let Me be.

Coping with change is simple. One way to cope is to compare what you are being asked to do with what you have been doing. Your brain can handle information that it knows and understands and doesn't like what it doesn't know. Making comparisons is one way to help your brain help you accept the change. Accepting that change is a normal part of life and is another way to cope. Stuff happens. It will always happen whether you accept it willingly or whether you are dragged off kicking and screaming. Third, maybe, just maybe, this change will prove to be better than what you have been

PREPARING YOUR MIND AND BODY

doing. That could be a real shocker, but who knows until you do it. Simple, but you are the one who may have to change. Here are some other suggestions to consider.

- Acknowledge your feelings about having to make changes to your daily living activities—playing golf, tennis, gardening. Write your feelings down and identify why specifically you are having doubts or are resisting having to change. Keep a private and personal diary.

- Prepare yourself for change. Make a plan. This book will (I trust) provide you with hundreds of practical suggestions about what and how you can make changes within your home and outside in your yard and for sports and the other ADLs you enjoy. Will every suggestion and idea apply to you? Absolutely not. But many could and, if so, include them as part of your pre- and post-surgical plan.

- You are still in control. Yes, you may have to do things differently and you are the one who can do it. Listen to your medical team, then do what they prescribe, telling yourself that you are not only willing to do it but are able to do it. Your team will be with you, from pre- to post-surgery.

- Talk to others. Be careful with this gem. Talking to folks who have undergone a similar procedure can be helpful so long as the conversation does not focus on *stinkin' thinkin'*. If what you hear is only the negative, then that will not be very useful nor helpful to you. It may be comfy, but not helpful in the long-run. Should it be all rosy and peachy-swell? No. If change is not high on your wish-list then listening to folks who reinforce your resistance will only make you more resistant and that can add to your stress level.

- Take responsibility. Your success, both before and after surgery, depends on you. You are the key for completing your prescribed exercises. You are the one who can decide what you want to eat and how much and whether you want to exercise or not. Make your decision, then live with the consequences, good or bad.

- Adjust in a methodical way. You have thought about having elective surgery. Maybe you have already scheduled it. Regardless, you should have

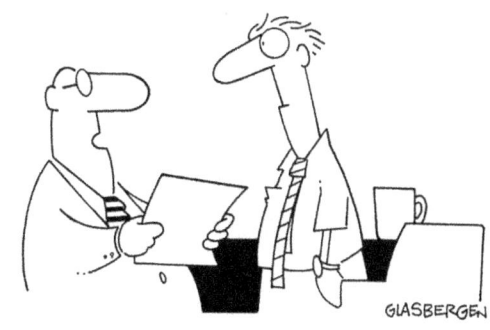

"I want you to find a bold and innovative way to do everything exactly the same way it's been done for 25 years."

time to make all or most of the adjustments to your daily activities. Do not procrastinate and wait until the week before your procedure. Start now and continue making any adjustments in a planned and organized way. This book should help you do that.

Everyone has the ability to change. Not everyone has the willingness to change.

> *"If it were done when 'tis done,*
> *then 'twere well it were done quickly."*
>
> —MACBETH (1.7.1-29)

What's to be Afraid of? You have your surgery scheduled. You have registered for a pre-surgery educational class. You have met with your primary physician and have the all-clear-go-ahead on your planned date. You are all set to go. You are counting the days to the big day (but who is counting?). You have some concerns. You are a bit anxious about your procedure. Why?

Change. We all have fears. Some fears pass. Other fears consume us. We learn to fear. Perhaps as children some event frightened us and we carry that memory and fear with us for many years, perhaps forever. That fear could influence whether you change or not.

Perhaps our parents or other adults taught us to fear something or someone and we carry that with us. Walking along a woodland path enjoying the sounds of birds and perhaps catching a glimpse of the song-maker puts us in a comfy zone until a snake or mouse or giant moose or mountain lion or other animal darts across our path and startles us. Or maybe you just walked into a spider web and have all that sticky crawly stuff on your face? Is the spider still on you? Where did it go? It was scary. Or maybe when you were younger you went into the basement to get something and as you started back up the stairs you heard a noise, a creaky-eerie noise. What made that noise? Who made that noise? Perhaps it was the boogey-man. Maybe it was the furnace. Someone, something made that noise and you ran up the stairs without touching the steps just a tad scared. It had to be the boogey-man. Passing event? Passing fear? Or do we carry that fear of a snake or something jumping out of the woodwork and scaring us half to death for many years to come?

Fear that is passing and brief can be no big deal. Sometimes fearing fear can take hold of us and create increased anxiety. It can affect our productivity at work for example. Perhaps it affects how we interact with people or at least men or women who look differently and act differently than we do. We see our behavior as normal. We see behavior that is not like us as different and, often, something as a negative. Something we fear. Fear and change can go hand-in-hand. If we fear something, we may not want to change. If we need to change, we may fear what that change will bring.

Does having surgery scare you? Does this cause you to worry? Congratulations! Join the club. You are not alone. You can manage your fear once you know that you are afraid of something and decide that it will not consume you. And besides, you are not the first person who has had your type of elective surgery, nor will you be the last.

Nevertheless, you may be concerned that you will have a bad experience with your upcoming surgery. Perhaps you did have a bad experience in the past and you are now more apprehensive. You may fear the result of the surgery. Will it affect your appearance? Will it affect your self-esteem? You may have friends who have had similar surgeries and their outcome was not as perfect as they hoped. Their rehab did not go as easy as they thought. My suggestion is to listen to your friend about his or her experience, then compare that person's physique and lifestyle with yours. You are not your friend. You are different. Their problems are not your problems. Their experiences, while entertaining, are not your experiences. Their tales of woe, real or not, may be nice to know, but not necessarily a need-to-know gem.

Ask yourself: Is your friend as active or inactive as you? Is their body shape and condition the same as yours? Do they (you) smoke? Do they (you) lead a more sedentary lifestyle? Did they (you) take the time to do the recommended pre-surgery exercises? Did they do the recommended post-surgery exercises and for how long? Sometimes we get in a bad habit of stopping our physical therapy or rehab exercises because we feel we have made enough progress and we don't need to do them anymore. Sometimes folks choose not to do the exercises while they are in the hospital, even with all the support personnel available to them. The exercises hurt. They are afraid to do the exercises because they fear it will cause them even more problems. Sitting in bed or a chair is easier. No exercise. No pain. Get up and exercise.

Friends are friends, but stinking' thinkin' is not what you need prior to your date with the operating room. If your anxiety is severe enough, whether because of a friend's comments or *just because*, it may cause you to cancel or postpone your surgery, though that decision may be more harmful to your overall health and well-being. If your anxiety consumes your life, seek help from your health provider. There are other options available to you.

Learn more about your surgical procedure. Yes, any surgery can cause problems. There is a risk. Driving your car can be a risk. Walking your little doggie on the sidewalk and meeting up with a much bigger doggie can be a risk. What is the risk you are concerned about? What are the positive outcomes to your body after surgery? You may have anxieties about how the financial impact your surgery will have on your overall finances. What will your insurance cover? Talk to your insurance-person. Talk with your hospital prior to surgery to set up a mutually beneficial payment plan.

If your fear and anxiety is making you more fearful and anxious, consider the benefits of having acupressure, acupuncture, massage therapy, meditation, Tai Chi and yoga. There are relaxation exercises you can do, with or without a physical therapist or another person. And they are free. You can make yourself more comfy with relaxation techniques such as slow and deep breathing. Listen to music. Maybe not the head-banger variety, but music that you enjoy and will relax you. Reading can help. You can do these at home. You can engage in more physical activity. Getting your body in better shape will make your rehab less worrisome and allow you to relax a bit more. How do you relax now? What makes you less anxious or less fearful? Do that. Channel your time and energy you spend worrying about whatever it is that you worry about and so something physical. Do your exercises. Go for a walk. Don't waste your time wondering if you can do it. Don't waste your time procrastinating. Spend your time doing it.

> *Almost bionic. I have had multiple surgeries and with every one of them, my surgeons assured me that the severe pain in my hands, hip, knee and foot would be gone once I had my surgery. They were correct. My concern, not an anxiety but a little concern, was how quickly will I be able to get back to what I am passionate about: gardening. I teach master gardeners and other gardeners in general about gardening: hydroponic- and soil-based gardening. I am a mentor to interns who will soon be master gardeners. Will I be able to stand and present a session for sixty to ninety minutes and respond to questions in a coherent manner? In the end, my little concern turned out to be a non-issue, not a concern at all. I was back gardening before I thought I could and as I continued with my rehab program my body got stronger and after a while, I wondered why I didn't have the procedure done sooner. Slow learner am I.*

Module Summary

Preparing Yourself. Start with you. That is what you can control. You can decide what you are willing to do and when you want to do it. You may be getting anxious thinking about all the things you need to do before and after surgery. You may not be as patient. You may be a tad grumpy. You will need to modify what you do and how you do it. You will have some restrictions about what you can lift or how much you can bend. You will not be able to drive so long as you are on opioids and other pain medications. You may need to rely on others to help you get around and do things for you, at least initially. You will be dependent, not independent. You can take some of the anxiety out of your mind with proactive-planning.

Start with your *head* and avoid the stinkin' thinkin' folks. Preparing your mind and body and adjusting your attitude and behavior for what the whole surgical process will bring is the hard part. You will be dealing with emotions and perhaps a little apprehension. You will be dealing with things and people that you probably do not know that well. Change. Apprehension.

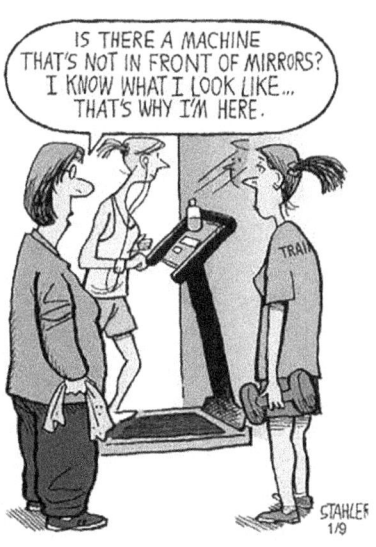

People tend to resist changing for many reasons. The top five fears include:

- Loss of control
- Uncertainty – focusing on the negative possibilities
- Immediacy-the change is too sudden
- Too radical – too different from your normal routine and habits
- Lack of competence – what if you cannot do it

Arthritis can affect any joint in your body and can occur in people of almost any age. It is an all-encompassing label used to describe different diseases and processes. Some non-surgical treatments for pain include aerobics, walking, meditation, physical therapy, riding a bike, lifting weights, stretching and walking in a pool. And you can keep your brain sharp and improve your memory by just walking. Balance exercises can help prevent falls.

Compare your current arthritic (or other) pain level. How bad is it? You probably experience that pain 24/7, whether you are sitting or standing or walking and maybe even while you are in bed. What is your preference? Would you rather continue having your on-going 24/7 pain or engage in some low-impact exercises that could alleviate that pain?

There is no question that if you have not exercised in a long time (or ever) doing so before your procedure can be a daunting task. You may be self-conscious. You be embarrassed. You may lack confidence. You may experience some pain. You may prefer to do a thousand other things, except exercise. Start slowly. Start easy. Start with what you can do now, then build from there.

> *Age is an issue of mind over matter.*
> *If you don't mind, it doesn't matter.*
>
> —MARK TWAIN

Your Notes

MODULE 2

PREPARING YOUR INSIDE WORLD

The focus and outcomes of this module are ...

■ Organizing for a safer home

■ Navigating up and down, in and out after surgery

Overview

You probably started to think about what you need to do to get your inside world more organized before you head off to the happy land of surgery. The more time you give yourself to plan and organize before your scheduled procedure the better your mental attitude. Less stress. Less stuff to worry about. And if you feel that cannot find the time to organize your home before surgery, how will you find the time to do it after surgery? When you are in your post-surgical recovery phase? Not good.

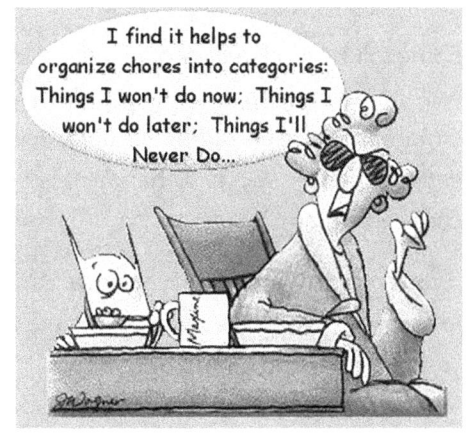

Preparation, organizing and execution are the keys to being able to get your ADL groove back after surgery. Prepare now before you get wheeled into the operating arena. Where will you go after surgery? Back home or to somewhere else? You may have decided to stay in an extended-care facility immediately after surgery where the nice folks there will cater to your every need. You may not need to do much preparation in your living space if you will do part or all your rehabilitation away from your home. Regardless where you go after surgery, you will need to move stuff out of the way, so it does not get in your way when you are walking around with your walker or crutches or cane or wheel-chair or knee-walker. Grab a helper-person to help you if necessary.

Sports Envy Have I

Are you involved with sports? Not necessarily as a professional (well, you could be of course), but someone who just enjoys playing golf or tennis or basketball or other sporting activities with your friends and team-mates. If so, doubtless, you have equipment and clothing to put away after the weather prevents you from playing outdoors or perhaps when the schedule for your team ends for the year. In any event there comes a time when you need to store your toys away for a period of time and having surgery is probably one of those times.

Your daily living activities often define your lifestyle, whether you are relatively active in that activity or not. Most folks would agree that exercise is critical for their health and well-being. Though beneficial, many folks tend to avoid it like the plague or having a root-canal or maybe having a colonoscopy. Time, work, social or family pressures can provide convenient excuses.

Some folks exercise daily or at least multiple times per week. Some folks exercise by walking, swimming, riding a bicycle or getting involved in an exercise-fitness class. Others are more energetic about exercising and engage in more physical sports, such as basketball or soccer or handball or squash and even in a serious weight-lifting or cardio-program.

If you are active in sports, you know there really isn't much you need to do to prepare for surgery. Who stashes all your sports equipment and clothes? If you are young, your parents probably do that for you. If you are an adult another adult probably does that for you. If you live alone, maybe you just pile stuff in a neat heap in the corner of a room. That works for you. And besides, who is going to tell you not to do that? And, of course, if you are on a team, your coach or the equipment manager does it for you. Your job is to use the equipment and let someone else tidy-up and clean up after you.

All things considered, folks who engage in sports or exercise classes have it easy, especially if surgery is on their to-do-list. Gardeners do not have it easy. Non-gardeners don't have much to do after their season ends or when their playing schedule ends; nor do they have much to do when their season begins. Not so with gardeners. Lots of hours. Lots to do before winter sets in and ends their season. Lots to do in the spring to start the season.

Do you work in your yard and garden? Do you grow veggies? Herbs? Flowers? Do you fertilize and mow and rake leaves from the lawn? Do you prune your shrubs and bushes? Make compost? Do you find yourself having to weed more than you want? Or, are you one of those free-spirits who let the weeds grow wherever they want and whenever they want? Gardeners do not have it easy. Sports-folks have it easy. Oh, sure, they may work up a sweat or glow when they play, but it is not like they play every day. An hour or two once a week? Tops. Okay, maybe a little more for some folks. By sports I mean those activities labelled as games, contests, races (with cars, people, horses or other animals).

What amazes me is how many sports revolve around the use and handling of balls. You could look that up. Of course, there are exceptions and not all sports require that you handle balls. Boxers, wrestlers, deep-sea divers, fencer-folks, archery-folks, low and high-hurdlers, pole-vaulters, white-water kayakers, down-hill skiers, ski-jumpers, speed-skaters, ice-skaters, roller-bladers, mountain-climbers and X-sports-folks do not physically handle balls, though some folks believe they have them (somewhere). Gun-folks who shoot at targets with rifles and pistols or bazookas don't need balls, but those who shoot with painted paint-balls need balls. So, what sports do require the handling of balls when sports-folks play? Lots.

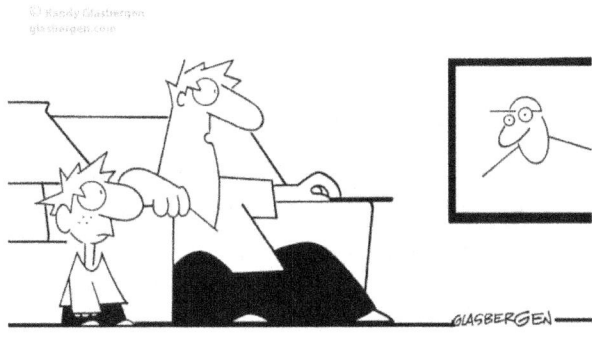

"Remember son, if at first you don't succeed, watch sports. If your team wins, it feels just like you actually accomplished something!"

Folks who play baseball, softball, football, soccer, tennis, basketball, racquet-ball, handball, broomball, paddleball, pickleball, fistball, flickerball, jorky ball (these last three cannot be a real sports, are they?), kickball, knuckleball, volleyball, ping-pong and wiffleball are just some sports that include the use and handling of balls. Those balls come in different colors, shapes, sizes and textures. Some balls are white, solid and hard while others are white, hard and hollow. Balls can also be yellow, orange, black multi-colored and every shade in between.

Balls can be soft, squishy, fuzzy, foamy and smooth. Some have vein-like ridges or raised dimples on them. Amazing. There are round balls and elliptical balls. Bowler-folks (I believe) are the only sports-folks who have holes in their balls. They stick a couple of fingers and a thumb inside their balls. Curler-folks (I believe) are the only folks who have a handle on their balls, though I am not sure those elliptical stones are considered balls. I think marbelers are one of the few who classify their balls by size (not sure if that is still a sport or not). The large balls they handle are called Bumbos or Bumboozers and their tiny balls are called peewees.

And just to be fair, some folks who may not consider themselves sports-folks also handle large 55cm or 65cm balls when they exercise. You often will see them in exercise classes. Folks sit, bounce and lay on them to stretch and do exercises on their tummies or on their backside. Some folks handle Chinese balls that are fondled and rolled around in one hand then another to relieve arthritic pain or just to chill-out. Does that qualify as a sport? Maybe not, but their balls are colorful and hard.

Inquiring minds may wonder what on earth do all those sports-folks do with all their balls? Depending on the sport, they squeeze, grab, grip, smash, swat, toss, hurl, roll, hit and kick their balls. Others handle their balls in a somewhat violent manner with weapon-like things called racquets, bats, paddles and sticks so they can smack, toss, hurl and kick them over a net or against a wall or at another person, friend or foe, it doesn't seem to matter. Lacrosse players use sticks with nets to hurl their balls. Polo players mount a horse and smash their balls with a double-headed mallet. Croquet-folks use a similar, but smaller mallet, when they smash their balls. Their level of play is not as intense and they don't mount animals.

Most sports-folks get rid of their balls as quickly as they can. Footballers run or pass their balls. Basketballers pass and dribble their balls. Soccer-ballers are always in motion and pass their balls with their feet. They can use their heads or chest but are not allowed to handle or touch their balls. Only goalies can handle their balls with their hands (and feet). Tennis players don't dawdle either and smack their balls back and forth rather quickly. Like everything else, there are exceptions. Golfers don't seem to be in much of a hurry and tend to stand over their ball looking at it for a while. Baseball pitchers seem to be the least anxious to get rid of their balls. They pause, rest, stare then finger, fondle and rub or massage their balls before they hurl them at their target. Seems a little odd. Not sure why they take so much time doing that. Anyway...

Sports envy have I.

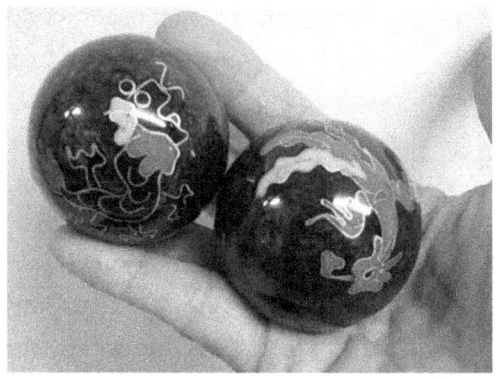
Chinese exercise hand balls are hard and smooth and can be a great exercise for folks who have stiff or arthritic hands. You can roll these babies around while standing or sitting in bed or a chair watching television. Multi-tasking.

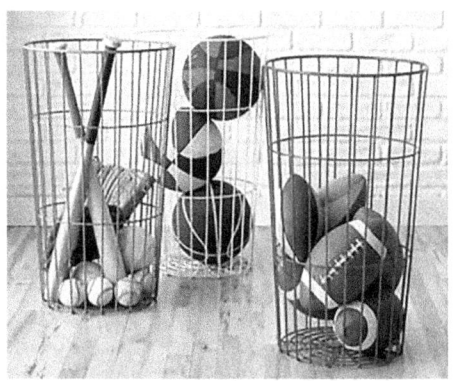
Are you kidding me? Come on. Is that it? No sweat? No kneeling? No heavy lifting? Apparently, there is not a lot of cerebral-thought or decision-making here. Just dump and run. **Done.**

It is not that I am obsessed with sports-folks or with the balls they get to play with or what they do with them for entertainment. To each his own. But as a life-long gardener, life seems a bit unfair. Why is that? Well, for starters sports-folks have little to do before any scheduled elective surgery. I already said that. Storing their balls (and equipment) before surgery does not take a lot of preparation, deep-thought or work. Gardeners do not have that luxury. Sports envy.

No question that golfers may have the most work to do. They wash, clean and dry their hard, white, dimpled balls before they stuff them in some bag. **Done.** Some also wash and clean the heads and shafts and rub them dry before stuffing them in that bag. **Done.** Tennis players probably don't wash their softer, fuzzy yellow balls, but just brush or wipe them before stuffing them in some bag. **Done.** What are we talking about here? Hours of preparation and clean-up? Maybe a couple of minutes, tops. Bless their hearts.

Who has the least amount of work to do? Runners, swimmers, basketball, baseball, soccer and pickle-ballers to name a few. What work do they do? They pack up their Speedos, shorts, shirts, shoes and gender-support-attire and their sports-weapon of choice and toss them neatly in a corner someplace. Maybe the clothes got washed. Others toss their balls into a basket or closet. And in many cases other people clean and stuff their equipment in bags or boxes. **Done**. My guess is the hardest thing for them to do is to remember where they stuffed all their stuff. Probably their spouse or partner knows where. Bless their hearts. Same deal for those who attend exercise classes. Those who do yoga or Tai Chi or play cards or board games have it even easier.

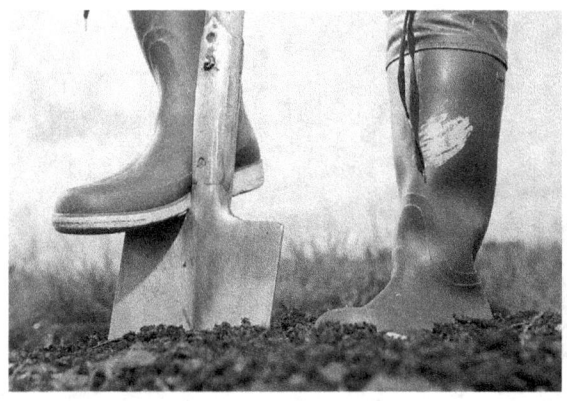

Sports-folks have toys they play with. Gardeners have lots of protective attire and labor-saving toys to help them with their daily-burden, especially if they have a good set of feet and arms.

Okay, probably all these folks do a little cleaning and maybe toss something if it is broken or cruddy looking, but that is about it. Five or ten-minutes. Tops. **Done**. Bless their hearts. I would like to meet just one gardener who only takes five or ten-minutes to prep their yard. Life is not fair. Sports envy have I.

We gardeners do a lot of work throughout the growing season, if not every day, then certainly multiple times per week. We get dirty, whether we want to or not. We sweat or glow, depending on our gender. We bend and stoop and kneel and crawl and weed and lift and push and haul heavy stuff to get our yards and gardens ready. We drag heavy bags of fertilizer and mulch and mow the lawn and tug and haul hoses around the yard so everything gets nice and watered so we can mow and fertilize all over again. We have to stay one step ahead of our neighbors.

And, if that doesn't tug at your heart-strings, we also have to do battle with all those creepy crawlers, such as spiders and earwigs and slugs and pill-bugs and cutworms and flea beetles (and don't get me started on Japanese Beetles) and things that crawl on you that you can't name and can't see and then there is the constant swatting of all those flying bugs that bite and get in your eyes and nose and hair and in your ears. Have you ever swallowed a bug?

And we are always on a 24/7 call to stop the invasion of those four-legged furry-critters who see our gardens as an outdoor buffet, open 24-7. And that is just for starters. Do sports-folks worry about deer and woodchucks and two-legged neighborhood kiddies who jump the fence to grab some berries and step on stuff you just planted and cause your blood-pressure to rise? I don't think so.

Gardeners and yard-folks in general don't handle balls so there is no need to clean and stuff them away. But we do have hoes and rakes and shovels and pitch forks and roto-tillers and hand tools and pots and containers that we clean and store before winter. We open and close our yards twice a year. We call that *winterizing* and *sprin-gerizing*. Well, I hope someone is blessing our hearts.

Gardeners are at the mercy of the elements. Gardeners suffer the effects of humidity, wind, drought, rain, hail, bugs on their bushes and soil diseases. Do non-gardeners worry about any of that? I don't think so. Well, on second thought, maybe just golfers are hesitant to come in out of the rain. If their court or course gets damaged, someone else will fix it for them, while they sit around and suck up a beverage or two and complain about when things will be great again so they can complain and make excuses about how they are playing. Any work around the yard is probably dumped on their spouse or partner or folks they hire to do all the heavy-lifting for them. Hello Happy-Hour. Bless their hearts. Sports envy have I. Well, perhaps one saving grace about gardening and yardwork is that at least we know enough to come in out of the rain and freezing cold. Bless our hearts.

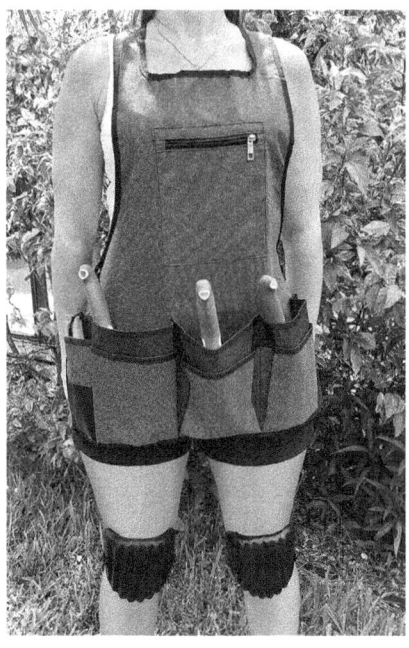

Not to be outdone by the fancy attire that some sports-folks wear, gardeners have their own fashion-forward attire as well.

Gardeners toil and moil in soil throughout their growing season and don't need to handle balls. They (we) struggle on, often alone with our plants, chatting with them, maybe giving one or two a name, feeding and caring for them, kind-souls that we are. Gardeners are neat and tidy. What we handle we clean, stack and store.

Of course, when all is said and done gardeners can eat what they grow. Can sports-folks who do not garden eat the balls they play with? I don't think so. Gardeners, for their endless toil and troubles, enjoy what they like to do. We get to enjoy eating fresh, pesticide-free food. We take charge and have control of what we eat. We are

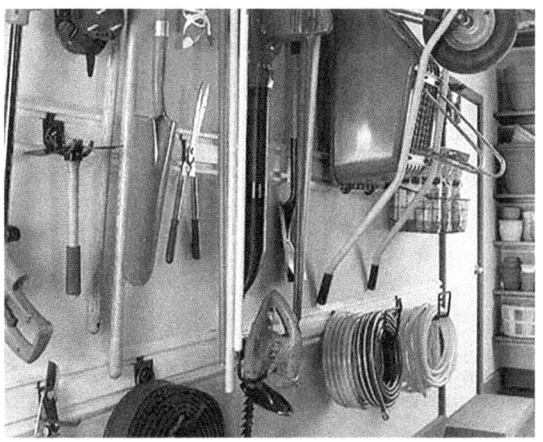

Gardeners have a lot of preparation to do before their elective surgery. Spring preparation, winterization, toiling and moiling throughout the growing season are normal, then everything is cleaned, stored and tucked away for the winter, ready to be untucked for spring and another cycle of toiling and moiling.

more independent than dependent. And when the season ends, we get to relax and play a bit. Bless our hearts. Maybe it is the sports-folks who have envy. So there.

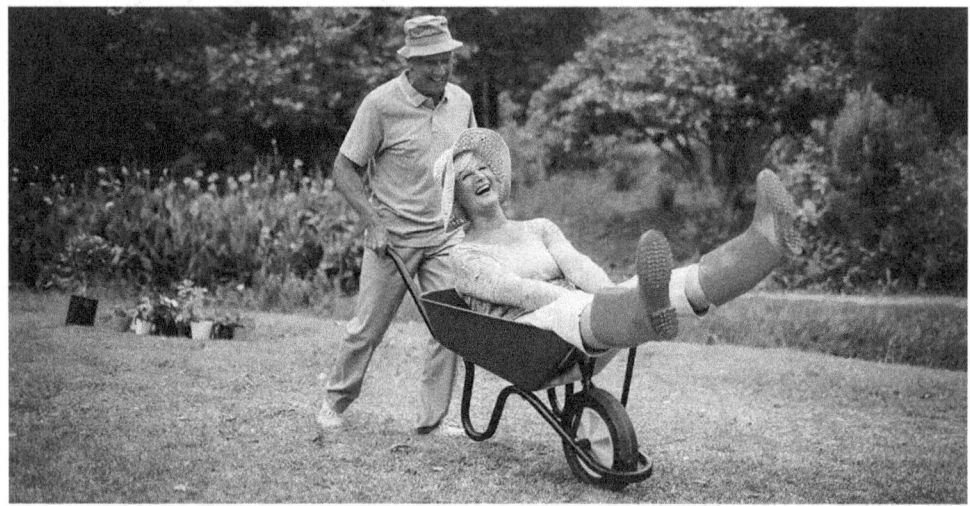

Backyard gardening is handy and eating fresh veggies dandy. We labor each day to pave the way for us to play and get a bit randy, which is better than sitting and eating handy candy.

Organizing Your Indoor Space

Your living space is already organized, right? If not, when you come back from surgery you may find that some things are in your way. That could cause you to trip and lose your balance.

Consider this checklist of suggestions if you will be somewhat incapacitated after your procedure. You may need an assistive aid. You may have trouble walking or climbing stairs. You will have to modify what you used to do or not be able to do them at all for a while. You may need to change what, how and when you do things. Organizing your indoors space can help you create a safer and more accessible world as you recover and long after your rehab has been completed.

- ☐ **Bars of soap.** Keep two bars in your tub-shower unit. All too often, that bar of soap magically slips out of your hand. You may not be able to bend down very far to pick it up (hip surgery). Having a second bar placed within reach solves the problem. Someone else can pick it up for you later or you can use one of those grabber-reacher-thingies when you are all nice and dry. If you are having shoulder surgery, it may be easier for you to use a soap container or something with a pump that you can squeeze or push with your unaffected arm.

- ☐ **Buy or rent a tub bench.** Think about getting a handy assistive-device called a tub transfer bench. It will help you get in and out of the bathtub. Part of it straddles the outside edge of your tub and the other part is in the tub, so you can more easily slide into the tub while keeping your balance. This could be handy if you need to use a wheel-chair.

- ☐ **Detachable shower head.** You will need to keep your incision area dry until given the all-clear from your surgeon. A detachable shower head should make it easier for you to take a shower while keeping your incision dry. And, depending on your surgery, you may be instructed to cover your bandage-cast-incision with a plastic bag or some other water-proof device. Taking a bath will probably not be recommended at all. Check with your physician.

- ☐ **Furniture Walks.** Keep the edges of your counters and furniture as free of clutter as possible. Remove towels or do-dad-things that slide easily. You need to walk when you have lower body surgery or almost any surgery for that matter to prevent blood clots. You may be using a walker or crutches or a cane. Doubtless, you will also be walking without these types of aids at some point. When you do, your tendency will be to grab, touch, and otherwise hold on to, say, the edge or top of your counter or table or other piece of furniture. You can risk falling or losing your grip on that piece of furniture if there is a loose towel near the edge.

- ☐ **Gas it.** If you drive, fill up the tank in your car before surgery. You won't be cleared or able to drive for a while (that depends on your surgeon). When you are cleared your car will be ready to go when you need to go.

- ☐ **Get up and out.** Get out of bed early in the morning and only use your bed to rest and sleep or do some of the prescribed exercises. Spend most of the day taking walks and exercising. Sit in a sturdy chair or recliner to keep your legs raised so you can ice the surgical area, to read, and to watch television.

- ☐ **Gripper-thingies.** Buy some gripper-thingies that will help you open a jar or bottle or whatever it is that you grab that requires you to twist your hand and wrist. There are resin and mechanical options, some with adjustable

Gripper thingies are handy devices that allow you to extend your reach or grip without having to hyper-extend your arms and shoulders.

jaws that allow you to open a wide range of jars and bottles. Buy a gripper-thingy that allows you pick up stuff off the floor, so you do not have to bend down to pick it up (hip and knee surgery). Check them out in your favorite store to make sure you can use them with your non-surgical hand. If you are right-handed, can you use the device with your left hand and vice versa? Tong-thingies can work as well. Put them in your bedroom and by your recliner. These are very handy for picking up things on the floor or on a bedside table or when they are above your reach. You can use them to put on your pants or slacks and pick up your socks and stuff that falls. Your physician may have been told you not to bend down or to cross your legs (hips).

- ☐ **Ice it.** Recliners and icing go well together. Does your refrigerator make ice-cubes? Icing your hip or knee or ankles or feet or other surgical area is important. Ice a couple of times a day. Keeping your legs up and getting plenty of rest will speed your recovery. If you are having shoulder surgery, chat with your therapist about what kind of support you should have in a chair or bed.

- ☐ **Launder your clothes.** Make sure you have several sets of clean clothes waiting for you after surgery. Do your laundry before the big day. Wear loose fitting, comfy clothing so you can easily get in and out them.

- ☐ **Long-handle sponge.** A long-handle sponge or brush is nice when you want to clean your back and other body parts, so you do not have to twist your body or bend down. Use it for your feet and ankles, especially if you are not supposed to bend or if you find it difficult to reach your tippy-toes or are not allowed to reach overhead and behind your head because of shoulder surgery.

- ☐ **Move it.** Move those small tables and chairs out of the way. Move them to the walls of the room. This will allow you to create a clear and safe path for using a walker or crutches or knee-walker or even a cane. Get stuff out of your way. And don't worry about how the room looks to your friends if they come to visit. And if you are that concerned about how your friends will react to your decorating, consider not inviting them over. Besides, when they arrive you will feel obligated to give them food and drink. Save your money! You need to rest and recuperate, not entertain.

- ☐ **Non-slip mats and rugs.** And make sure you have a non-slip mat for your tub or shower. Your feet will get wet. The tile in your shower or tub will get wet. You do not need the risk of slipping and falling. And when you come out of the tub or shower have a non-slip rug there waiting for you. You could easily slip on the tile in your bathroom if you are not careful. Remove any loose rugs. If you need a walker or crutches after surgery, you don't need a rug to grab the legs of your walker or crutches, which could cause you to fall or stumble. Roll those babies up and set them aside, out of your hallway or pathway where you will do your in-home rehab.

> *TIP*: Check with your medical facility. Many offer a free in-home service to help you identify what should be moved, removed, replaced or fixed before your procedure. Some may demonstrate the safe and proper way to enter and exit a shower or tub. Freebie services are good.

- [ ] **Other trip hazards.** Remove electrical cords and magazine racks from your walking path to avoid accidental falls. Again, do what you can to widen your path to accommodate a walker or crutches if you will need to use those after surgery.

- [ ] **Organize stuff.** Toss stuff. Maybe this is a good time to let go of some stuff that has been collecting dust and taking up space since the beginning of time. You will find that tossing stuff and moving stuff is great physical exercise and good for your brain and mental attitude. There is a certain amount of satisfaction that says, time to let it go. It can be a great pre-surgery distraction. Find it. Grab it. Toss it. Donate it.

- [ ] **Organize your kitchen.** Are you the one who does the cooking or will you have help? Regardless, arrange the pots and pans and cooking utensils that you know you will use often so they are nice and handy to you. Avoid having to bend down after surgery. Avoid having to stretch and reach up to get something from that upper shelf. If possible, place what you need towards the back of the counter or in shelves or drawers that are easy to access. Again, don't worry about what the neighbors might say if they decide to invade your nap and rest time. Put up a sign on your door:

> **Welcome! And thank you for stopping by to visit me.**
> **Come on in!**
> **I only serve high quality food. Did you bring any?**

- [ ] **Prep Your Meals.** Are you planning to eat after surgery? Cook and freeze or refrigerate several meals that you can easily prepare and eat after surgery? Plan your menu and prepare your meals before surgery. By the way, if you live alone you may have decided to spend some rehab time in an assisted living facility where you can have your meals prepared for you and have trained personnel to help you with your physical therapy and exercises. If you choose to stay at home, alone, consider contacting the folk who can home-deliver your meals. Meals on Wheels is one such organization. There are also grocery stores, fast-food and other organizations that offer home-delivered meals. Check with them before surgery to see if that service is available in your area. Having food delivered during that first week or two can be a big help. Granted, that will cost you a few bucks, but better to do that than set back your rehab process because you strained or injured yourself.

> *TIP:* You may experience constipation after surgery, which is normal, especially if you were given opioids to reduce your pain. High fiber foods can help. Consider stocking foods such as oatmeal, black beans, prunes, apples, pears, and baked potatoes with skin, broccoli, raspberries and blueberries, and air-popped popcorn or something you can pop in a micro-wave with little preparation.

- [ ] **Pre-packed, frozen foods.** Fresh is best, but convenience might favor the fresh stuff. Buy some frozen fruits and veggies. Stock up on some canned soups that you can open easily and heat in a pan without a lot of preparation. Ramen is quick and easy and the packaging is easier to open compared to some boxes, cans and those hard plastic wraps-containers.

- [ ] **Park it.** Do you have room for a small table next to your chair that will not be in your way? Use it for that book or magazine you are reading or that cup of tea or glass of water. Make sure it is out of your walking area, so you don't smash into it. And get up every hour or two and walk around. Get your body moving. It will help with circulation and digestion and help you wean yourself from your meds. Even a five-minute walk from room to room can help.

- [ ] **Pillows for Shoulders**. Sleeping after shoulder surgery will be an adventure. Use pillows to support your surgical arm-shoulder while you are sitting in a chair or lying in bed. You need to raise your arm to not only support your shoulder but also to reduce the swelling and pain. Chat with your favorite physician or therapist about best positions and which pillows to buy.

- [ ] **Practice**. Do you have a walk-in shower? A tub? Practice getting in and out of both before surgery, without relying on help from someone. This will give you confidence and what you need to do to avoid any awkward movements. If you are having upper-body surgery, can you easily get in and out of your tub or shower area? If it is lower-body surgery that is on your to-do-list, practice getting in and out with a stiff leg—the soon-to-be surgical leg. Initially, you will not have full flexibility with a repaired hip or knee or ankle or foot. Practice.

- ☐ **Recliner chair.** You may want to invest in a recliner. Granted, a good recliner is not cheap. It can be a good long-term investment and a recommended piece of medical equipment. It is also a great sleep-aide, whether you are watching television or not. Buy one *without* a handle on the side. Many recliners allow you to push back with your back and butt. If you have shoulder surgery, say on the left side, and the handle is on the left side, you will not be able to push the recliner back. Side arm handles are useless. Get a chair where you can use your back and butt.

- ☐ **Spare bed.** Is your bedroom on a second floor? Are you comfy being able to navigate up and down those stairs, especially during the first week or two? If so, fine. If not, consider renting a bed that you can park in your living room or where you will have enough room to get in and out and around the bed. Check with your medical facility or the VFW. They may be able to loan you a bed for a couple of weeks or so.

- ☐ **Shower chair.** A shower chair sits inside your tub. It can help reduce your risk of falling. You can sit and shower and rest while doing so. If you have a bandaged leg or foot, sitting on this type of chair, while (perhaps) having your surgical leg outside the tub resting on the edge of the tub, should alleviate any issues about standing or keeping your balance while showering. Remember: tile can be slippery and nasty when wet. Again, you probably will not be allowed to take baths until cleared to do so by your surgeon. Keep some large trash bags handy for when you need to shower and cover your affected leg before you get all wet and soapy. Avoid having an infected incision. Keep it dry.

- ☐ **Sock and Stick aids.** These devices can provide you with greater accessibility when dressing. Dressing sticks can help you put on your pants if you have lower-body surgery and allow you some flexibility putting on a shirt if you have shoulder surgery. Sock aids are great for putting on socks without having to bend down.

(A) DRESSING STICK

(B) SOCK AID

- ☐ **Surgical Aides.** Beg, borrow or spend some money buying some post-surgical aids that will help you navigate in and around your bathroom in a safe manner. Do you have a walk-in shower? If so, consider installing grab bars in the shower so if you decide to take a stand-up shower you will have something sturdy to grab on to (just in case). Do you have a grip bar on the edge of the tub which will help you get in and out safely and without pain and reduce your chances of slipping and falling? Some organizations will provide you with these aids for free. You can use them for thirty to sixty days. Check with your local VFW or with your hospital.

> *TIP:* Do not buy a grab-bar that sticks to the wall. The nice person at the store may have told you how easy it is to install, but they can be dangerous (not the nice person, the grab-bar). The adhesive may not hold you if you suddenly lose your balance or fall. Get it installed by screwing it directly into the stud wall. Can you do that? No? Call a carpenter-person or other professional. Yes, that will cost you some money. Weigh that cost against falling and, possibly, breaking some body part that you did not want broken.

- ☐ **Toilet Seat Seats** There are several options to consider. You can add a cushion-type seat that fits on top of your current toilet seat. You will need this if you have fractured your sacrum or coccyx. You can also rent or buy a portable commode that you place near your bed or where-ever it will be most convenient to you, especially during those first weeks after surgery. In addition, consider installing an adjustable frame unit on your existing toilet unit that includes both arms and legs, which will provide you with greater stability getting on and off.

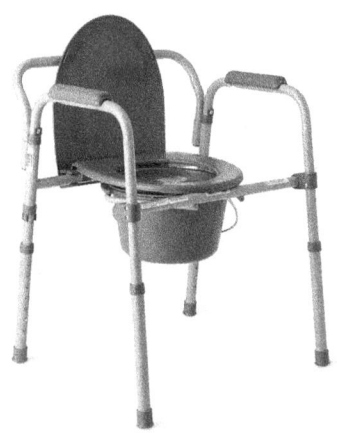
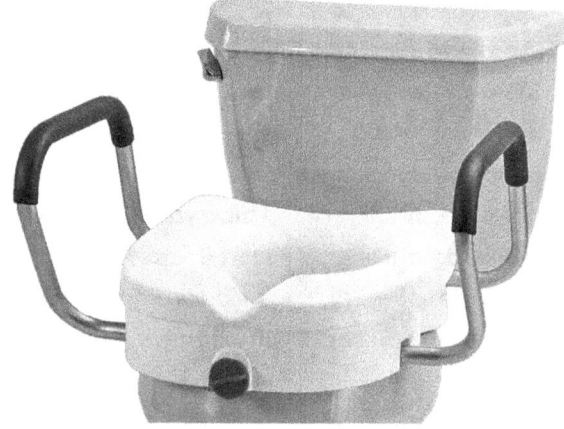

One option is to rent or buy a portable toilet unit or commode that you can move around where ever and whenever you want. You may want to consider placing this near your bed or at least somewhere in your bedroom so you do not have to walk very far, especially if you are in a hurry.

You can easily attach an adjustable unit with arms and legs on to your existing toilet seat. In this photo you will also see a cushioned or raised seat (optional) that sits on top of the existing bowl, thus reducing the need to squat down lower than is necessary.

- ☐ **Toilet Seats.** At the risk of being décor-impaired, forget about those low-lying, closer to the floor type toilets. Forget about what the style of the day is. Try getting down and back up from one of those babies after having lower body surgery (hips, knees). Not good. Toss them. Replace them. Your health and recovery are more important than what happens to be in fashion. Toilet seats are for sitting not for squatting (though that may not apply to all cultures). With hip, knee and ankle-foot surgeries you will need to stretch out your leg far enough to avoid bending your leg too close to your body. Replacing your current toilet with a raised seat will cost you some bucks, but now you have something much more practical for as long as you remain in your house. It will make it easier for you to get on and off the throne.

- ☐ **Air conditioning-furnace check-up.** If your rehab will be during the warmer or hot months in your area, have your air condition-person check things out for you. Likewise, if your rehab will be during the winter months make sure your furnace and heat system are working properly. You want to be as comfy as possible during those first weeks after discharge. You don't need any added stress calling in repair-people while you are in recovery.

- ☐ **Bed sheets and blankets.** Tuck in your bedding at the end of your bed, but untuck it along the sides, especially the side that you intend to use when you want to get in and out of your bed. This will allow you simply toss the bedding aside without having it grab at your feet. As I mentioned above, if your bedroom is on the second floor, you may want to consider setting up camp on the first floor and sleep in a recliner or spare bed for a while and avoid having to navigate up and down stairs, especially if doing so will create stress or cause problems for you.

- ☐ **Collect Stuff.** Do you take vitamins? If cleared to do so by your surgeon, keep them handy along with any other meds that you want to use. And have your toiletries handy—toothpaste, toothbrush, comb, hair-brush, etc. Have a bottle of water within reach so you do not have to get up and down every five minutes, though walking around every hour is a wise practice. Drink plenty of water whether you are on opioids or not.

- ☐ **Collect More Stuff.** Get all the heavy stuff out of the way. Now gather all the little stuff that you know you will want and be able to grab at arm's length—books, audiobooks, video games, cross-word puzzles, movies, some stationary and pens, tissues, lotion, lip balm, medications, back scratcher, the television remote thingy. Put it in a nice bag or bucket with a handle that you can keep by your chair, out of your way, but within easy reach. If you use a walker, buy a basket that you can hang on the front. Fill it with the stuff you just collected.

- ☐ **Create a Hit List.** Depending on your procedure, you may need some assistance within those first few days or weeks. Who can you grab to help you do things and take you places when you need to see your surgeon for follow-up appointments, for going to the store or the mall and for doing chores around your house or yard? Write their names down with phone numbers and e-mail addresses so you can reach them when you want and identify what you would like to have them do for you—drive, mow your lawn, clean your house. And make sure you have the contact information for your medical team and other people who can help you in an emergency if necessary.

- ☐ **Deliveries.** Are you expecting a package or delivery of something? Buy it and have it delivered *before* your surgery because you may not be able to bend or lift it from your front door or steps after surgery. And you don't want your package sitting outside your door for any longer than is necessary and risk having it borrowed by a stranger.

- ☐ **Ice and snow removal.** Are you having surgery in the winter? Does it snow where you live? Make sure someone clears your driveway and sidewalk so you can get into your home safely. Walking on snow is a problem, but usually less of a risk than walking on ice. Make sure the areas where you walk are ice-free (and snow-free).

- ☐ **Pamper up.** Get a haircut before surgery. You may not need another one for at least a month after surgery and by that time you could be cleared to drive and get about town on your own.

- ☐ **Set Security Lights.** If you have not already done so, plan to set some lights in different rooms and especially rooms that you may need to frequent right after surgery, such as your bathroom. Having a night light could prevent a stumble or crash into a piece of furniture. Setting security lights with timers lets folks know that someone is home. Set the timers to go on-off at different times so it appears that you have moved from one room to another.

- ☐ **Social Time.** You may be a more reserved or a quiet-leave-me-alone-person. Or, you may prefer to be the center of attention and what better way to have folks focus on you than to share the details of your surgical procedure. You may want to invite folks over for whatever reason. You won't (or shouldn't) be drinking alcoholic beverages while you are on meds after surgery and chubby-comfy-food is not a good food choice. Of course, your friends will ask you how you are doing and after you have spoken a sentence or two about your procedure, they will, no doubt, launch into their own surgical woes and all the negative things that have happened in their lives and of the lives of folks they know. That type of conversation may not be good for your mental-recovery state. In case you feel badly about not inviting folks over so you can chat about everything and nothing, go ahead and invite them. On the other hand, give yourself an easy out. Ask them if they are afraid of snakes or big dogs. See if they still want to come and visit. If so, fine. Consider taping a sign or two on your front door that has a welcoming message:

> Beware! Big-Butt Dog tends to Bite and bark.
> Come on in!
> Use caution when entering.

Or, how about this gem and relationship-builder?

> Welcome! Thank you for visiting me.
> Are you afraid of snakes?
> They do not always curl or crawl on your lap or neck.
> Come on in!

Navigating after Surgery

Assistive Aids. If you have been using an assistive aid prior to surgery, such as a cane or walker, you probably already know how to navigate within your home, up and down stairs and in and out of vehicles. Generally, if you are scheduled for upper body surgery you may not need to use any assistive device. Your physician will indicate what, if any, device would be most appropriate to you.

If you are having lower-body surgery for a hip or knee you may only need a walker or cane. Foot surgery is another matter. There are different types of surgery and some require that you cannot put any pressure or weight on the affected foot for a minimum of two weeks. Even with a boot or other protective device you could have weight-bearing restrictions and probably will need to use crutches or a kneel walker. Using a cane or walker may not be advised. Your physician will recommend that you not only keep any weight-bearing off your affected foot but also what device would be most applicable to you and your situation.

Motoring around after lower-body surgery, such as a hip, knee or foot or ankle procedure, can be a task. Navigating up and down stairs and getting in and out of chairs or vehicles can be more of a challenge, at least initially. Practice using any recommended assistive device before surgery, so you can do them easily after surgery. Better to learn before surgery rather than afterwards.

Navigating up and down steps and stairs after foot surgery would require that you use crutches, which can be a tad challenging. Normally, you would be advised to go *UP* with your good leg and come *DOWN* with your bad leg. Your good leg is the one that did not experience the joys of surgery. The bad leg is your surgical leg and while you are in the early stages of rehab it is typically not considered your good leg (yet). Your surgeon may disagree with this last point.

> *I have had four lower body surgeries and the first thing I do when I come home from the hospital is to climb the stairs to the second floor and rest a bit in bed. I am back home. I am in my little bed. I spend an hour or so resting and glad that I am alive and well. Then I go back down and walk around a bit then sit in my recliner and usually ice my surgical area. Climbing stairs is good exercise for your knees and hips. You may be afraid or nervous about climbing stairs after hip or knee surgery. Don't be. Your physical therapist at the hospital or medical center can help you practice going up and down stairs with a cane or crutches if necessary.*

Transferring from Assistive Devices. When you are released from your medical-care facility you will be wheeled to the front door by a nice assisting-person. You probably will be in a wheel-chair and then will need to transfer from that assistive device to a vehicle. And when you return home you will need to get out of that vehicle, navigate into your living space and then you may want to sit or stand or go up or down a set of stairs. You may need to use the bathroom. Regardless, you will need to learn how to transfer from one assistive aid to a chair or bed. Ideally, you would have practiced getting in and out and up and down with the assistive device before your procedure, ideally at the medical facility. Your physician's assistant or a physical therapist should have demonstrated how to use that device and given you some time to practice. They haven't done that yet? Ask them to help and demonstrate how to use the device. In any event, you will need to learn how to transfer from Point A to Point B.

- **Devices and Cars.** Practice getting in and out of a car while you are in the hospital. Many facilities have a mock-car in their rehab room. If so, great; if not, then practice with your own vehicle before surgery. First, push your passenger-side seat as far back as possible. You will not be driving, so the passenger side is yours for a while. Second, tilt that seat back so you are almost in a reclining position. When you are ready, back into the seat and use the door or car-frame for support. Swing one leg in at a time. Get help doing that if necessary. Get settled and have someone else shut the door for you so you avoid having to stretch and strain yourself.

- **Chairs to Walkers.** First, make sure the chair you are sitting in is firm, with armrests. Scoot forward on the chair so you are sitting on the edge. Lean forward and push down on the armrests and stand on your good leg. Do not put pressure on your surgical foot if you have had foot surgery. Stand and reach for your walker with one hand, then the other.

- **Walkers to Chairs.** Balance yourself with your walker, then back up to a sturdy chair until your legs touch it. Extend your surgical leg (foot) out in front of you, keeping it off the floor. Use one hand to grab on to the armrest, then the other. Slowly lower yourself into the chair, keeping your operated foot off the floor. Settle into your chair.

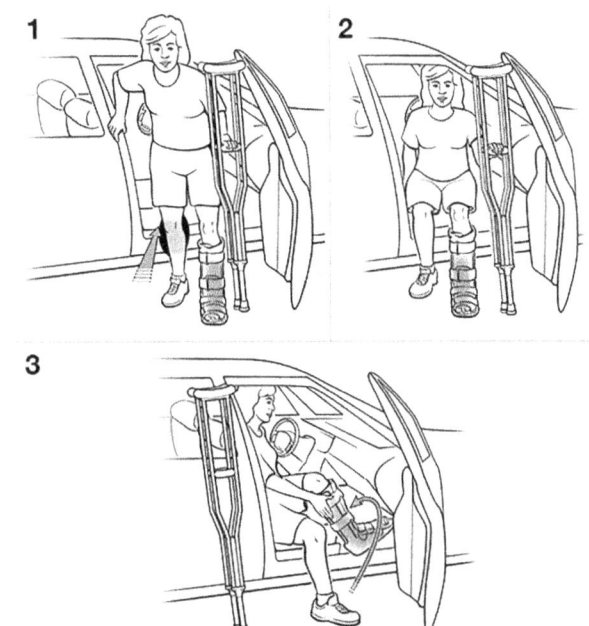

Whether you are using crutches, a walker, cane, wheel-chair, knee-walker or another device, back up to the car seat. Move (or have someone move) your seat all the way back and set in a reclining position if that allows you to get in with less discomfort. You may need to steady yourself on your device and the door frame (or have someone support you) before you swing your leg into the car.

- **Walkers to Curbs.** Before stepping down from a curb, bring your good leg to the edge of the curb. Set your walker down on the ground below the curb, first. Maintain your grip on the walker and push your weight down through your hands. Keep your surgical leg out in front, lower your good leg to the ground and start walking. To climb up a curb, place the legs of your walker against the curb and push down with your hands. Keep your surgical leg in front of you, lift your good leg on to the curb and bring the walker up to the curb and start walking.

- **Walking with a Cane.** Navigating with any assistive device takes practice. If you need to use a cane, hold it in the hand opposite of your surgical side. If your surgery is on the right side of your body, hold the cane in your left hand. Move the cane a few inches ahead of you then move your surgical leg forward at roughly where your cane is and put some weight on your cane to keep you balance. Using your cane properly can help keep weight and pressure off your surgical leg. One of the better canes are those with a pad or *feet* that allows the cane to stand upright.

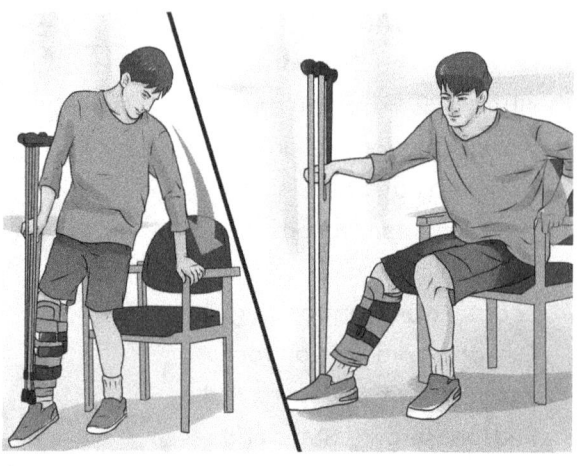

- **Crutches to Chairs.** Getting in and out of a chair or a toilet seat with crutches (or a walker) is easy. Walk up to either and turn so you are facing away from the chair or toilet seat and use your crutch on the same side as your affected limb. Steady yourself with your walker if you are using one. Extend

*Steady yourself with your device and back up to a steady chair until you feel the chair with the back of your **good** leg. Use the arm opposite your surgical leg for balance while you lower yourself onto the chair. Keeping the crutch or cane on your surgical side acts as another leg, a substitute leg, and takes the place of your **bad** leg.*

your affected leg and with your opposite arm grab the arm of the chair and slowly lower yourself down. Always use a sturdy chair with arms. As I mentioned above, modify your toilet seat with an easy to install adjustable unit with arms and legs to facilitate getting up and down with crutches or a walker. A higher seat is easier to navigate, getting on and off, than a lower seat.

- **Wheel-chairs to chairs.** If you are about to get into a car, make certain your coach-helper-person has opened the door as wide as possible and has moved the car seat back as far as possible. This should allow you to have optimal space. Fold the footrests and make sure entry into the vehicle is as free of obstacles as possible. Move the chair close to the vehicle, lock the

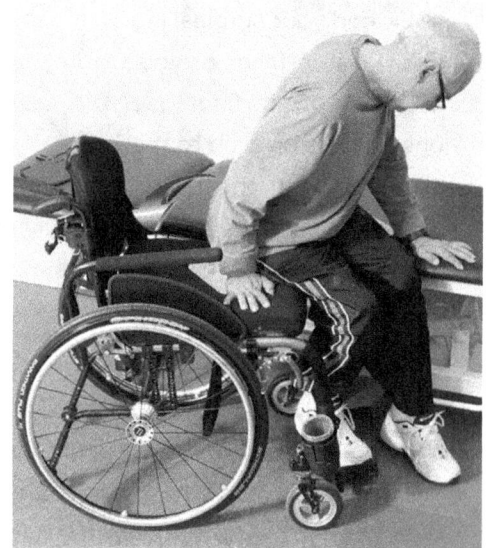

If you are using a wheel-chair before your scheduled surgery, you already know how to get in and out of chairs and cars. If using a wheel-chair will be a new experience for you, practice as much as you can before your surgical date. Keep your wheel-chair close to the chair or bed when you want to transfer from one to the other.

wheels and scoot yourself close to the edge of the wheel-chair seat. If available, use the handle above the vehicle's door to lift yourself up and out of your chair and into the vehicle's seat. If no there is no handle, your coach-person will need to assist you.

Transferring to and from a wheel-chair to a toilet seat is a bit easier if you have a raised seat with arms, allowing you to hold on to something for support. The sturdy arms can help you to raise yourself, turn around and sit, then allow you to stand and return to the wheel-chair in a more comfy and safe manner.

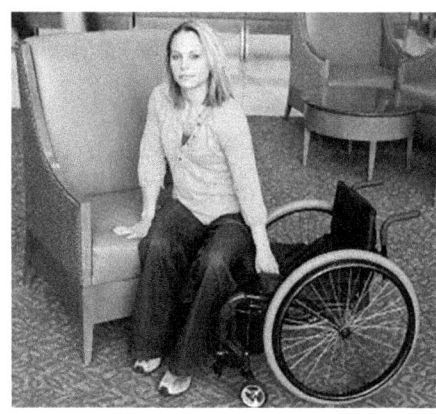

Does your wheel-chair have arms to help you get in and out? If so, great; if not, practice before surgery.

Transferring to different types of chairs or to a bed or bench may require that you have relatively good upper arm strength and balance. Pre-surgical exercises would be highly recommended (re: **Module Six**). Transferring from a wheel-chair to a sturdy chair will require that you keep them both close together and at the same relative height. If they are not close together or are at a different height you may need assistance from your coach-person. Make certain the wheels on the wheel-chair are locked so the chair remains stable while you transfer to a seat.

Navigating with crutches. Do you have to climb a step or two to get into your house? Most homes have at least one step at the front door or in the garage. If so, practice using your walker or crutches to navigate this step.

Using assistive devices, such as a walker or cane or knee-walker are easy to use on flat surfaces. You may need to use them for hip and knee procedures, but probably not for upper body procedures, such as for shoulder, elbow, wrist or hand surgeries. Normally, if your surgery requires an overnight stay you will be given time to practice using the devices recommended for you. If you are having foot and ankle surgery, chances are that you will be in and out in the same day and, therefore, may not be given much (if any) time to practice. Talk to your care team about using crutches and practice using them *before* surgery, *before* you get to the medical facility. They can give you tips and suggestions and identify if you are doing them incorrectly.

You will probably need crutches for foot and ankle procedures. Surgery for a *posterior tibial tendon disfunction, PTTD*, is just one example. Learning how to use crutches effectively can require a bit more practice. Do you remember the first time you were

GETTING YOUR ADL GROOVE IN GEAR WITH PAPS

forced to jump or dive into a pool? The height may have only been a foot or so but at the time it may have seemed like a ten-foot drop. Whether you are climbing up or down a flight of stairs, or just a few, or even stepping over a curb you may find yourself being a bit tense or nervous. The rule is: *Up* with the *good leg*, the non-surgical leg. *Down* with the *bad leg*, the surgical leg. Take one step at a time.

Crutches can be a tad tricky when you need to navigate steps and stairs. Note the proper positioning in the illustration below. One key point is not to use your arm pits to support your crutch. Push down on the handgrips with your hands, otherwise you will have a nice new sore spot, your armpit, in addition to your surgical sore spot. Be careful out there. Make sure you do your pre-surgical exercises to tone up your arms. Chat with your surgeon and physical therapist who can prescribe a series of personalized pre- and post-exercises. Practice. **Module Six** and **Appendix Six** include illustrations and descriptions for some of those exercises.

- **Flat Surfaces with Crutches.** Avoid uneven surfaces as much as possible and as you move forward on a flat, smooth surface, use your good leg to balance yourself while you move both crutches at the same time. Keep your crutches under your arm pits and about a shoulder width apart. Again, avoid using your arm pits as a weight-bearing technique and instead, push down on both hand grips. Step forward with your good leg and keep your surgical leg off the floor-ground.

- **Steps and Stairs with Crutches.** If you are in a chair and want to get up, place both crutches in one hand on the hand grips. Use your other hand to grasp the armrest. Move your butt to the edge of the chair, then lean forward and push up with both hands and your good leg, keeping your surgical leg off the floor. Get your balance, place crutches under your arms, place your weight on the hand grips and avoid placing your body weight under your arm pits. If you want to sit down in a sturdy chair, walk up to the chair then using small steps turn around until you feel the chair against the back of your good leg. Place both crutches in one hand and with your other hand reach

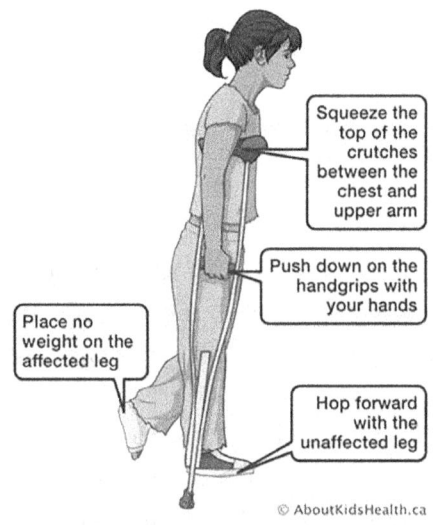

Do not use your arm pits to support your weight. Use your hands on the handgrips. Using your arm pits could result in another element of pain, which you may not be keen to have.

PREPARING YOUR INSIDE WORLD

back for the arm rest. Bend forward at the waist, keeping your balance, and sit back into the chair, keeping your surgical leg off the floor.

Ideally, your stairs have a hand-rail to support your efforts. Again, basically it is up with the good leg, down with the bad (affected) leg. Be careful up there. Using crutches to go up and down stairs is more complicated and requires practice *before* you need to use them.

- Bring your good foot to the bottom step, then bend your knee to bring your surgical foot behind you.
- Push your weight through your hands onto the hand grips.
- Step up onto the first step with your good foot.
- Use your crutches and your good foot to raise your body to that step.
- Repeat, going up one step at a time, slowly, maintain your balance and rest before going up the next step, keeping your surgical foot elevated, off the step.
- With practice you may be able to use only one crutch to go up the stairs, using the crutch on your surgical side, again going one step at a time.

> **TIP:** *This may not be possible or practical for you, but if you have access to a nice sturdy helper- person have them stand behind you as you venture up the stairs. Have them stand two-steps behind you and just in case you lose your balance or feel a bit dizzy, they could prevent you from falling backwards. Regardless, be careful. Practice going up and down your stairs before surgery if at all possible.*

- Before traveling down steps, bring your good foot to the edge of the steps.
- Straighten your knee to bring your bad leg forward, but do not put it down on the step.
- While balancing on your good leg, slowly bring the crutches down onto the next step by bending your good knee.
- Push down through your hands onto the crutches, lowering your good leg down to the next step and proceed slowly until you reach the bottom of the stairs.

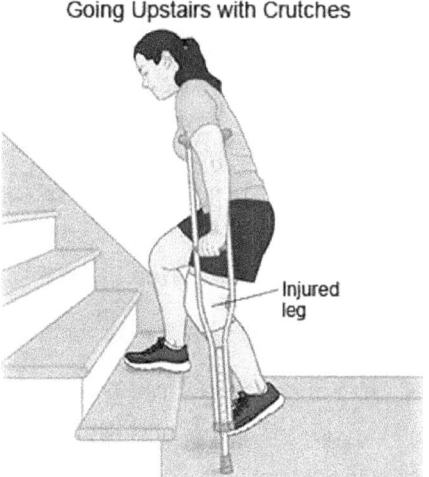

Going Upstairs with Crutches

Injured leg

Are you still a tad nervous about using crutches to go up and down a flight of stairs? You may not have a choice but using crutches to go down or up a flight of stairs may not be high on your wish-list. One or two steps, fine; but more than four, forget it. Regardless, you could navigate any stairs with a little *cheating*.

Bum Bumping Stairs. Going up and down stairs, without crutches is much easier, though perhaps not as dainty to someone who might be watching you. Use your butt.

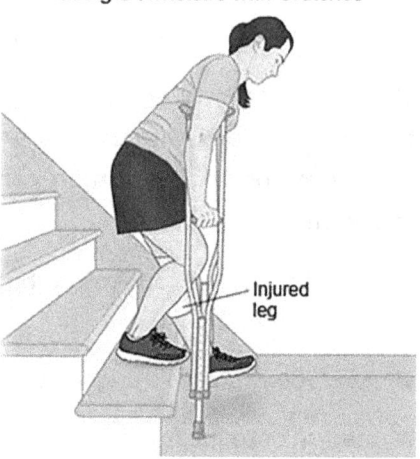

Navigating up and down a stairway can be frustrating and disconcerting. Practice. Have your physical therapist or other member of your care-team show you how to do it before your surgery on a short set of steps with a hand-rail.

- To come down a set of stairs, come to the top step and use the handrail to lower yourself down on that first step.

- Then, gently bounce your butt and body down each step until you reach the bottom.

- Make sure your favorite coach-partner has your crutches waiting for you.

- Raise yourself up with your good leg and the hand-rail.

- You could, if you are all alone, bounce down and pull your crutches behind or beside you as you descend or ascend the stairs. Just be careful.

- To come up a set of stairs, have your coach place a step-stool or sturdy chair at the top of the stairs prior to your *mountain-climbing* adventure.

- Back up to the stairs until your good foot touches the stairs.

- Reach back and sit on the step that is most comfy for you, probably the third step from the bottom.

- Keep your surgical leg out in front of you and off the ground and lift or bump yourself up to the next step using your arms and your good leg, continue until you reach the top step.

- Use your arms to lift yourself up from the top step and on to the step stool.

- Lift your yourself from the stool to the sturdy chair and swing your legs around so you can then stand with your assistive device—crutches, walker, cane, knee walker.

PREPARING YOUR INSIDE WORLD

Safely raising your favorite body up from the top stairs and getting into a vertical position, using your arms, is another important reason for toning up your upper body (arms, shoulders). Remember: you cannot use your surgical leg (especially with foot-ankle surgery) to help you get up because you will probably need to place too much weight on that leg and, as a result, you could injure yourself. Tone up those arms and shoulders if you have had lower body surgery.

> *By failing to prepare,*
> *you are preparing to fail.*
>
> —BENJAMIN FRANKLIN

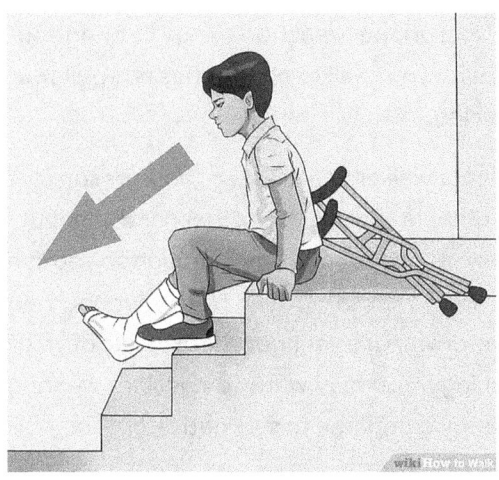

Going down or coming up on your butt is an alternative to using crutches on stairs. And, for some, it can dramatically reduce any stress or anxiety when you navigate those steps in your home. It may not look glamorous, but it sure can help you navigate both up and down a set of stairs. And it could also be fun.

Dressing, Undressing. At some point you will want to change whatever you are wearing to wearing something else. Shoulder or rotator-cuff surgery may present the bigger challenge for you when you want to dress and undress. Here are some suggestions for dressing and undressing.

If you are having a hip and lower body procedure, putting on clothes from the waist up should not change from what you were doing before surgery. Put on your shirt, blouse, dress, whatever just as you did before. Wear loose-fitting garments that are easy to put on and take off and maybe have an open front that you can button or zip up. Consider clothes (and footwear) with Velcro straps. Tying shoes will require that you bend down, not a good move (hip surgery). Use slip-on shoes or slippers. You can use helpers such as a gripper-thingy, a long shoehorn (at least eighteen inches) and your assistive device-walker, crutches to assist your efforts if you need to balance yourself. (Recall the information about the dressing-stick mentioned earlier.) You may also need to have a bit more patience. Got some?

You can have someone put your socks on for you or you can use a sock-aid. A sock aid works best with socks that stretch or have been worn and washed so they are not as tight as a pair of brand-new socks. While you are sitting on the edge of your bed or a sturdy chair, slide one sock on to the sock aid, lower it to the ground, insert your foot and pull up on the rope handles. Do not bend down. The rope handles on the sock-aid take the place of you having to do that. If you have a wide foot, I suggest you buy a five-inch wide sock aide. A slightly wider aide is better than one that is too narrow for your foot.

You may prefer to put on your pants or panties first, before your socks. Regardless, for getting in and out of your pants, Speedo-bathing suit or undies, place your surgical leg in first, then your unaffected leg. Always put your shoes or footwear on after your pants are on. Otherwise, your footwear may hang up in your pants and you may find yourself in a tug of war with your foot and garment. Pull your garment up as far as possible while you are still sitting down. Use a gripper-reacher-thingy to bring your socks or other garments to you. Stand up with your walker or crutches and pull your garments the rest of the way up. Start walking.

To remove your clothing, stand in front of your walker or a dresser-table for support and balance. Keep one hand on the walker or table and use your other hand to unbutton or unzip your lower garments one at a time, one leg at a time, enough so you can now sit on the edge of your bed or a chair. Remove the clothing from your good leg first, then your surgical leg last. Do not bend down. Use your good leg to slide off your pants-panties-shorts or use a reacher-thingy. You may want to consider wearing 100% cotton clothes. They may be a bit heavy compared to synthetics, but they will provide you with a bit of warmth during your recovery.

Getting dressed and undressed after upper body surgery, e.g., rotator cuff, is easier to do if you have practiced putting a shirt or blouse or bra on before surgery. Recall the dressing stick illustration shown earlier in this module. Ask your physician's personal assistant for suggestions about other clothing to consider. You can use some of the items mentioned above to help you with your pants, socks and shoes. In addition, you may want to include these items regardless whether you are having upper or lower body surgery. I mentioned these earlier. Here they are again…

- Detachable shower head so you can keep your incisions dry until cleared by your physician
- Shower chair and a shower grab bar (screwed securely into the stud wall)
- Shirts, blouses or pants with large buttons, Velcro fasteners or zippers
- Use open-front blouses, shirts, jackets, dresses

- Women should wear bras that can be opened in the front, though you may not want to wear one for at least the first few weeks because they can be uncomfortable if you had shoulder surgery
- Wear larger, loose fitting shirts, sweat-pants with elastic-waist bands

Module Summary

Maintain as positive an attitude as possible before and after surgery. You need to prepare for your surgery. Get help as needed. Your rehab and recovery after surgery will take time. Have patience. Do your exercises. You should have plenty of time to complete your pre-surgical exercise program, get your mental groove in gear, organize yourself and your home, make any adjustments as needed and get ready for your big day. Make a plan. Execute your plan.

Surgery in your shoulder area can be a bit of a challenge when you want to dress-undress. Use your good arm to place the sleeve in your surgical arm and around your neck. Slip your good arm in the other sleeve and fasten your shirt-blouse with large buttons or with Velcro. Reverse the process when you want to remove the shirt-blouse.

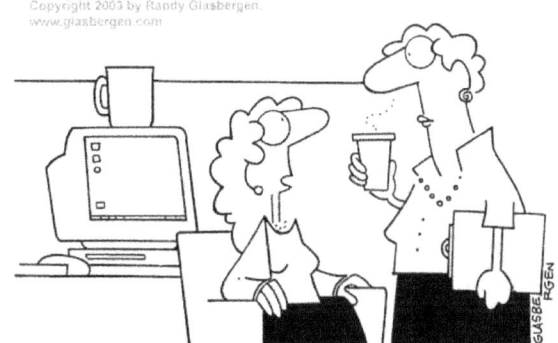

"On Mondays, I get ready to plan my week. On Tuesdays, I plan my week. On Wednesdays, I revise my plan for the week. On Thursdays, I put my plan for the week into my computer. On Fridays, I think about starting my plan for next week."

One of the best activities you can do prior to surgery is to have a plan. Be proactive. Your plan can act as your guideline, with timelines and a checklist, for what you may need to do and when and how you will need to do it before you land on the operating table and after you return home and resume your active daily living activities.

Pro-active Plans (PAPs). Planning to prepare for surgery can include many different activities and decision-points. Forget perfection. If your goal is to have a perfect plan you may end up spending your time planning your plan and little time implementing your plan. Your first attempt at planning, your first draft if you will, is for getting it down. It is not for getting it good or perfect. Keep your plan fluid to allow for new suggestions and changes in what you are able and willing to do. Will you be able to do everything yourself? Will you need help? Who can help you? Prioritize what you must do and, depending on your time, what would be nice to do.

Start preparing your home well before your day of surgery. Clearing out clutter and moving stuff can reduce your stress prior to the big day. Create a hit list of folks who you can rely on to help you when necessary. Practice using any assistive devices that your favorite surgeon has recommended—walker, knee walker, cane, crutches, wheel-chair. Exercising will make your rehab more effective and safer.

- Keep the edges of your counters and furniture free of clutter
- Buy some gripper-thingies to help you pick stuff up and open jars and bottles
- Practice using your dressing stick and sock aids
- Practice getting in and out of your shower or bath-tub without using your affected leg
- Practice using crutches before you need to use crutches
- Practice going up stairs with the good leg and down with the bad (surgical) leg
- Practice bum-bumping up and down your stairs
- Practice getting in and out of cars
- Practice getting dressed and undressed without using your affected leg or arm

Organizing your home may seem to be a waste of time. You may think it is organized already. Practicing may seem to be a waste of time. Better to organize and practice before surgery and feeling comfy and confident, rather than waiting until after surgery. You will have enough to do and think about after surgery and organizing your indoor space should not be one of them.

In addition to canes and crutches and walkers and knee walkers and wheel-chairs, there are other devices and options to consider.

- Use chair raisers to help raise your chair to the same height as your wheelchair.
- Chairs with removable or arms that drop down can provide you with more sideways transfers.
- Some recliner chairs include a battery-operated vertical lift option that can help you rise and transfer to your wheelchair or walker with little or no effort on your part. You push a button and your chair moves like magic.

- Sliding or transfer boards can act as a bridging device between your chair and a wheelchair. Make certain they have slip-resistant undersurface.

Your Notes

MODULE 3

PREPARING YOUR OUTSIDE WORLD

The focus and outcomes of this module are the following:

- Returning to your outdoor ADLs after surgery before surgery
- Better accessibility in your garden
- Integrated Pest Management
- Ergonomic tools

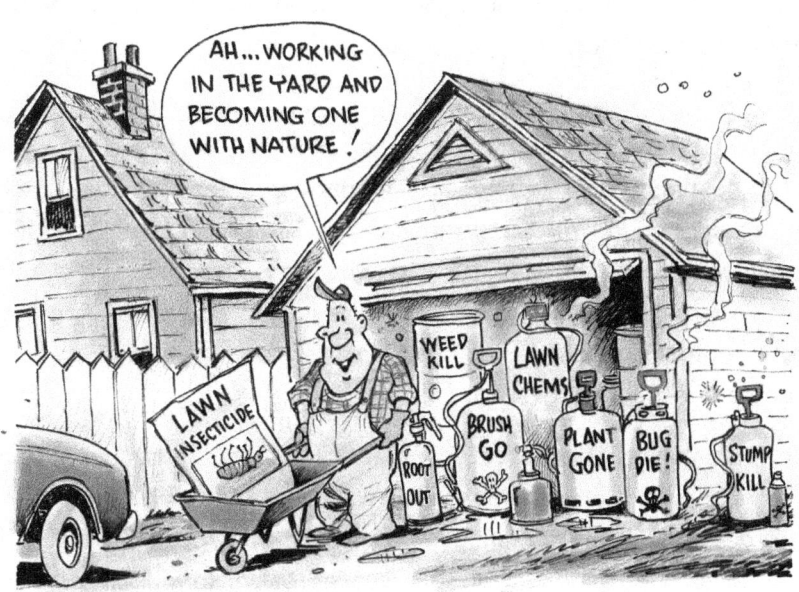

Overview

This module includes suggestions that you can implement before surgery and other ideas that you can easily do while you are recuperating, depending on the type of surgery you are having. Some of these ideas you can do yourself and others may require the help from kiddies or other helper-persons, especially those who can differentiate between using a hammer, saw and other basic tools. You will agree with some of those ideas, others maybe not so much. Regardless, each idea is workable. Each could be used to modify your existing yard and garden if you choose to spend the time, energy, and money to do so. All, if implemented prior to your surgery, could help you return to your yard and gardening ADLs with less maintenance and manual labor after your procedure.

Planning for after Surgery before Surgery

Do you have a yard? A garden? Do you like to grow some of your own veggies, herbs and flowers outside where you can get lots of Vitamin D and rosy cheeks? If you have no desire to even think about gardening or playing catch-'em-catch-'em with those cute little bunny-rabbits, then feel free to skip this module. If you are a gardener and like to grow some of your own food, pesticide and herbicide-free, the suggestions in this module may be beneficial to you. If you are an avid golfer or tennis player or someone who engages in other sports or ADLs and still enjoy working and prancing about your yard, then read on. Though the suggestions are practical and can provide you with better accessibility, there may be suggestions that you would classify under *is-he-kidding me*?

The focus in this module is primarily on your veggie and herb gardens. Planning what you want to do in your garden (and yard and patio and deck) next season begins while you are still working in your current season. This allows you to identify which varieties have produced well for you, which have attracted more than their fair share of bug critters and whether you need to adjust the spacing between and among rows. Planning takes time. Plan to set aside time to plan as soon as you have planned your elective procedure. Be proactive, not reactive.

Depending on the type and extent of your gardening efforts and the input from your favorite surgeon, you probably want to know approximately how long your rehab process will be and how you will manage your gardening activities. Give yourself time to plan and move stuff around to make your recovery easier so you can garden sooner and when you want without having to run around and re-organize things at the last minute, or worse, attempt to do them while you are still in your rehab-recovery phase. Plan, organize and implement according to when you have scheduled (or will schedule) your surgery.

Fall for Winter. If you plan to have your surgery in the winter, then plan and organize yourself, your home, your sports gear and your garden in the fall. Do you need to transplant flowers? Trim some bushes? Spread lawn fertilizer? Clean and store your sports equipment? Depending where you live, if you start to organize your outside world on or about Labor Day you should have enough time to make modifications to your garden and do any sports or non-sports preparations before the cold weather arrives.

Winter for Spring. If you plan to have your surgery in the spring, can you organize and do what you need to do during the winter months if it is not too chilly where you live? Will you have time to do that in the fall? If you are planning on a late spring or early summer surgery date, can you do what you need to do in February, March or April?

Spring for Summer. If you plan to have your procedure in the summer, organize your outside and sports world in the spring. For example, if your surgery is in June or July, prepare in April and May. If surgery is scheduled for late summer, say August or the first part of September, prepare in June or July. Check to make sure your tools and any sports equipment are in proper order and ready to go when you are ready to go after you finish your post-surgery rehabilitation.

Summer for Fall. Likewise, if your procedure is in the fall, spend the summer or at least the latter part of summer doing what needs to be done.

Organizing your outside world will be dependent on the weather, regardless where you live. Scheduling your surgery could be dependent on when you plan to return to gardening, when you plan to smack your balls around and when the golf course or tennis courts open for the season. You may be able to schedule your procedure and complete your recommended rehab protocol prior to the next planting-growing-playing season in your area.

> *I have scheduled my various surgeries in the winter, usually January. I do this because it is a slow time for me as a master gardener. I cannot garden outside here in Zone 4 during that time (but I can and do garden hydroponically inside). And it allows me to have my surgery, start and complete a major portion of my rehabilitation process before spring thaw and outdoor gardening time.*

Winterizing Your Yard. Whether you like to grow veggies or flowers, prepare for spring by preparing for winter. Some of us in the sunny-climes in the northern part of the United States refer to that period as the snow-bird season. There are other words we use, but winter should suffice for now. For each growing season you have a nice long list of things you need to do. In the spring, you need to prepare your soil-based garden for your tried and true plants and maybe some new veggies, herbs, and flowers. You may be gardening in containers. You may be amending the soil. You may be hiring someone to roto-till your garden. You may be thinking about sprucing up your pathways with more wood mulch or other material. You may be thinking about buying mulch or composted manure and potting soil for your containers as soon as it goes on sale. And, of course, you should have your garden plan all set for where you want to plant what and how many to plant of what. Then after a summer of enjoyment you need to clean up your garden and containers. Spring preparing in the spring and winterizing in the fall.

When winterizing, spread any unused fertilizer and work it into the soil—by hand, with a roto-tiller; hire someone to do it. Mark out your rows for what you intend to plant where. Buy bright plastic stakes and nylon string to mark your rows. I do not recommend using twine or jute, because it could rot or partially disintegrate by spring. In the spring, you will need to rake out the rows before planting. The snow/rain over the winter will pack the soil, raking will loosen the row for seeds or plants that you intend to put in. Do not work the soil if it is wet. Doing so will create nice hard lumps and clumps that will remain throughout the growing season and cause you frustration and perhaps a bit of stress.

Trim your trees and bushes. Repair any serious cracks on your patio or driveway or repair any loose boards on your deck. You will be in rehabilitation for a period after surgery. You do not need to trip and fall and sprain or break something. Fix what needs to be fixed. Replace what needs to be replaced.

You may be living in a Zone that allows you to garden the entire year or certainly longer than we can here in the upper mid-west or along the frontier with Canada. If so, do as much cleaning and preparation before your growing season begins. Regardless, winterize your yard and garden at the end of your growing cycle and certainly before you travel to the

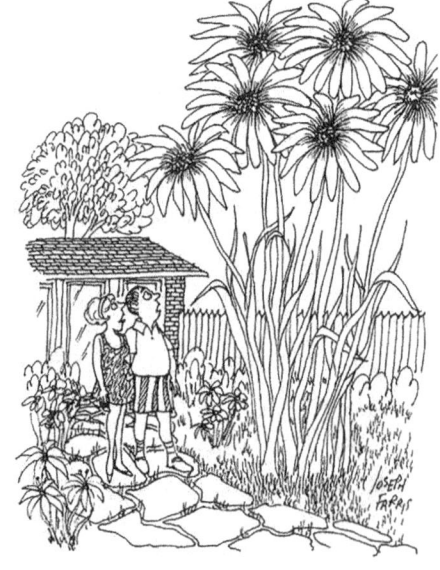

Isn't that where you spilled the fertilizer?
(**Saturday Evening Post**, May/June 2004.)

hospital. Winterizing is important because you need to remove diseased and dead plants. Pull out those weeds before they set seed, otherwise you will be pulling out more during the next growing season. Pull out any plants that you consider to be invasive or otherwise plants that you no longer want to live alongside plants you do want.

> **TIP:** Do not compost weeds that have seed heads. Unless your compost bins reach a temperature of at least 135-degrees for several days, the weed seeds will not die; they will germinate when you use that composted material for your next growing season.

Catch-22. Pruning most trees and bushes are best done during the dead of winter. No threat of bug-critters or diseases. Cutting down, chopping up, mowing down plant debris for your compost bins or for your favorite trash-recycling-pickup-person is all part of the winterizing program. It gives your garden that clean and tidy-bowl look. It gives you a feeling of satisfaction. Planted. Harvested. Cleaned-up and done until the next year or next growing cycle.

There are at least two schools of thought about this aspect of winterizing. One group recommends that you clean up everything, which then better prepares you for the next season. They do not recommend vacuuming or steam-cleaning or disinfecting your yard and garden, but the implied tidy-bowl intent is there. Another group recommends that you clean up everything that is diseased and leave the part that is not diseased untouched and left standing in place.

Leave some litter for the critter. The good bugs and bees and other critters need a place to winter over. Dead grass stems, left standing, are one good place critters can winter-over. If you do cut down the non-diseased plants, leave at least a twelve-inch stem standing for the critter-bugs. Leave a pile of leaves along the edge of your garden or in a corner or two for other critters. How much is a pile? The equivalent of a thirty-three-gallon trash bag should suffice. This provides many critters with protection and by spring your pile will be dramatically reduced from any rain or snow and partially decomposed. Use what is left for mulch or as partially composted material to work into your soil or containers. And as an aside, by not cleaning everything up in your yard, you avoid a lot of extra work. Use the time you save to go to other pre-surgical tasks.

Some native bees need bare soil or sand to winter over. There are approximately 400 bee species in Minnesota alone. And if you tend to roto-till or plow your garden, do it very early in the fall before days and nights get too chilly. The critters are starting to dig down and settle in for the long winter to come. Ripping up the soil later will destroy their nests and the channels they make to burrow and re-emerge in the spring. If you want to attract mason bees, set up their nests late summer. They will find them in the spring.

This is also the time to divide any perennials. Plant your flower bulbs. Deep water any evergreens, shrubs and shade trees thoroughly. But you already know that.

Green Manures. Many gardeners and many farmers tend to keep the soil bare over the winter. Nice and neat and tidy. Not such a good practice as it turns out. Wind can easily pick up your valuable top-soil and fling it past your yard into the next county or state. Don't let that happen. Think about planting a cover crop. Cover crops form a type of living mulch. They grow quickly and keep weeds in check. If you plant a cover crop and let it grow and die, then remove the dead stuff, it is still called a cover crop, an ex-cover crop. If you turn that cover crop into the soil to provide organic mass to the soil, it is called a green manure. Same plant. Different process. Different name.

Some green manures to consider include the legumes, such as hairy vetch, clovers, beans, and peas. Alfalfa, like legumes, take in nitrogen gas from the air and convert it into a form that your plants can use—nitrogen (N). The process is called *nitrogen fixing* or *fixing nitrogen.* Farmers use this effectively when they practice crop rotation between soybeans and corn. Grasses include annual ryegrass, oats, rapeseed, winter wheat, winter rye, and buckwheat. You need to plant these early enough in the late summer or very early fall so they can germinate and create a nice thick cover to keep the weeds down. When does it get chilly-cold in your Zone?

On the other hand, you can spread the seeds in early spring and let them germinate. When you are ready to plant your veggies and herbs just roto-till or push the cover crop aside and plant in that space. The remaining cover crop, which is your aisle or pathway, will help keep weeds down and, depending what you plant, can attract pollinators. For example, calendula, lacy phacelia, alyssum, and crimson clover are just a few possibilities that produce pollinator-friendly flowers. Not too crazy about that idea? Till them into the soil and they become a green manure. Your plants will benefit either way.

Is your soil mostly clay or *hard?* There are several mustards and daikon radishes that will not survive cold weather. Plant as directed. They grow extra-long roots that easily penetrate heavy or dense soil and create air channels. Plants grow in air, not in soil.

> ***TIP:*** Be careful about which daikon radish you select. Not all are edible. Read the description on the package or in the catalog. The radishes advertised as breaking up the soil are not always of the edible variety. Check them out before you buy so you know what you are buying.

No-Till Option. Yes, you can till in your ground cover as green manure, or not. One very low maintenance option is to not till the whole area, which I mentioned above. Allow the plants, now dead from the winter and now called *residue*, to remain as a cover to prevent some weeds from germinating. You can pull back some of that cover, till or turnover a row(s) and plant your plant or seeds in that space. You can create the same basic effect with grass clippings or leaves or a heavy layer of straw. Add what is available to you in the fall, allow it to compress over the winter, then separate it to plant individual plants or a row or block of seeds and plants. Keep the remaining material in and around your plants throughout the growing season. By mid to late-season that material should decompose, adding new soil to your garden. Springtime: No tilling. No double-digging. Less weeding. Less work. Less maintenance. Less stress. Fewer bad words need to be uttered.

Coconut Coir. If adding green manures or leaves or grass clippings or straw is not something you can do because they are not available, consider using coconut coir in the spring just after planting the plants. Coir is a renewable and sustainable resource. It is made from coconut husks and is usually available in many garden centers, hydroponic stores and online.

In the spring, use the product as a mulch on your tomatoes, peppers and eggplants and other veggies and flowers. It does a respectable job of keeping the weeds down and keeping many diseases, such as *Septoria Leaf Spot* a bay, at least for much of the growing season. The product is sold in compressed bricks or bales. You use it by soaking the brick or bale in water and spread it about one inch around your plants or mix it into your soil or containers.

Coconut coir acts as a substitute for peat. It retains moisture when mixed in with your potting soil or garden soil. You can use it in containers and around your flower beds. The problem, if it is a problem, is that you need to soak the entire brick or bale before you can use it. Yes, you can cut up the bale with an axe, chain saw, jack hammer or other device and soak what you think you will need at the time. Use warm water and as the material softens break it up with a hand tool, such as a trowel to hasten the process. When it is all nice and soaking wet and mushy, spread it as you would any mulch. Apply it about one-inch thick to allow water to reach the roots while keeping the weeds at bay.

Too messy for you? You can also buy the product in bags, ready to use—open the bag and spill out what you want where you want it. The product is not compressed and can be easily spread or integrated into your planting area. You do not have to soak this version. You can just spread it then spray it with some water, so the wind does not carry it to the next state. It is a bit more expensive than the brick or bale versions, yet it may be more convenient to use.

> *TIP:* Instead of bagging up your leaves and giving them to your trash-person, use the leaves to cover the bare ground in your flower and veggie areas. The leaves act as a kind of cover crop. They protect the soil from flying away to the next county and it allows the critters you see and the microbes that you do not see to decompose them. Got lots of leaves? Chop them up with your lawn mower and leave a very thin layer on your lawn. No bagging. No extra work. Leaves contain many of the nutrients your lawn and trees need. Bagging just fills up landfills.

Compost-Mulching. After you have made your garden all nice and tidy and kept some litter for the critter, add composted material, such as composted manure, to your flower beds and throughout your garden. What if you do not or cannot garden next spring? If you leave your garden bare, the weeds will take over and you will be a bit upset that they are growing like, well weeds, and you are not able to control them. You might find yourself using some colorful language. Spread a good layer of compost over your flower and veggie areas, two to four inches would be ideal. The compost will pack down over the winter so that by spring it may be about an inch thick. This should be enough to keep most weeds down at least in the early and late spring.

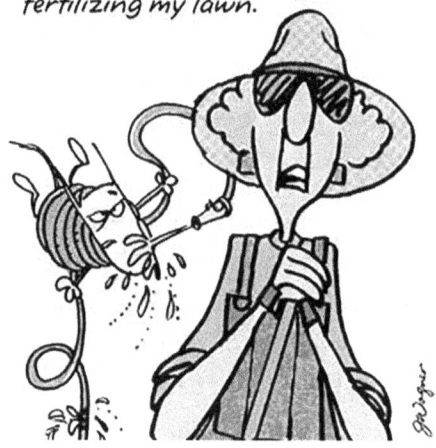

They say that now's the time to fertilize your lawn so it'll grow extra tall and thick this summer. Which is precisely why I won't be fertilizing my lawn.

Add mulch in your flower beds or around your bushes. Lay it on thick, at least two- to three-inches. Snow and rain will release the nutrients within the composted material benefiting your plants. As I mentioned, you can turn under any remaining material or simply leave it for weed control. The compost will keep some of those early-rising weed seeds from germinating.

> *TIP:* Before you plant warm-season crops, such as tomatoes, peppers and eggplants, make sure the soil is warm. If you added mulch or other material in the fall, spread it away from the rows you want to plant, leaving the rest on the *aisle*. Cold or cooler soil will set warm-season plants back a bit, resulting in slower growth and a longer mature-harvest time.

I plant four varieties of potatoes each year. In some years I plant them directly in the garden and in other years I use wire cages-containers. Each circular wire container is six feet in diameter by two feet high. Use wire that is one-half inch or smaller to keep out the critter mice and voles. I plant three or four eyes in each container. I fill the bottom third with my own mix of potting soil, compost, composted manure, bone meal and peat, add the eyes and cover them with about four inches of the same mix. As the plants grow, I add more composted material and/or composted manure. I fill the areas between the containers with leaves saved from the previous fall. By early August the leaves have decomposed into soil. When I harvest the potatoes, I lift the wire and harvest the potatoes. No digging. No mice or vole problems. If you think you have too many leaves from your yard, distribute them around your potatoes (or other veggies).

Save newspapers, cardboard, grass clippings, straw (never hay; only marsh hay), or use weed fabric to prevent weeds from sprouting all over your soil-based garden.

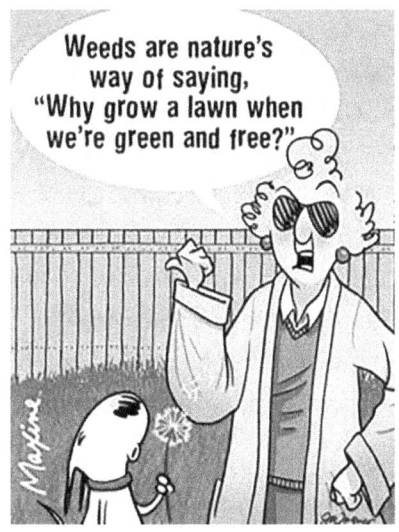

Pulling weeds requires physical stamina and mental stability so you don't go ballistic and hysterical whenever you see one of those rascals. Weeds are what people-folk call plants they do not like or are growing in the wrong place. A plant called 'Creeping Charlie' (aka ground ivy, gill-on-the-ground and creeping Jenny) and dandelion are undesirable weeds to some folks and a desired ground cover or edible food product to others. Go figure.

Mulch the ground under your elevated bed to reduce the need to bend down to weed. Weeds have a knack for growing where you don't want them to grow and to grow better and faster than the veggies, herbs, and flowers you want to grow and enjoy. If you do not want to use them in the fall, store your bags or pile of mulch or compost near your raised beds or garden area so you can spread them without having to haul them from your garage or a place far-away during your rehab period.

Don't have leaves or other material for keeping the weeds at bay? One option is to use a product called *Preen*. You can only use Preen with plants, not seeds. The product will prevent your veggie or herb or flower seeds from germinating just as they would weed-seeds. Another option is to use the square-foot gardening discussed later in this module. Planting your plants closer together can prevent weeds from taking over. This is a good water conservation practice, though you may have problems with slugs who like to live in nice cozy, warm and moist places. You will need to check your plants for mold or diseases that thrive in closed-in, moist environments.

If your garden is overloaded with weeds, or maybe more weeds than you want to handle, consider SEDIFY (someone else does it for you). Bring in some needed help. If not, and you have lots of folks stopping by to ask how you are doing before they launch into their woes and tribulations, consider putting up a nice little sign:

> Free Weeds.
> Pick Your Own.
> Give them a Home.
> Plant their Seeds.
> Give yourself a Treat
> And keep my yard Neat.

Animal Manures. Only use manures that have been cooked-cured for at least one year to eliminate or minimize any weed seeds. Horse manure compared to cow manure can be loaded with weeds. Horses have two stomachs and, as a result, the weed seeds do not always get digested or destroyed in their tummies. Moo-cows have four stomachs and generally their product is weed-free after it has been cured. Chicken and bunny-rabbit manure is considered *hot* and can burn your plants if applied to closely or too heavily. Better to cure it and/or apply it late in the fall or very early in the spring before you set out your plants. Organic-growing issues aside, take care about applying animal manure: it is one cause of E. coli that you may have heard about (re: **Appendix Three**).

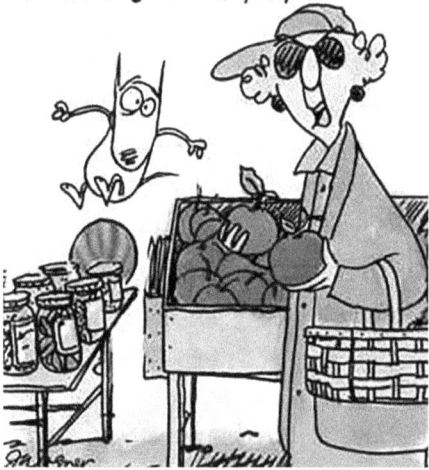

They call them "organic" vegetables. But what they really mean is "grown in poop."

Pathways. In a traditional garden your pathways will probably be what your garden is made of—soil. Soil is dandy when it is dry and hard or firm to walk on. If not, using a wheelchair on soft, loose, fluffy soil could be difficult. If wet and muddy, that could be more difficult. A cane or crutches could poke through wet or loose soil, making those devices sink and perhaps cause you to lose your balance or at the least mess with your confidence. Kneel-walkers? Ditto. Walkers? Ditto.

You can use boards and flat stones and wood mulch on your pathway, but first lay down some weed fabric to prevent them from sinking into the soil, especially after the soil is wet and you walk on it. Or spread mulch a few inches thick and have the kiddies in your neighborhood walk on them to pack it down. They may like to stomp around on your path.

I recommend wood mulch or bark mulch, not wood nuggets. Nuggets have a nasty habit of floating away on you during a heavy rainfall. Re-cycled wood mulch—cheaper and better. Bark is usually bug-free. Insects bore through the bark on their journey to the tasty wood lying underneath. They usually are not fond of bark as an edible item so you should not have to worry about attracting ants.

If possible, modify your pathways so they are thirty-six inches wide, level, and include turn-around areas either somewhere in the middle of the row or at the ends, especially if you will need to use a wheel-chair. You can create a safer path with a variety of materials, including grass (sod). Grass can provide a more solid base for you and you would not need to mow it. If the grass grows long and goes to seed, so what? It is going to stay within the aisles of your raised beds. No raised bed? Use edging or an edging tool to contain it. If you can, practice walking on the paths with your assistive device to test its firmness and your stability well before your surgery date. Then if you need to make modifications if necessary.

Extending Your Season

Regardless of your growing Zone, choose varieties that will grow well and are easy to maintain, especially if you will be recovering from surgery during that time. Check with your local extension agent if in doubt. Master gardeners could provide you with suggestions as well. Cool weather crops are great to plant during the cooler months.

Depending on the variety, these veggies can withstand some reasonably chilly temperatures: beets, 'Winterkeeper', and carrots, 'Merida', for example, can survive even if the temperatures drop to 15F. Collards, 'Champion', kales, 'Winterbor,' 'Siberian', parsley, 'Italian plain leaf,' parsnips, 'Gladiator', and spinach, 'Tyee', 'Melody,' could survive at a minimum temperature of zero-degrees F (*Webgrower* Winter Gardening).

You can protect your plants from chilly and downright cold weather with plant protectors, such as baskets, burlap or canvas sacks, boxes, blankets and buckets. There are other options that can protect your plants and extend your growing season. Most of these extenders will need to be set up prior to your surgery. If you cannot do these yourself before surgery, you may want to call in the troops to help you. In short, SEDIFY, or Someone Else Does It For You, may be a viable option to consider.

Cold Frames. This is a handy way to start seeds and harden off your seedlings. Do this at the start of your growing season. You can use cold frames to protect your flowers and other plants until your weather warms up. You can build a cold frame from a wide range of materials—wood, concrete blocks and straw bales. The windows can be glass, plexiglass or heavy-duty clear plastic stapled to a wood frame. Plant your seeds or place your seedlings inside the frame and close the window to trap in the heat.

During the earliest part of your season and especially if the weather is cloudy you could keep the window closed all the time. Monitor the heat within the frame. On cloudy days the temperature inside may be just fine for your plants. If it gets too hot when it is sunny (though the outside ambient temperature may still be chilly) your plants could cook and die. A thermometer would be handy to include inside the frame. Generally, during sunny days or when the temperature gets too high (above ninety-degrees) you can release any excess heat by simply keeping the window open by the width of a piece of wood that is an inch or two thick. Close the window late afternoon to retain the heat over night.

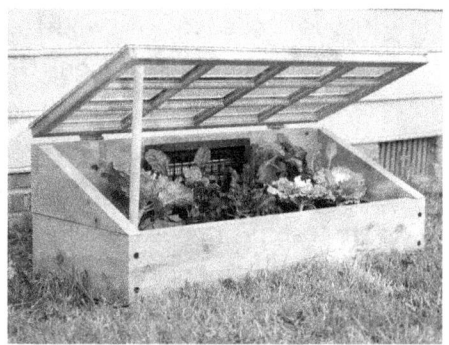

You can buy or build a simple cold-frame. Ideally, you will want to place it along the south side of your house to maximize exposure to the sun.

High and Low Tunnels. Tunnels are easy to set up. You can use them at the beginning of your growing season and in the case of high tunnels you could keep the frame up all year-round.

The concept and purpose for both tunnels are the same. Both provide protection from the elements, especially cold and frosty weather. The main difference is the height of the tunnel. Low-tunnels are, generally, no more than eighteen- to thirty-six-inches high. They are not made for you to walk inside the tunnel. High-tunnels are much higher and you could walk in and

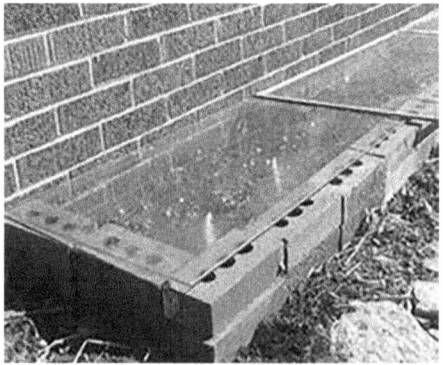

Simple and very functional. Got some bricks or cinder-blocks hanging around? Use them to build a cold-frame.

through the tunnel. How high? As high as you are tall is one option (or you could stoop a bit).

You can easily make your own low or high-tunnel unit with half-inch PVC pipe. You can create a frame around an area with wood, or not. You can bend and place the PVC pipe inside or outside the frame. Some folks will attach the pipe to the frame with a metal clamp. You can also insert a two-foot section of rebar into the ground (nine to twelve inches). You will then have at least twelve-inches above ground to stabilize your PVC tube. Simply insert one end of the PVC pipe over one end of the rebar and bend it so you can slip it over the other rebar. The length is up to you. If you have a ten-foot long raised bed, include the rebar-PVC pipe at both ends and at least one in the middle of the bed to support the plastic or netting or floating row cover.

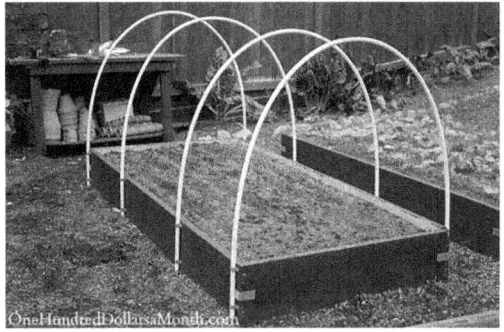

For starters, buy a ten-foot PVC pipe, one half-inch in diameter. Once you bend and secure it over the rebar, you should have an internal height of about forty-eight inches, which will allow you to grow a wide variety of veggies. Initially, you would use clear plastic over the frame. This will trap heat inside, much like a cold frame, protecting your plants. As the weather warms and your plants grow, remove the plastic and switch over to a floating row cover. The plastic cover keeps your plants warm. The row cover keeps bugs and critters away from your plants and allows rain to come through to your plants. You could also replace the row cover with netting to keep critters away from your berries. You do not have to remove the PVC frame, unless you want to. Keep it up all year-round and cover it with plastic or row cover or netting for the appropriate time of year.

Create your own high or low tunnel with half-inch PVC pipe bent over to accommodate the width that you want. I suggest a forty-eight-inch width so you can work both sides of the tunnel by either lifting the plastic or floating row cover. You should be able to weed and harvest your crop. You can attach the PVC pipe to a frame with brackets or place the pipe over rebar which you push into the soil to anchor the pipe. In this photograph the PVC pipe is secured to the outside of the raised bed with "C" clamps.

Floating Row Covers. You can extend the season of some veggies by protecting them with floating row covers and low-tunnel hoops. Row covers can protect plants down to 20-degrees F and low-tunnels can keep plants growing inside 15- to 20-degrees warmer than the outside temperature (ambient temperature). Frost blankets or floating row covers are great products to use in your soil-based garden.

Floating row covers come in different densities, widths and lengths. The heavier the density, the greater the frost protection and less light is transmitted to the plant. They are placed over an entire row or block of plants. They can increase the air temperature under the cover from four- to eight-degrees or more, depending on the density. Row covers allow rain-water to reach the plants.

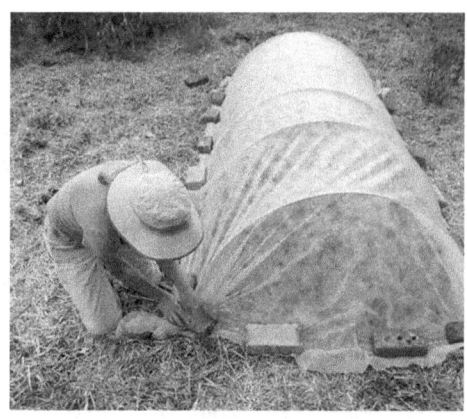

Floating row covers are light enough to lie on top of your plants without crushing or damaging them. Most come with pins to anchor the sides to the soil. Keep enough slack in the cover to allow the plants to grow up and out. In addition to frost protection, you can use the covers to protect your plants from insects, such as thrips, aphids, flea and other beetles, birds, deer, bunny rabbits and other critters who see your garden as an open buffet. If you use the lighter varieties, you can keep them on your plants throughout the season to prevent insect critters from laying eggs on your produce. This is a great way to thwart the cabbage moth from laying eggs on your broccoli or cabbage.

This floating row cover includes rust-proof galvanized steel hoops to support the blanket at a specific height. Not all row covers come with pre-formed hoops. Check that out before you buy. Many covers include pins to tie down the edges; others include drawstrings at the ends; and still others require that you use bricks or stones to anchor the sides and ends, as you see in this photo.

Some blankets include drawstrings to close off the ends and others come with rust-proof galvanized steel hoops to keep the blanket at a specific height. Check the manufactures' specifications on the packaging, but generally a product with a weight of 0.55 to 0.99 will protect plants from three to eight degrees (F) above the ambient temperature down to about twenty-eight degrees (F). Blankets weighing 1.5 ounces may let in as much as 70 to 85% of sunlight and protect your plants down to twenty-four degrees.

If frost is not an issue for you, consider a product that transmits 90% of sunlight. These products are generally .45 ounces or lighter. You need to decide which tradeoff is better for you: transmit more sunlight at slightly less frost protection or warmth, or, transmit less light to your plants and provide more frost protection to the plants. Compare the different weights and decide what will work best in your Zone.

PREPARING YOUR OUTSIDE WORLD

TIP: Do not use plastic that touches your plants. Plastic will transfer the cold to your plants. Not good.

Cloches and Hot Caps. These options can be easily set in place after surgery when you are able to walk in your garden. Set these out if you can bend down. Otherwise, SEDIFY.

Cloches are bell-shaped glass units that you place over each plant. Some units have vents that allow excess hot air to escape, but they may not allow enough water to reach the plant. They trap solar radiation and keep moisture from evaporating (generally). You will have to monitor these to make sure they do not *cook* the plant.

Got a glass cutter? Want a hobby while you rehab? Cut off the bottom off one-gallon jugs. Select those that have a narrow top and handle. Discard the cut bottom and simply place the jugs over the plants. Cloches allow you to set your plants out earlier than you normally would set them out. Though the ambient temperature may still be cold, the glass-jug traps the heat from the sun. Excess heat can exit through the top of the jug. You just created a mini-cold frame.

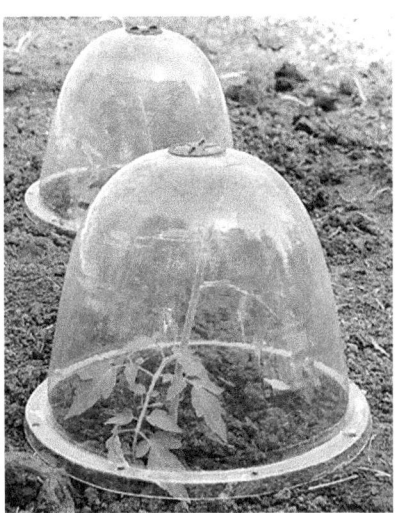

Cloches and hot caps act as mini-greenhouses. Set cloches and hot caps over each plant. They will warm up the air and soil temperature to allow your plants to grow during the cooler (colder) spring-time weather. This unit includes a vent to allow hot air to escape.

Stagger-planting is another option. Section off your planting area in thirds. Initially, plant a third of what you want to grow, say peas, then plant another third (of peas) a month or so later, and perhaps a third planting a month or so after that. Plant your first batch before surgery. Have your surgery. Then, depending on your procedure and progress, you may be able to get in a second or third planting after surgery. By then you should be in better post-op condition to weed and maintain your garden. Stagger-planting will allow you to have a continuous crop throughout your growing season, yet not overwhelm you with lots of stuff coming in at the same time. You will be organizing your home and yard before surgery and you may not have time to do everything you think you want or wish to do.

Container Options

Okay, you are not so handy. Not to worry. Go with containers. You can purchase nice fancy ceramic containers of any color and size and shape. Make certain that your container has drainage holes to drain off excess water. If it is ceramic without at least one drainage hole, don't buy it. If you buy resin containers, make sure it has drain holes. Otherwise, drill several one-half inch holes in the bottom.

Clay containers will suck up the moisture from your soil-mix. As a result, they typically require more frequent watering. If possible, position your beds and containers close to a water source. They also may require more fertilizer than plants grown in your regular garden. Rain, especially a heavy rain, tends to dilute and wash nutrients from the soil out the drain holes. Containers are nice and heavy. Once you set a container down and fill it with a soil-mix it can be difficult to move. Consider buying container dollies or a pot-mover trolley.

Plastic or resin containers will hold moisture better than clay or earthenware. They may not be as trendy as a ceramic container, but they will be lighter and easier to manage. Generally, the newer types can be filled with potting soil and left full over the winter, without cracking or splitting after winter gives way to warmer weather.

> *TIP:* If you are a tad skeptical about whether your containers will crack over the winter, cover them, soil and all, with a large trash bag to keep out the snow and rain.

Plastic or resin containers should not split over the winter. Ceramic pots can split. Clay pots can split. Usually, containers with tapered sides fare better over the winter than straight-sided versions. You can remove the potting soil in the fall (clay, ceramic) and add that to your compost bin or spread it in your regular garden or fill in low spots in your yard.

You can garden after surgery once you are fully recovered or at least are cleared to pick up heavy bags of potting soil. If you still want to use containers, then empty the soil, and position the containers where you want them, so you do not have to move them. Then add your soil and plants when you are physically able to do so. Not all plants need to be planted at the same time. Stagger your plantings. You can then harvest over your growing season.

Do not put broken pieces of pottery or whatever in your containers. That is an old story. Folks suggested that to lighten the weight of the container. It does nothing for the plant.

Drain holes in the bottom or along the sides of your container will release excessive water. Filling your containers with a lighter soil mix works in place of adding Styrofoam pellets or broken pieces of whatever (Gilman, *Decoding Gardening Advice,* December 2011).

> ***TIP:*** Never, as in never, use soil from your yard or garden for your containers. Use potting soil, which is lighter and should be free from any insect eggs and soil pathogens. Your soil has all those nasties. Oh, you say, not in my garden. Yes, in your garden. Don't do it. Mix in some peat or coconut coir and a slow release fertilizer and mulch with grass clippings or more coir and you should be fairly maintenance free for most of the season, adding water of course through out that period.

If you use containers now or plan to use them to help you garden after surgery, consider those plant varieties bred especially for containers. They are compact and take less maintenance and for the most part they are comparable in taste and yield like the taller determinant and indeterminate varieties. The lower maintenance could be a plus for you during rehab. The bush green bean variety "French Mascotte' is one example that grows well in a container. Other possibilities to consider are a carrot variety called 'Chantenay Short Stuff', and a cucumber 'Bush Slicer', eggplant 'Little Prince', pepper 'Pizza My Heart' and a tomato variety called 'Roma Inca Jewels'. There are more options, of course. Seed catalogs often list their compact and patio container varieties in a separate section.

Just as with a regular soil-based garden, if you grow your veggies in containers practice botanical rotation. That is, if you planted a tomato or pepper or eggplant or potato (Solanaceae family) in container **A**, do not grow any varieties of that family in the same container for at least three years. This will help you control some insect and soil diseases. More on botanical rotation later in this module.

> ***TIP:*** By the way, if you choose to purchase ceramic or the more expensive containers, buy them towards the end of summer or growing season. Most garden centers have them on sale, as in discounts to 70% or so. The nice folks at the garden center do not want to inventory them over the winter. They want you to inventory them over the winter in your yard. Buy them on sale.

What do you do with the soil in your containers at the end of the season? Toss it? Don't. You can re-use that soil year after year. You can mix in granular fertilizer if you like to replace some of the nutrients. You can remove some of that *old* soil and mix

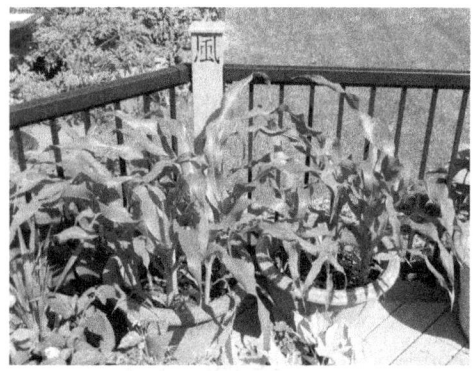
You can grow any plant in a container, including corn, such as this variety from Burpee Seeds called, 'On Deck'. Set your containers so you have easy access to them. You may need to reduce what and how much you grow. Your rehabilitation period is important, so adjust your yard and garden efforts accordingly.

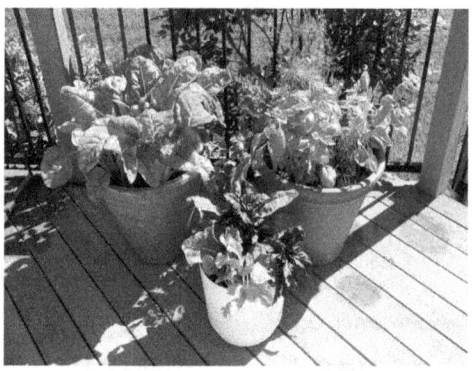
Grow all types of leafy green veggies, herbs and flowers in containers. Here you see chards, basils, arugula and rosemary. How large is small? The two-gallon containers in front could be considered smaller when compared to the fifteen-gallon clay containers in the back row. If you can easily lift and move it when filled with soil or water, then call it a small (manageable) container.

in some *new* potting soil. You can use it on your flower beds or spread it around any low areas in your yard. But don't toss it.

Spoiler Alert. Are you tired of moving large, heavy containers around your patio or deck? Cheer up. Think smaller. You can garden hydroponically in containers as small as 32-ounces. Limited space? Consider having one unit on a counter. More room? Consider multiple containers on a table or other elevated units, such as benches or something you build or have built for you.

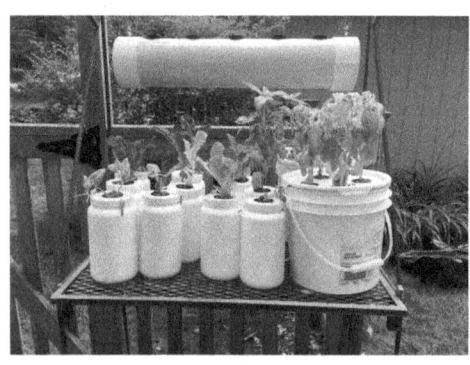
These small containers include half-gallon, 3.5 gallon, and a 2.5 gallon four-inch by twenty-four-inch PVC tube. Grow a mix of flowers, veggies and herbs (or whatever you like). The bucket was once home to cake frosting (food-safe, from a local bakery). Use warm to hot water to wash away the sugar and your bucket is good to grow.

You can paint the outside with acrylic paints to create your own masterpiece. The seniors and kiddies in my various master gardener projects enjoy painting these smaller units. Some folks may prefer to splash some paint on the container, call that modern art, while others paint images such as flowers or geometric designs. Your container. Your creativity. Do it. Have some crazy fun. You can read more about hydroponic gardening in **Module Four.**

TIP: Do not pile extra soil around the trunks of trees and create that pyramid-look. This could result in a tree that will die before it reaches its full potential. You will see this done on city streets or public parks to keep the weeds and grass away from the trunk so the maintenance folks can mow the area without cutting into the bark of the tree.

Stock Tanks. Resin and galvanized stock tanks are easy to work with and are great for container gardening. Drill several drain holes in the bottom of the tank. Fill the bottom third of the tank with a sand-loam mix or drainable soil. Then fill the rest of the tank with a mix of potting soil, composted manure or your own composted material. Resin tanks come in different sizes and three sizes that are ideal of growing veggies and herbs (and flowers) include a 100 gallon tank, 52.5"L x 37"W x 21"H; a 110 gallon tank, 53.5"L x 36"W x 20" H and a 150 gallon tank that measures 58"L x 39"W x 24" H. The prices range from about $70 to $150. These heights should defer most four-legged critters. There are shorter and smaller tanks. Your local farm store or garden center should be a good source for you.

Galvanized tanks contain zinc. You may be a tad nervous about planting herbs or vegetables in galvanized pots because of the health hazards often associated with zinc. At one time, cooking your dinner in a zinc pot was considered not a wise move. Zinc can be toxic if it is consumed or breathed in. However, any danger from growing veggies in a zinc tank-container are very low, according to the folks at *GardeningKnowHow.com* (April 2018).

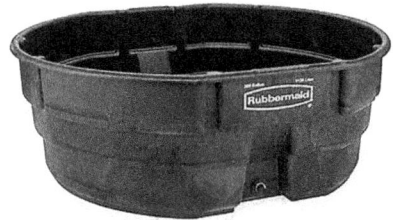

Resin tanks can make great raised beds. You would need to drill a few drainage holes, but otherwise you buy it, haul it home, set it where you want it, fill it with a good mix of potting soil and composted manure and you are good to go. No hammers or saws or carpentry-experience needed.

Each of these options allows for easy access and minimal bending. The one drawback with almost any raised bed or large container is that they are a tad heavy when filled with soil. Set them where you can forget them. You need to remove most of the soil if you decide it should live somewhere else. Do not drill holes in the sides at the bottom—mice critters may decide to take up residence in the tank. Drill them in the bottom of the tank and cover the holes with wire mesh, then add your soil-mix on top.

Straw Bale Gardening. Straw bales are a type of container. This method is not organic and if that is not a critical point for you, then it could be an alternative to consider.

If you cannot modify your existing garden or don't want to for whatever reason you could still garden with straw bales on any surface. Setting up the bales is simple: buy the number of bales you want and plop them down wherever you want—driveway, lawn, soil, rocks or concrete. Easy.

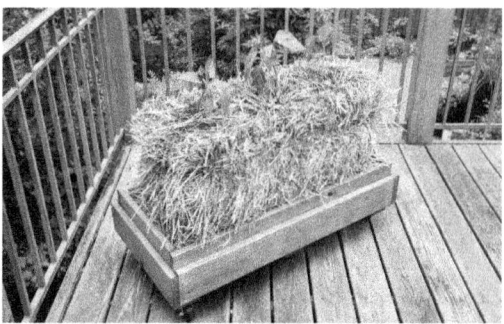

Straw bales can tend towards the messy side as they decompose. You may want to build or buy an enclosed frame to catch the falling straw if it lives on your deck or patio.

Setting up the growing cycle is a bit more involved. You will need to add a high nitrogen fertilizer prior to setting out any plants. Soak the bales and they should start to decompose within a few weeks. When the bale starts to decompose (rot) it is ready for your plants. The decomposing bales will provide a nice toasty-warm environment for your plants. Keep the bales moist. Once the bales are conditioned properly you should realize success.

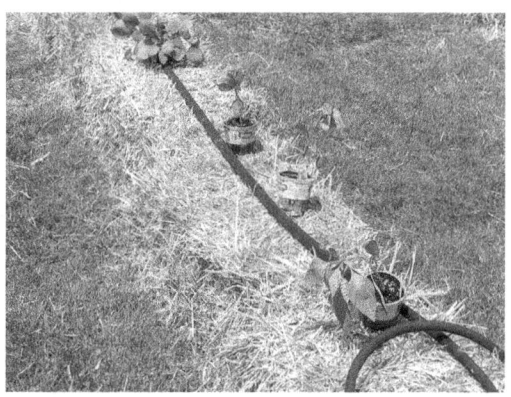

Straw bale gardening method with drip irrigation. In this photograph the seedlings are still in their original pots and would be removed prior to setting them into the bales, once the bales start to decompose (rot).

The bales can only be used for one growing season, though at the end of your season you can spread the residue as mulch or composted material in your soil-based garden or flower beds. Straw bales are for plants, not for setting seeds. Seeds will fall into the bale and be lost.

The bales can be a tad pricey if you live in a metro area. Drive out into farm country and see if a friendly farmer will sell you the bales at a reasonable price. Only use straw bales, not hay bales. Hay bales have lots of weed seeds, straw bales do not. Straw is the stem of the mature-dead plant. No weed seeds live there.

Growing Plants. You have some ideas for extended your growing season—cold frames, containers, tunnels and stagger planting and a few varieties that are cold hardy. Time your plantings so you can get your garden somewhat established before you trot off to see your surgeon and after you have completed the first part of your rehab protocol process. Here is a very short list of cool-weather veggies and herbs to consider (re: **Module Four** for more options).

- **Brassicas** or **Cole**-crops include broccoli, raab/rapine, kailaan (Chinese broccoli), cabbage, collards, kale, kohlrabi and turnip greens.

- **Leafy Salad greens** include escarole, chicory-dandelion, all types of leaf and butterhead lettuces, spinach, chards and Asian greens. Other varieties to consider include peas, mache, mustard greens, arugula, cilantro, beets, carrots and onions.

- There are several **perennial herbs** that you can include as well. These include, but are not limited to, garlic chives, onion chives, mints (plant mints in containers to prevent them from spreading), oregano or marjoram, sage, French tarragon and thymes.

> *TIP:* Aside from where you live and garden, if you grow Cole crops plant them as you would tomatoes—deep and up to the first layer of leaves. Cole varieties, especially broccoli, have a habit of growing a bent stem. This does not affect the yield, but you may not like to see them bent. To keep them straight and upright, plant them so the bent stem part is below the ground.

Grow Vertically. You can grow your plants horizontally, on the ground, as you probably do now. Now, think vertically. If you can reach above your head (careful if you had or will have shoulder surgery), consider adding a trellis to your elevated bed. Use stakes, trellises, wire cages, wood or metal rods to support your plants as they grow. Recycle a baby's crib or even the bottom metal frame of a single or double-bed. These can work great for supporting cucumbers, peas, and even pole beans. Save your back and limit the need to bend down.

If you feel a strong urge to plant vining crops that produce heavier fruit, such as melons or winter squash, place your vertical supports at an angle. This allows you to grow vertically while the angle supports the weight of fruit. If you have access to wood pallets, set them as an *inverted-V*. Set steel posts between the pallets and lean the pallets against the posts.

Companion Planting. Have you heard about companion planting? There are a lot of articles and books on this subject. And there are a plethora of myths surrounding it. Part of the appeal of companion planting is the belief that one plant can impart its fragrance or flavor on to another different variety (a different botanical family). Planting basil among tomato plants is one belief. Nope. Cannot happen. Basil cannot enhance the flavor of a tomato or vice versa. That may work in the kitchen when cooking and preparing these varieties, but it does not work in the garden.

Nor can plants *transfer* their antibug deterrents to another plant. But they can deter some insects by their *proximity* to another plant variety. The real value of companion planting is the deliberate mixing of different scents plants give off naturally. This can confuse the bad critters. When a plant grows it emits a fragrance (or smell or stink, depending on your perspective). When attacked by insects or a disease, it can emit a different fragrance, which can draw in other insects who then take the opportunity to snack on your plants.

The mixing of fragrances can confuse the *bad bugs* from finding the plant, especially your favorite plant. Including fragrant herbs next to tomatoes or peppers could *confuse* the insect critter so they may not be able to *find* your plant. Planting nasturtiums around the base of summer squash could confuse the female Squash Vine Borer so she doesn't lay her eggs at the base of the stem. Planting onions next to or among Cole crops could reduce damage from the cabbage worm. Will this be 100% effective? No. But it can dramatically reduce insect damage.

> ***TIP:*** Not overly excited about cabbage worms munching on your broccoli? Plant broccoli raab instead. Some varieties have a higher natural chemical that seems to deter the cabbage moth.

Our general practice is to plant rows or blocks of the same variety. Mix it up. Include herbs and flowers among your veggies. Another aspect of companion planting involves planting a short maturing variety with a longer maturing variety, such as planting a longer maturing tomato variety with one that matures quicker. You can do this with winter and summer squash and any other variety. Companion planting also means planting a lower growing variety with a taller variety. Lettuces between tomato plants are one example. As both grow, you will harvest the lettuce first thus providing more space for the tomato as it grows and develops.

Companion planting and integrated pest management complement each other. Both can help reduce damage from insect and soil-based diseases. Spraying pesticides should be your last resort (if at all).

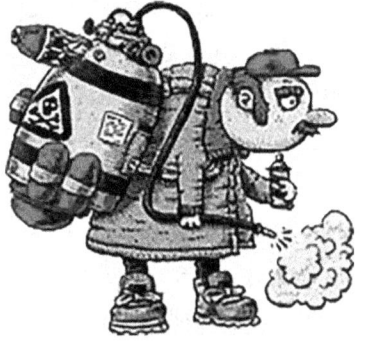

*Know what you are trying to kill before you reach for the chemical. Pesticides are non-discriminatory. They can kill both beneficial and harmful insects. And, depending on the pesticide you use, the residual effect of that product can remain when you harvest the plant. And that pesticide now resides in your body. Nice thought. (re: **Appendix Three**).*

Integrated Pest Management (IPM). According to the National Center for Environmental Health Division of Emergency and Environmental Health Services, "Integrated pest management (IPM) is a science-based, common-sense approach for reducing populations of disease vectors and public health pests. IPM uses a variety of pest management techniques that focus on pest prevention, pest reduction, and the elimination of conditions that lead to pest infestations. IPM simply means (1) don't attract pests, (2) keep them out, and (3) get rid of them, if you are sure you have them, with the safest, most effective method."

Basically, "IPM is a comprehensive, systems-based approach to pest management with the goal of providing the safest, most effective, most economical, and sustained remedy to pest infestations. IPM reduces the risk from pests while also reducing the risk from the overuse or inappropriate use of hazardous chemical pest-control products (*www.cdc.gov*)."

Great. So how can you do this in your own backyard? You can reduce damage from insects by rotating what you grow from one section of your garden to another. Insects that damage Brassicas (Cole) crop varieties, such as broccoli, cabbage, etc., will not (generally) attack plants from another botanical family, such as Solanaceae (tomatoes, peppers, eggplants, potatoes) or Allium (onions, garlic). The adult female insect critter lays eggs and in the spring the critters emerge as caterpillars. By not rotating, by planting the same variety in the same space each year, you create a convenient underground elevator for the caterpillars. Their preferred food source is right there, all nice and handy. By rotating, you deprive them of that convenience.

Likewise, soil-based diseases attack varieties from one botanical family, but not necessarily a different family. A good rule of thumb is to establish a three-year rotation cycle to reduce damage cause by insects and diseases. One-hundred percent elimination? No, but a dramatic reduction, nevertheless. Less work. Less insect or disease damage. Less pesticides. Less herbicides. Safer food. Healthier food.

Another IPM technique is to plant plants that attract beneficial insects to your garden. Plant Lacy Phacelia or Alyssum. Or consider setting up an insectary area near or within your garden to attract the beneficial insects. Plant these varieties in blocks, versus having just one or two of each variety. Yarrow, dill, fennel, zinnias, sun flowers and wild carrots will attract parasitic wasps and robber flies. These insects attack caterpillars that are attacking your veggies, which means you would not need to spray or use chemicals. The caterpillars are then fed to the young of those wasps and robber flies. A very nice sight to be sure. (*Permaculture News* 2014). Less maintenance. Less work. Less stress. Less frustration. And, no, the parasitic wasps and robber flies will not attack you.

In an article titled, *Organic Pest Control: The Best Plants to Attract beneficial Insects and Bee*, the case is made for thinking about the Three-P's: "The three 'P's' of beneficial insects are pollinators, predators and parasites. Pollinators, such as honeybees, fertilize flowers, which increases the productivity of food crops ranging from apples to zucchini. Predators, such as lady beetles and soldier bugs, consume pest insects as food. Parasites use pests as nurseries for their young. On any given day, all three 'P's' are feeding on pests or on flower pollen and nectar in a diversified garden. If you recognize these good bugs, it's easier to appreciate their role and understand why it's best not to use broad-spectrum herbicides." An illustrated listing of some of these beneficial insects can be found in my book, *Hydroponic Gardening The Very Easy Way*, available on *Amazon.com*.

"The use of such herbicides and pesticides can be detrimental to the complex relationships between plants, pests and predators —*all the more reason why natural insect control works better*. Because pesticides, even organic varieties, make no distinction between helpful and hurtful insects, in the end their regular use can have many negative impacts, including the suppression of the soil food web and pollution of waterways. Instead, encouraging the presence of predatory warriors that will defend and protect your garden plants from common pests is not only an environmentally sound management strategy, it also encourages biodiversity and plant pollination (*Mother Earth* 2019)."

Accessibility Options. This section includes a wide range of ideas designed to increase your mobility and accessibility, so you can continue to enjoy the outside world in a safe manner. You may have included these ideas already. If not, consider them as designs that could make your post-surgery gardening experience more comfy and stress free. Choose those that will work for you, given the space you have and your financial situation. Some ideas may only apply to your first post-surgery year. Others could be longer more permanent modifications. You may need to enlist the help of professionals or at the very least folks who can help you.

There are many types of accessible gardens. For many of us, gardening is therapeutic. Yet, as we get older or have some sort of disability, or are limited thanks to arthritis or other ailment, whether that is a short- or longer-term condition, gardening can present a challenge. We become frustrated because we cannot do what we did five or ten years ago.

The concept behind accessible gardening practices is to allow you to enjoy and maintain your garden, regardless of age, illness or disability. Here are some very traditional and alternative options to consider as new or as a reinforcement for what you have already been doing.

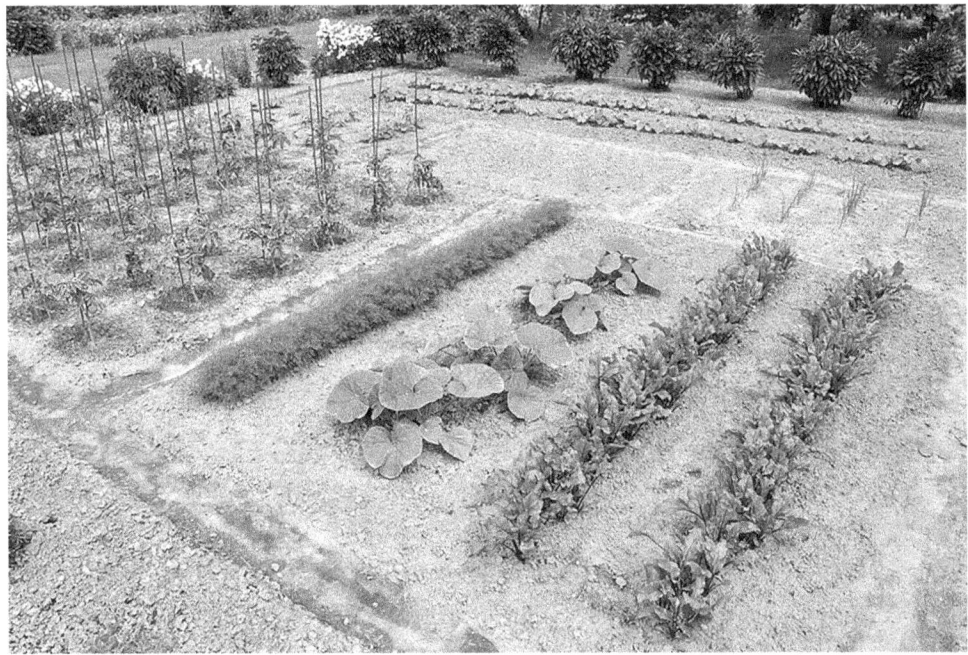

Row planting can provide space for pathways, allow room for the plants to develop and decrease fungal problems by allowing better air circulation. Plants planted in a traditional row design are very common.

Planting in Rows. Plants growing in nice tidy straight rows. Very typical. Very traditional. Planting in rows allows you to access plants from either side and gives you space for walking. Maybe your pathways are about eighteen-to-twenty-inches wide. You will be in rehab after surgery. As you read earlier, you may want to consider planting less in your next growing season and have wider pathways so you can more easily maneuver through your garden with a walker or wheelchair or knee-stroller. Wider pathways allow you to maintain your garden while standing or, if you can, kneel and crawl along as you yank out weeds and chat with your plants.

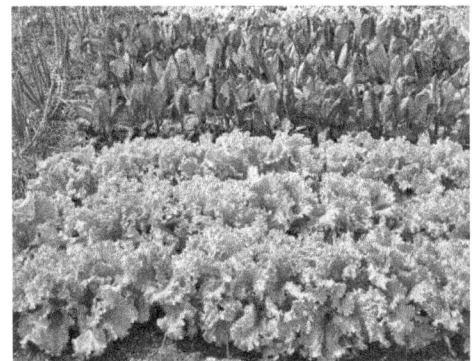

Planting in wide rows or blocks vs. single rows can be an efficient way to realize higher yields in a space while keeping the need to weed at a minimum.

Planting in Blocks. If you are growing salad greens, you can plant them in rows and in blocks or sections. Simply take a small handful of seeds and spread them, broadcast them, in that block or section after you have prepared the area. Yes, they will all grow every which way but if you are harvesting them while they are small and tender, you simply gather them up by the hand-full for your next meal. Usually, when you harvest them while they are young, you will not have a problem with weeds. Depending on what you are growing, as your plants mature, they can shade out many weeds and reduce your maintenance efforts. Then as you harvest a section within that block you can loosen the soil and prepare it for re-seeding and start the process all over again (re: stagger planting above). Or, heavily mulch the area and keep it fallow for the rest of the season.

Mandala Design. The premise behind this method is that you can access any edge of your garden from a central point. Plants are set in circular or semi-circular sections and radiate out from that central point or path. This design can be at ground-level or in an elevated bed. The word, *mandala*, comes from the Sanskrit word that means *circle*. Mandalas represent the link or connection between our inner world and outer reality.

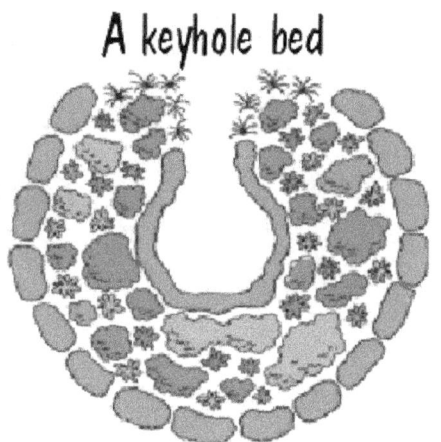

A keyhole bed, aka Mandala, is a handy way to garden from one spot or garden with minimal movement.

If this design is elevated, you should not have much of a problem. If it is at ground level, you could have a problem kneeling, especially if you have issues with your hips or knees.

Square Foot Gardening. Mel Bartholomew created this concept many years ago. His motivation was to grow and harvest higher yields in smaller spaces. You create a

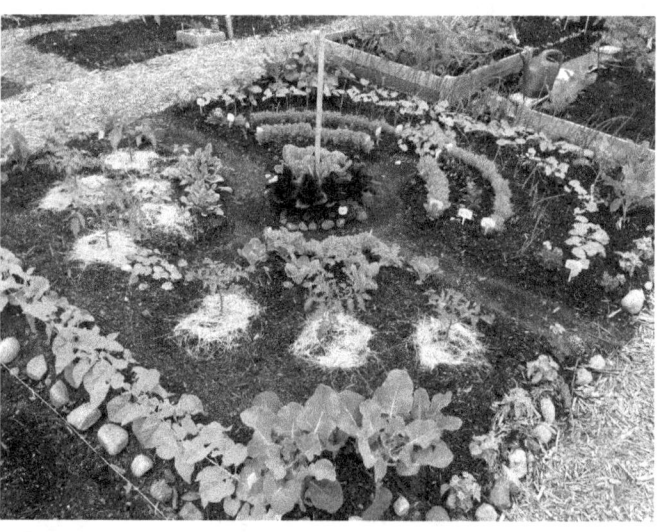

Mandala design includes a semi-circular pattern and easy access to all sections of your garden. This type of garden design can be as simple or as ornate and creative as you want. In this community garden, the gardener can access the plot from the pathways outside the garden and the access path within the plot, all within arm's reach.

PREPARING YOUR OUTSIDE WORLD

grid system in your garden or raised or elevated bed. Each grid is twelve-inches by twelve-inches, hence the name square-foot gardening. The basic premise is that a specific number of plants can be planted in each twelve-inch by twelve-inch space. For example, you could plant nine beets in that space or four bush bean plants or two basil plants. Or, you could plant one bush tomato plant in that twelve-inch space. Or, plant nine to twelve onions per grid or one potato per grid and so on. Planting in grids allows for

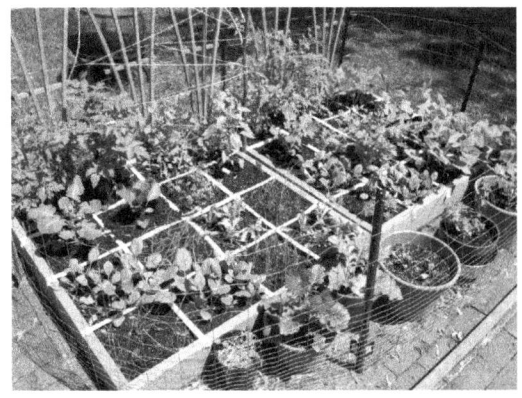

Lay out a grid system to help you plant each variety in a specific square. You can use twine or lath to mark off each twelve-inch square. This bed is four-feet, front to back, allowing the gardener to reach in to maintain and harvest.

SQUARE FOOT PLANTING GUIDE

Arugula 16	Dill 9	Leeks 6	Rutabagas 4	Fennel 2	Bok Choy 1	Melons 1	Rosemary 1
Carrots 16	Onions 9	Bush Beans 4	Basil 2	Kale 2	Brussel Sprouts 1	Okra 1	Sage 1
Leaf Lettuce 16	Parsnips 9	Pole Beans 4	Calendula 2	Parsley 2	Cabbage 1	Oregano 1	Summer Squash 1
Radishes 16	Spinach 9	Garlic 4	Celery 2	Potatoes 2	Cauliflower 1	Hot Peppers 1	Winter Squash 1
Beets 9	Turnips 9	Kohlrabi 4	Corn 2	Swiss Chard 2	Chives 1	Peppers 1	Sweet Potatoes 1
Cilantro 9	Peas 8	Head Lettuce 4	Cucumbers 2	Thyme 2	Eggplants 1	Pumpkins 1	Tomatoes 1

Number denotes # of plantings per square foot

You can find these types of guides on the Internet. In this example, you could plant sixteen leaf lettuce plants (vertical growing habit, such as Romaine) but only four head-lettuce varieties, such as 'Iceberg'. If you include tomatoes, consider the determinant-bush-patio types. They will take up less room (less spreading) than, say, an indeterminant or heirloom variety.

easy access, less weeding, higher yields per allotted space and less maintenance while you recover from your procedure.

There are several online resources that allow you to use this concept. Identify the dimensions of your garden, then select a variety, say kohlrabi or kale or peppers. The software will automatically insert an illustration of that variety and the number of plants you can include in that twelve-inch grid. Very nice and easy to use. One resource is *www.gardeners.com*.

You can get a lot of product in each grid, much more than with traditional row planting. Before your surgery, mark out each square with nylon string or strips of wood. Then when you are ready to plant, before or after surgery, you just plant the recommended number of seeds or plants.

Raised Beds. A raised bed is any framed structure that sits on the ground. The frame can be made of wood or blocks or recycled resin-type materials and filled with soil up to the top of the frame. The shape can be square, rectangular, triangular and any reachable height. You can create a round shape, a spiral shape, an L-shape, a pyramid-shape, and so on. You can include a door or gate to facilitate entry without having to step over the sides.

If you choose wood, choose the untreated options. As of this writing, the chemicals used to treat wood are not always considered food-safe. Untreated wood should last about ten-years or so. Buying cedar or redwood will extend the life of your bed by about five years or fifteen-years total and yes, it is more expensive. One option for extending the life of your bed is to line the inside of your untreated wood bed with a commercial grade landscape liner or fiber.

A bed made from stone or cinder block could last for close to forever. Using cinder blocks will change the pH of your soil a bit, but that should not be much of a problem. Have your soil tested for the first two years to identify whether the pH has changed or not and, if so, what you can do to amend it. Most plants will grow well within a pH range of 6.0 to 7.0. West of the Mississippi River, soil is generally alkaline (sweet, a high pH). Using cinder blocks for your raised bed can lower the pH a bit during the first few years, which can be good. Using peat or pine needles, for example, can lower pH levels or acidify your soil, which can also be good. East of the river the soil tends to be more acidic and folks often use lime to sweeten or raise the pH level (a low pH).

The height can vary from, say, six-inches to 30-inches. You can buy raised beds as a kit, easy to assemble (more or less), or buy the components—wood, or resin boards, concrete blocks—and build them to whatever specifications you want, height, length, width. Depending on the height you choose, raised beds are great for keeping out some critters, like bunny-rabbits. A height of twenty-inches should be high enough. Lower beds may not be a wise choice for you if you have problems bending down or getting down on your hands and knees to garden. The length of each bed is not as critical as the width or height. The limiting factor is the size of your growing area.

If you include multiple beds, keep them at least twenty-four inches apart, or preferably thirty-six inches apart if you have the space. This will allow you to access each bed with a wheelbarrow, cart, a walker, a wheel-chair and even with a scooter or stool.

> **NOTE:** If you use a wheel-barrow or garden cart or wheel-chair, measure its outside width (the wheel hubs) and space your aisles accordingly.

The overall inside dimensions in the photo shown below are two-feet wide and twenty-feet long. Decorative concrete blocks are the material. The flat blocks on the larger portion of the bed allow you to sit and garden. Use the uncovered area of the blocks to plant flowers that attract pollinators. If you use a garden cart to haul material, make the aisles three-feet wide. If you do not intend to use a cart or wheel-barrow, two-foot wide aisles should suffice. In any event, before you set your aisle width, measure the widest cart or wagon you plan to use within those aisles and set your aisle-width accordingly.

Spiral raised beds are another example of a raised bed and can be fun to do with the kiddies. It can also add a little art and creativity to your yard. You can use a

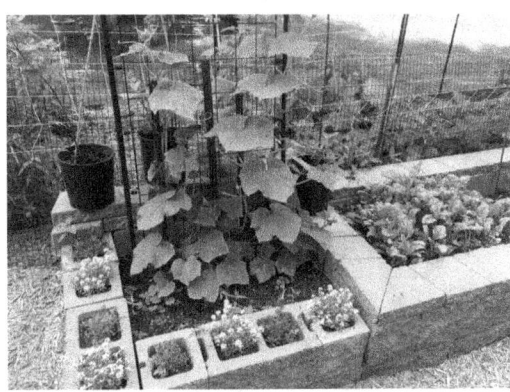

Don't waste the space. If you use concrete blocks, set a cap on top so you can sit while gardening. If you do not use caps, plant pollinator plants into the open sections in order to attract more beneficial insects to your garden and plants.

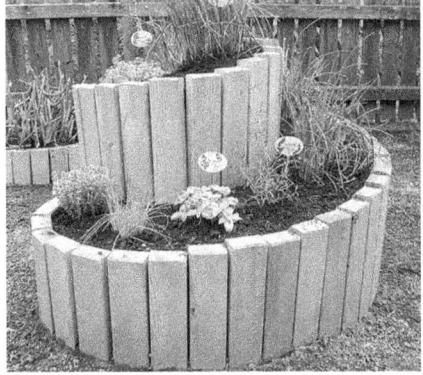

One example of a spiral vertical raised bed. You can make spiral beds from different types of materials. Look for rolled-up wood edging that is fastened together at your favorite garden center.

variety of materials. Wood edging is one option. Commercial-grade edging is another option.

Depending on the length of your rolled-up edging, lay it out in a circular design for your first tier. Fill in the first tier with soil or your own mix of potting soil, compost, composted manure, peat and perhaps a slow-release fertilizer. Next, lay out the edging on top of the soil of the lower tier and fill it in with your soil mix. The height depends on your ability to reach in and weed and harvest the plants you intend to grow.

There are two basic measurements to keep in mind. If you can walk around your raised bed and easily reach into it, you can make the width a maximum of forty-eight inches. Generally, you can reach into your raised bed twenty-four inches from one side, twenty-four from the other side. If you cannot walk around your bed, but only have access from the long side, make the width a maximum of twenty-four inches. Again, this should allow most people with easy access without having to stretch too far.

You could increase the height of a spiral raised bed so long as you can reach each level easily. You may hear spiral beds referred to as pyramid-type beds. Careful if you are having shoulder or upper-body surgery.

One point of having raised or elevated beds is for ease of access and accessibility, without having to get on your hands and knees. A second point with raised beds is

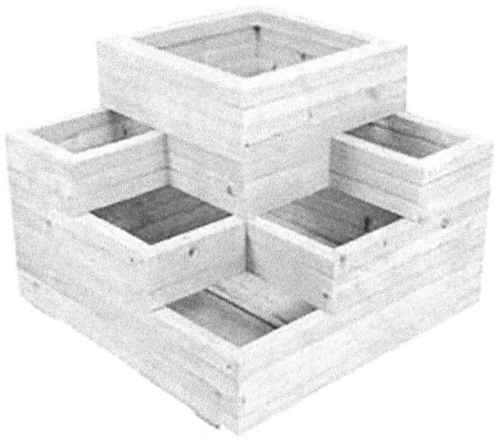

A bit of carpentry skill will be required with these two options. Tiered, vertical growing can dramatically increase your yields and productivity. This design could be tucked into a corner with access on three sides, or with access on four-sides. Consider SEDIFY.

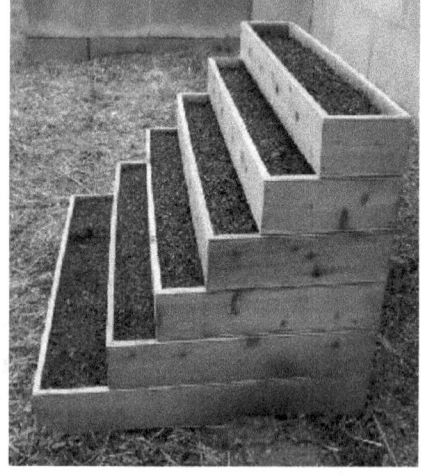

A tiered raised bed that is accessible from three sides. This design uses straight, untreated lumber, one-inch wide and can be placed against a wall or fence.

that you should not need to walk in them. In fact, once your bed is set up and filled with a soil mix, stay off it. If you absolutely, positively must walk in there for whatever reason, place some stepping-stones as a permanent fixture for that bed. When you walk in a raised bed, you will be compacting the soil. Compacted soil will require that you dig it up with a shovel or pitch-fork to loosen the soil before planting. More work for you. Stay off. Put up a sign as a reminder to stay off.

> *Please don't tread on lil' ol' me*
> *With your big foot or sore knee,*
> *You'll squash the lil 'ol' pea,*
> *And squish the lil' ol' lettuce,*
> *Unless you also let us*
> *Squish and stomp on thee.*

Elevated Beds. Are you a Handy-Andy? Or a Mr. or Mrs. Build-it or Fix-it person? I like to think of an elevated table as a piece of furniture that, ideally, you can move around or disassemble for storage if necessary. If you think you will be moving these babies around, for whatever reason, do not attach the upper section to the lower section. It may be too heavy, depending on the size and material you use. And, if practical for you, add wheels to the legs so you can more easily move them around when and where you want.

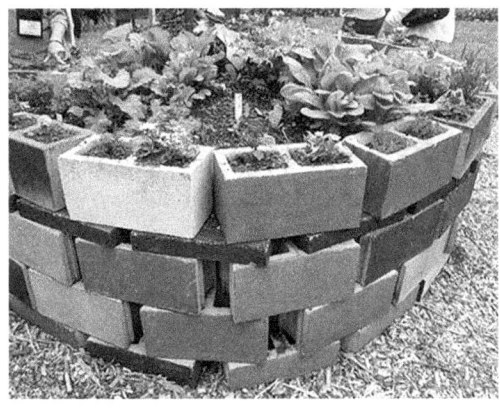

Okay, so maybe you are carpentry-impaired. Can you handle bricks or blocks? Your raised bed can be of any manageable length but keep the width to four feet so you can maintain it within easy arm-reach and be able to walk around it. Make it out of the materials you have on hand. Cinder blocks, painted or not, are relatively inexpensive and manageable.

An elevated bed is basically a raised bed with legs set on a table-like platform. You can also set it on two or more sturdy resin, metal or wooden saw-horses. Usually they are waist high, say about thirty-inches, or whatever waist-high is for you, which allows you access from all sides without having to bend down or crawl about on your hands and knees. You could also make the height about twenty-seven inches to accommodate a wheel-chair.

Your elevated bed can be as simple or elaborate as you want. If you use wood, paint it for outdoor use. This will help preserve the wood. As with raised beds, if you choose wood, go with untreated pine and paint it with a product that is food-safe. If you have the bucks, choosing cedar works and should give you a few extra years. Line the inside of both treated and untreated lumber with a commercial-grade weed-fabric. This should extend the life a bit further and help prevent premature rotting of the wood. This can be a fun project for you and the kiddies. Let them take a bit of ownership. If you are not handy, then SEDIFY.

What is sitting around your yard that is not being used? Got an old wheel-barrow that you have not used in a while? You can toss it. Or, use it as an elevated bed.

Build an elevated bed from wood. Make it rectangular, square or L-shaped.

Wheelchair Gardening. This design could be an option for you or someone you know who will use or now uses a wheel-chair. There are products such as the Vegtrug Patio Garden which you can purchase as a kit or already set up for you (check on that before you buy). The sides slant inward, which is great for sitting on a portable bench or even for moving a wheelchair closer to your plants. There are several straight-sided beds you can buy or build, but the Vegtrug (or similar products) with its tapered sides allows you to garden without having to twist your body when you want to cultivate or harvest your produce.

Test out any elevated bed with your wheelchair at your local garden center

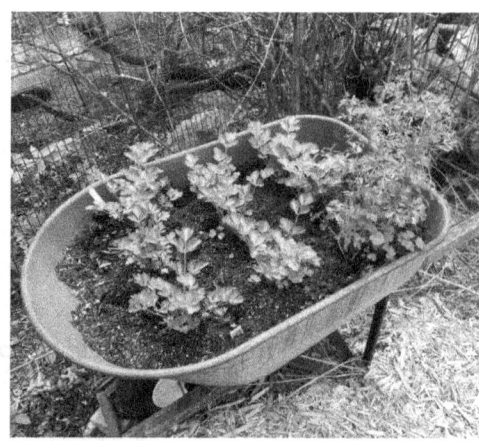

Is this an elevated or a raised bed? Regardless, beds are not limited to any specific shape so long as it allows you to have easy access. Got an old and underused or misused wheelbarrow? Don't toss it (yet). Use it as an elevated bed. Drill holes in the bottom for drainage. Here, celery and cilantro are growing in an old wheelbarrow. You can also grow basil, peppers, eggplants, carrots, beets, cucumbers and kale in an old wheelbarrow. If the wheel is still in good shape, keep it so you can move the unit around when and where you like.

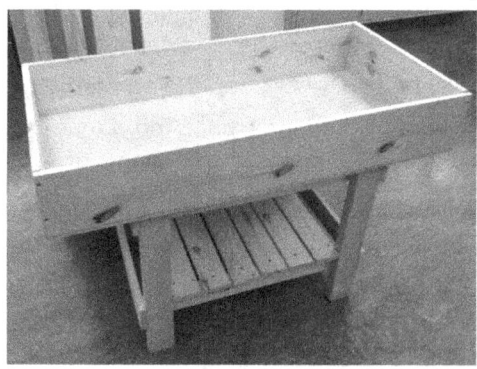

Elevated bed with solid top-section which you can use with various containers or lined with weed fabric and filled with soil along with several drainage holes. Designed and built by Dr. Tom Michaels, University of Minnesota. A bottom shelf can provide extra support to your unit and give you a place to stash stuff. This design allows you to move the unit. The top section is not fastened together, but set on the bottom section.

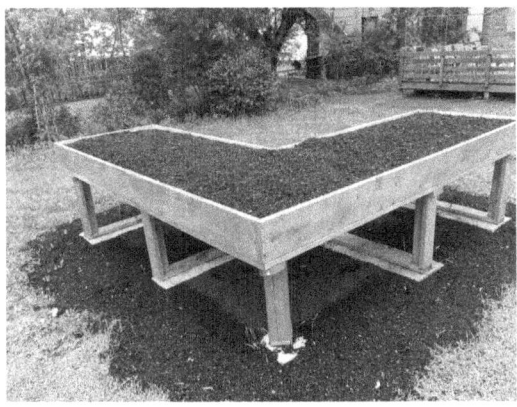
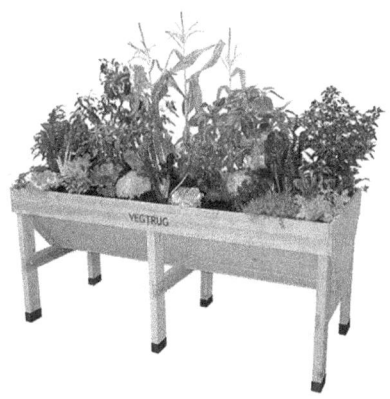

An L-shaped table with access all around the unit. Greg Towne, master gardener, is the designer, creator, and handy-man-person who built this versatile design for a senior project. This design is here forever, or close to that. The top section is fastened to the bottom and filled with soil.

Relatively easy access and functional. Vegtrug Raised bed with inward slanting sides is a great design to consider. You can garden straight-on without having to twist your body and is fantastic for wheel-chair access.

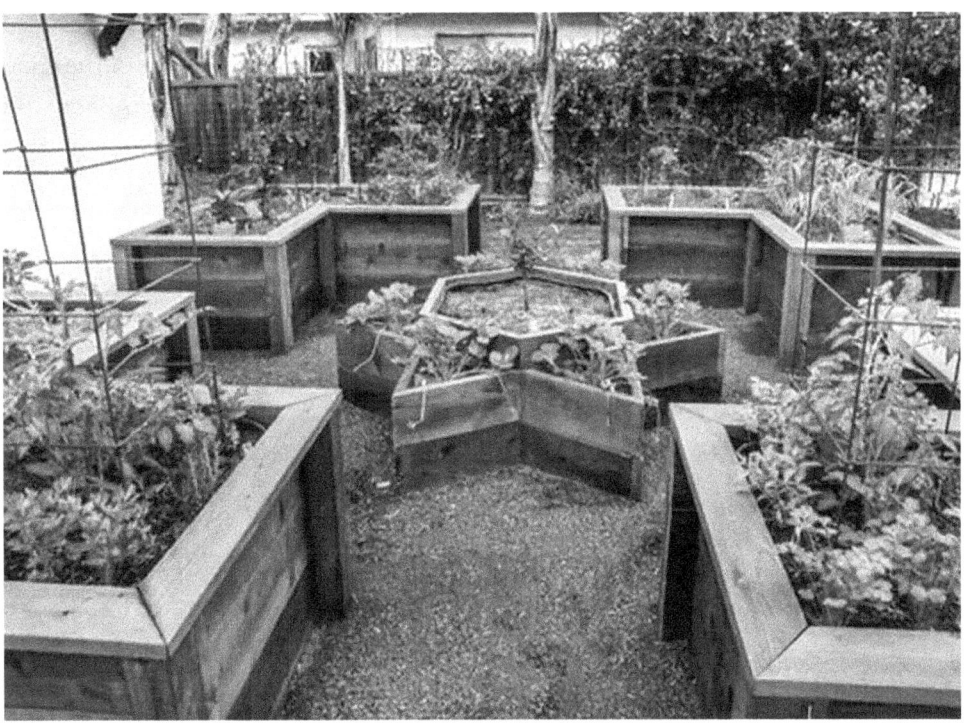

Examples of accessibility for one or more gardeners. This design includes a star-shaped wheel-chair accessible area. Perhaps a tad elaborate for your backyard to be sure. School yard garden? Community Garden? Senior living facility? Raised beds do not need to have straight, rectangular or square shapes. Easy access for all types of assistive devices. Use your creativity.

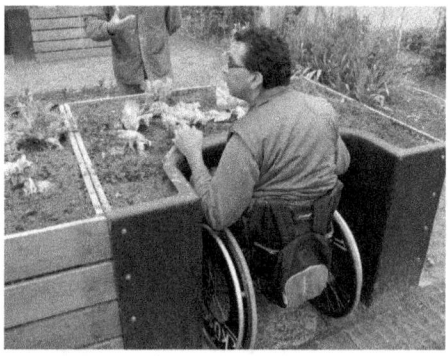

Do you need to use a wheelchair while you continue to garden? U-shaped, star-shaped or a Vegtrug-design could be very workable for your backyard or a communal garden for seniors and gardeners in general. This could be considered a type of Mandala-garden design.

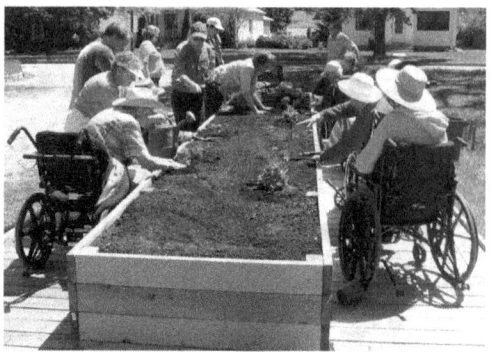

The key to wheelchair gardening is to have a hard, solid surface to roll on with accessibility from all sides of your raised or elevated bed. Keep the height at a level to avoid having to bend or crouch. Note that the sides are not tapered.

or big-box store. Some of you may find it easier to garden face-forward versus gardening from your side. Others may prefer to garden sideways. You will need to reach into the garden if you choose a bed that has straight sides. Straight-sided beds could prevent you from getting close and personal with your plants. Your knees or the chair will block you. Will that put too much pressure on your shoulders or back? Beds that slant inward, away from your knees, should help and you can use both hands and arms to plant, weed, harvest, and so on. Gardening from the side may limit your efforts to using one hand-arm at a time. You may tire more quickly. Having to use a wheelchair should not keep you from gardening. Review your options and include those that make the most sense and are practical for you to implement.

TIP: Hang your gardening tools on the elevated bed. They will be easy to reach and you would not have to haul them back and forth when you want to garden.

Ergonomic Toys and Tools

Ergonomic Tools. No doubt you have heard about these tools. Maybe you own some. Keep in mind that what is ergonomic to you may not be ergonomically practical for

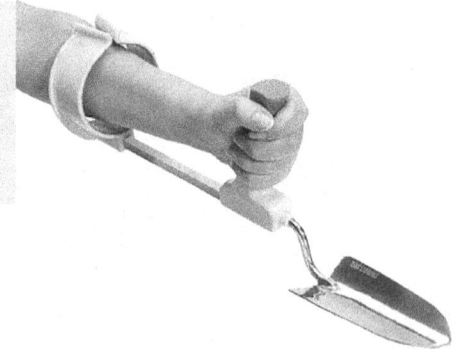

Peta Easi Grip Garden Trowel provides hand and wrist support for digging or planting in soil. The handle and brace could provide extra digging power for you.

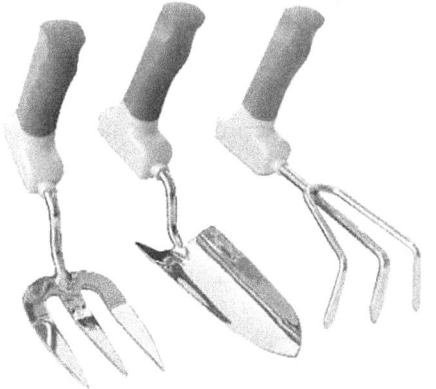

There are many ergonomic hand tools available for you to choose from. Select hand tools that are comfy for you to use.

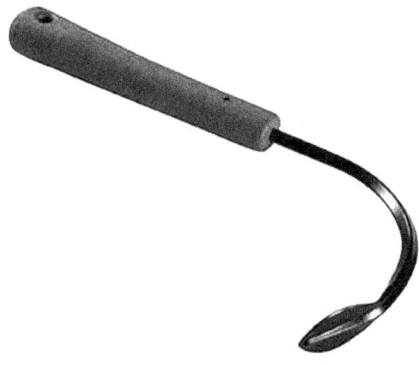

The Cobra Head Weeder can help you garden with a bit less muscle power and to dig out weeds or to cultivate in narrow, tight spaces.

someone else. An ergonomic tool for you is one that you can use with less force, less repetitive movement, is less awkward to use and does not require you to contort your body. What does that mean? A tool that strains your neck or shoulders or elbows or wrists or hands, for example, is one that is awkward to use. Other examples of a tool that is awkward are those that require you to bend or stoop or twist or reach too far.

A tool that you can say is ergonomic is one that fits the task you are performing, fits your hand without causing awkward contortions, does not require excessive force and is not a safety or health risk to you. A tool that is labelled as ergonomic in the store or online will not be ergonomic to you if it creates the issues I just mentioned. A tool is not ergonomic to you if after (or while) using it causes some tingling or swelling or numbness in your hands or in your joints; or, if it causes muscle fatigue or sore muscles. Caution: you could experience these symptoms while you are using the tool or after a few days.

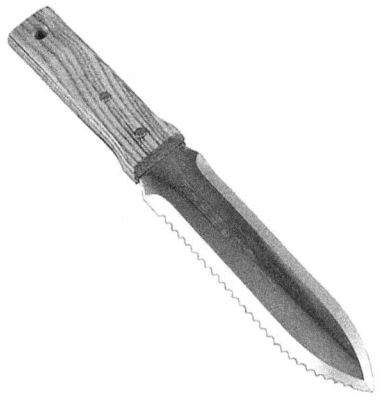

A tool that is not comfy to use and causes you pain with extended use can result in damage to your muscles, tendons, nerves, ligaments, joints, cartilage, spinal discs and other body parts. The best way to find out what works for you is to visit your favorite local garden center

Japanese Hori Hori knife with ruler for planting bulbs and serrated edges for digging-cutting out weeds and for slicing up slugs and other creepy crawlers, if you are so inclined to do so. Check to see if gripping the handle causes you discomfort.

and touch and feel the tools you want to buy. Play with them a bit. How do they feel? Comfy? Fine. Not to worry. You will not get arrested for playing and fondling them. Make your purchase where you prefer, making sure that you get the exact brand name, model number and so on. Here is a checklist of suggestions to consider when looking for a non-powered tool.

- ☐ If you are buying a single-handle tool, such as a screwdriver or a garden trowel, check the diameter of the handle. It should be between 1.25- and 2-inches in diameter.
- ☐ Double-handle tools, such as pliers or pruning shears or cutters, should not open more than 3.5-inches when the handles are spread apart. When the handles are closed, the closed grip should not be less than 2-inches. Select a tool that is spring loaded so that the handle automatically returns to the open position.
- ☐ Look for tools with a cushioned or soft handle or coated with some type of soft material.
- ☐ Do not buy a tool if it has sharp edges or finger groves on the handle.
- ☐ Tools with bent handles are often easier to work with than one with straight handles.
- ☐ Buy tools that you can use with either hand.
- ☐ Select a tool with a handle length longer than the widest part of your hand, which usually is between four- and six-inches. If the handle is too short for you, the end of the handle will press against the palm of your hand and cause pain or a blister or an injury.
- ☐ If you are left-handed, purchase left-handed tools or make certain you can easily use a right-handed tool before you buy it.

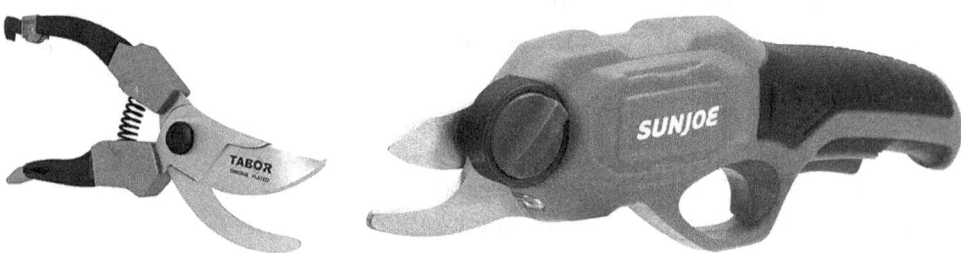

Do not buy anvil-type pruners, which tend to crush the branch or twig rather than cutting it cleanly. The by-pass pruner on the left is a better style to choose. Note the angled handle. You can use the SunJoe cordless pruner with one finger. A bit expensive but a good tool for pruning small twigs and brush.

Two companies to consider are Fiskars and Felco. There are others. Sun Joe Cordless markets an electric pruner, which could be a tad pricey. It could be a great addition to your tool-box, especially if you have hand or wrist or problems using other types of pruners or shears.

Long-handle tools. I am a fan! These types of tools can help you dig and cultivate and cut down weeds while standing upright. You may need to bend just a bit, depending on your height of course, but bending will not be as severe as with the shorter handled tools. Pick up one of these babies. Does it feel comfy? Too heavy for you? If so, don't buy it. That said, if it is difficult for you to bend, long-handled tools may be right for you.

Stools and Kneelers. Sit on it. Rest a while. If you have some physical difficulties or find it hard to get down to work in the soil as you used to, take a break. Digging, cultivating, planting can put a strain on your back, shoulders, arms and if you are lifting stuff you may notice strain on your knee joints.

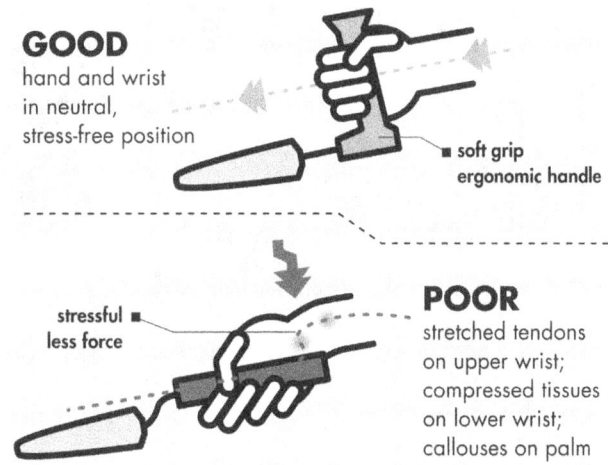

Pick up and play with the tool before you buy it. How does it feel? Comfy?

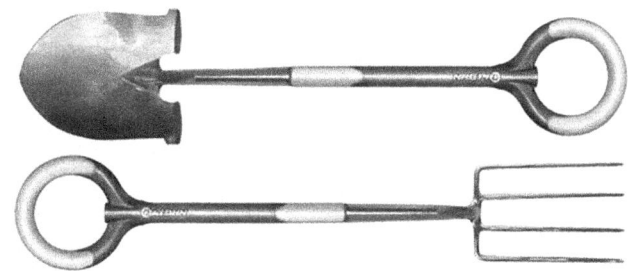

Radius Pro Garden Fork and Shovel with ergo-friendly handles. Longer-handled tools could provide you with greater ease of use than shorter versions. Test them out before you buy. What works better for you?

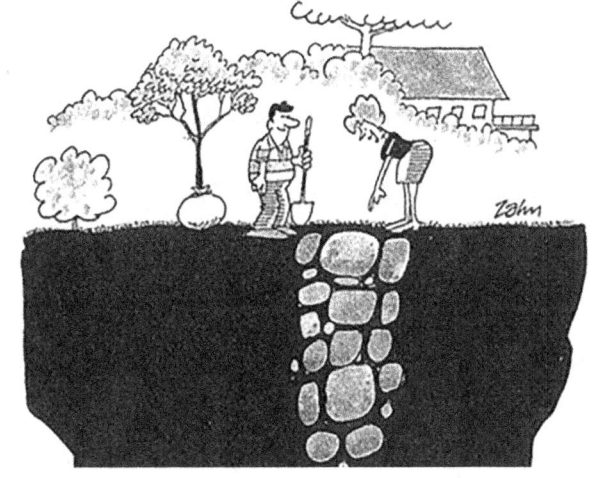

*Let's plant it right here (**Saturday Evening Post**, July/August, 2001).*

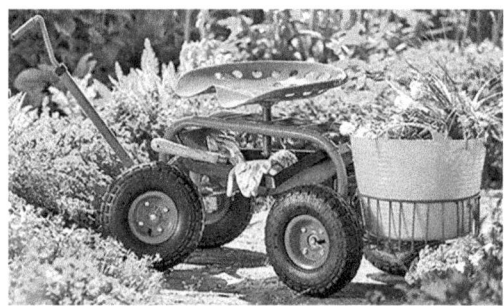

You may prefer a racier model that allows you to zip around on hard or softer surfaces. Inflated tires, swivel seat, a steering handle and a basket in the back for plants or hand tools. You power this bad-boy with your feet, which could be a major problem if you have had lower body surgery—hips, knees or feet. Note the handle so you could always pull or push it along or, grab someone who can push or pull you along so you can enjoy the ride.

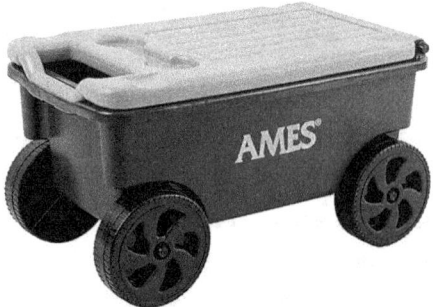

Ames Lawn Buddy Cart provides you with a comfy seat and storage space for your hand tools, gloves, hat, a bottle of water and whatever else you can stash inside.

Sit on it and stand up periodically to avoid any numbness in your legs. Consider a stool with wheels or a sturdy chair (not the over-stuffed living-room variety, but something easy to carry or pull around). Gardening can be easier if you can sit and swivel around a bit. Consider a product called Deluxe Tractor Scoot or the Ames Lawn Buddy Cart or other brand that feels comfy on your bum-side.

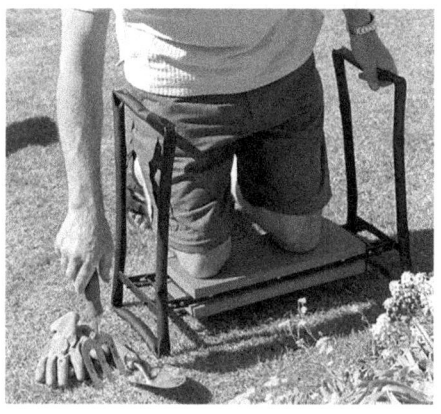

This is a dual-purpose device. You can kneel or sit on it. This type of garden kneeler will protect your knees a bit with a cushioned pad. The tall handles make it easier for you to get up and down without losing your balance. This kneeler doubles as a seat when you invert it and sit on the pad. The handles fold down flat to save storage space.

pH and Plant Care

Growing veggies, herbs and flowers in containers (or beds) allows you to grow a wide variety of varieties before and after surgery. Your garden soil has a specific pH—alkaline, acidic, or balanced. If you want to grow an acidic-loving variety such as blueberries, you will experience absolute failure if your garden or beds-containers have a pH that reads more alkaline (sweet, high pH) than acidic (sour, low pH). Test your soil. Send a soil sample to the Extension Service at a University. Note the pH levels of commonly eaten (and grown) foods.

Potting Soil. Most store-bought potting soils will allow you to grow almost any plant. Use a lighter soil mix in any of the options identified above—raised beds, elevated

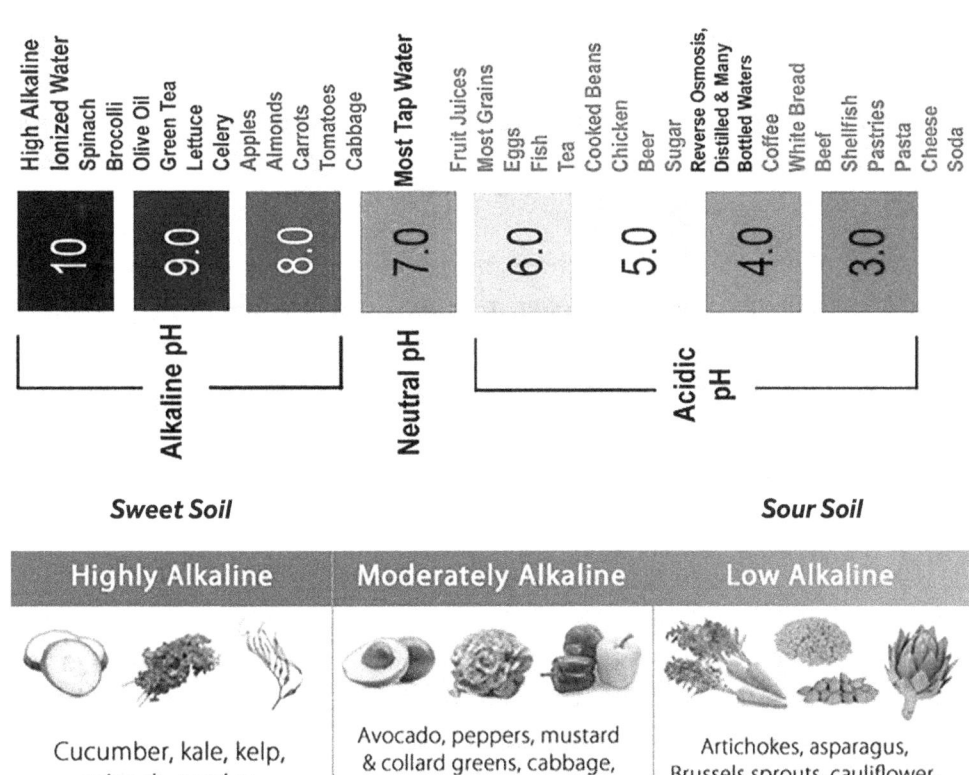

What's in your soil? If your soil is sweet, you should be able to grow the veggies listed under 'Highly Alkaline'. If it is sour, consider those under 'Low Alkaline' (or acidic).

beds, and containers. As I mentioned, do not use soil from your garden. If you do, any soil diseases (and they are in there), bad bug eggs and larvae (and they are in there), and any other nasties will transfer to your new beds and containers. Your garden soil may be too sandy or too heavy because of clay. Or, if you live within city limits, your soil may be contaminated with toxic chemicals or construction debris or who knows what. Potting soil is an excellent option for you. Buy it or make your own recipe.

Ideally, you can use a garden mix composed of 45% black dirt, 45% composted matter, and 10% sand. You can also use a sterile potting mix or composted manure with your own compost if you have it. Another option is to mix one-third peat, one-third composted material, and one-third potting soil. If you prefer to use fertilizer, mix in a slow release variety, such as 14-14-14 from Osmocote. You should not have to worry about fertilizing your plants in containers or beds for at least a couple of months. By then you will have recovered from your surgical procedure and can resume gardening at a more involved and active pace. Bagged potting soil usually identifies the pH level of the product.

Watering Options. You may have an automated overhead sprinkling system now. If not, think of this suggestion as a longer-term benefit to you, well after your rehab is finished. If someone you know is handy, they could install a system for you, No Handy-Andies in the neighborhood? Contact a professional. Once installed, set the timer and zone watering times. If it is the way you want it, you should not have to worry about watering your crop. No more dragging hoses. Cost for installing a system may or may not be within your targeted budget. Get at least three estimates (for any project).

An alternative is to use a drip-watering system. You can use drip or soaker-hoses on your straw bales, inside your tunnels, low or high or next to your plants in each row. Set that up way before your surgery date because this type of drip or soaker-hose system will require that you do a lot of bending down or crawling along on your hands and knees. You can set the system in place with U-shaped pins to secure them in the soil. SEDIFY is an option.

> **NOTE:** Depending on the water pressure in your area, a drip or soaker hose could cause a slight problem. The plants closest to your outlet will have plenty, maybe too much, pressure. The plants at the far end of the hose may not get as much water.

Another myth that needs clarification is over-head watering. Hauling hoses and sprinklers around may not be high on your wish list just before you go off to work and especially after surgery. Those are some reasons why you may want to consider an over-head system. These watering systems by themselves do not create diseases. Almost everything you have read about over-head watering leaves out one teensy tiny and important detail: *when* the watering occurs.

Generally, you probably water your plants when it is convenient for the you, not the plant. You work. You are in a suit or some nice clothes. Or, you are wearing some high-heeled sneakers. Likewise, when you come home from work or from wherever and need to water you do so because, well, you haven't been around all day and maybe around dinner time is the time when you can do it. I am not disputing that. There are times when you can water and times when you cannot. Simple.

The best time to water is early in the morning. Granted, that may not be the best time for you. With an overhead system, you can set your timer to start at, say 03:00 or 04:00 in the morning, and have all zones watered by, say 06:00. Your water pressure will be higher during that time before your favorite neighbors wake up and get ready to start their day. Watering during the heat of the day is not a good practice. Too much evaporation.

If you have containers to water, keep the soil mix about one inch from the lip or top of your container. Use enough water to fill that space between the soil mix and the top. Let it soak in. Go on to the next container and repeat. You want to water deeply, not shallow. Shallow watering can mean a shallow root structure which can mean your plants will dry out quicker.

And just in case your favorite neighbor or friend or the article you read says NEVER to water overhead ask them if they have heard of a concept called (wait for it), *rain*. Yes, *that* rain. Unless I miss my guess here, rain does not come up from the ground (broken water lines or overflowing rivers or lakes or high tides notwithstanding). Rain is overhead watering. Period.

Rain comes at any and all hours of the day and night. You cannot stop the rain. Ideally, it will rain in the morning and give the plants all day to dry out. Leaf-type diseases will be minimized and perhaps even eliminated, maybe. Keep proper spacing with plants within the row and between rows. When air circulation is good, leaf-type diseases can be minimized. You have no control over rain or any other weather-related issue. Minimize (or eliminate) overhead watering as best you can, especially if you expect to have a couple days of rain.

Rain: the key is *when* you water that causes the problem, not the act of watering.

Module Summary

> *Knowledge is knowing that a tomato is a fruit,*
> *wisdom is not putting it in a fruit salad.*
>
> —MILES KINGTON

Prepare to garden after surgery before surgery. Consider no-till as an option to minimize your work-load after surgery. Simply move any mulch or compost away from the row or area that you want to plant. Then plant.

Composted material can help your soil, but it will rob it of the Nitrogen needed to break-down the material. Adding extra Nitrogen will help. Plants cannot take up any solid material. Therefore, for compost to provide any nutrients to your plants it needs to be broken down into a soluble form by the microbial bacteria and creepy-crawlers found in the soil.

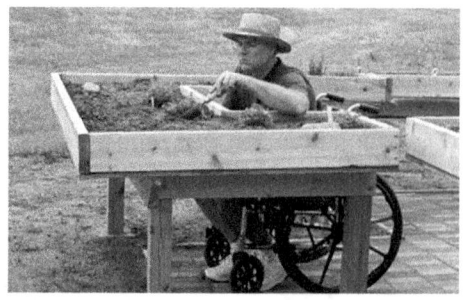

*A Mandala **U-shaped** elevated bed with wheel-chair accessibility.*

You can extend your growing season with cloches and hot caps, low or high-tunnels, cold-frames, floating row covers and stagger planting. In addition, plant cold-weather varieties that will survive cooler weather and light frosts.

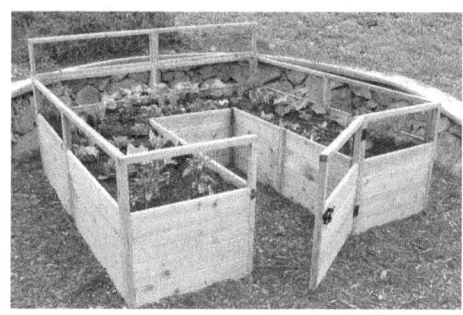

A Mandala design for a raised bed with an access door.

Companion planting is fun to do and can confuse insects who target your plants. No plant can impart its qualities to another plant. That is, basil will not improve the flavor of a tomato growing on the plant. Plant different varieties with different fragrances (smells) to confuse the insects' ability to find lunch. You will not eliminate insect or disease damage, but you can minimize it with this and other integrated pest management (IPM) practices, such as botanical rotation.

Before you reach for the chemical spray can, know what you are trying to kill before you spray the world. Most chemicals are non-discriminatory. They kill both the good and the bad bugs.

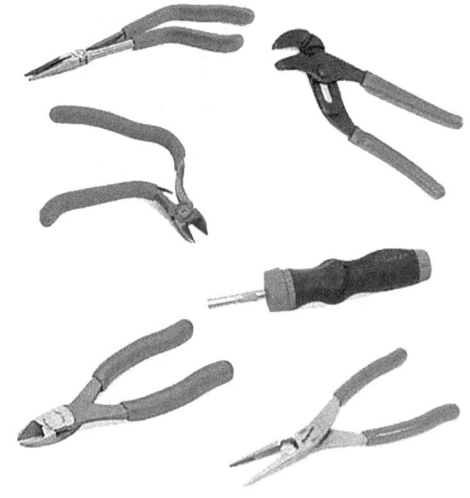

You can improve accessibility to your garden by planting in rows and blocks with wider aisles, by incorporating a Mandala design, the square-foot method, raised and elevated beds and using containers. Limited space? Grow vertically.

Tools advertised as ergonomic should fit your hands without causing you pain or discomfort. If they cause pain, they are not ergonomic to you. Handle them at your favorite garden center. If they feel right and are comfy for you, buy them there or online.

Make any elevated bed wheel-chair friendly if needed in your garden. Consider the Mandala-keyhole design shown on the previous page with wheel-chair accessibility.

Test your soil for its pH level. Most plants will grow well in a 5.5 to 6.5 range.

Ergonomic tools are ergonomic if they fit your hand without causing you pain or blisters or having you make contorted moves.

Rain and overhead irrigation systems are two examples of over-head watering. You can control when you want your system to start and stop; you cannot control when rain will start and stop. Rain is overhead watering.

Your Notes

MODULE 4

PREPARING YOUR WATER WORLD

The focus and outcomes of this module are ...

- Accessibility and sustainability

- Year-round alternative to soil-based gardening

- Creating low-cost, low-maintenance, eco-friendly hydroponic system

Overview

What is the one thing you really do not like to do when you are out and about in your yard? Is it weeding? Chasing away the four-legged critters? Amending your soil? Worrying about asbestos or other toxic-goodies in your soil? Not being able to play in your garden because it is too wet and muddy? No one to help you? What sinks your motivational boat?

Have you ever had a plant die on you? Especially one of your house plants? What happened? One day you notice the plant looking a bit tired and droopy and you start to think that maybe it needs some water. So, you water it. The next day you do not notice any improvement so what do you do? You add more water. Then, zip. What happened? You drowned it. You over-watered it. You suffocated it. Nice going. Congratulations.

Well, cheer up. In this module you will learn how to grow veggies and herbs in water, straight-up. 100% water. No soil. No dirt. No worries about drowning. No soil diseases. No weeding. No dirty hands or fingernails. No creepy crawlers climbing on your forearms or down your neck. No worries about the weather when you garden indoors.

No worries about doggies marking their territory on your salad greens. No gardening experience needed.

Hydroponic Gardening

*Join the growing trend
And away with soil send.
Reduce your daily toil
And grow sans soil.
Not a choice of either-or,
But to reduce the chore.
Grow veggies and herbs galore
With less trips to the store.
Grow 'em inside or out
With great taste no doubt.*

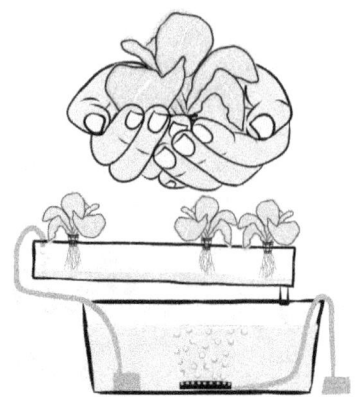

Hydroponics. Active Systems require electricity for the pump and filter, providing the aeration-air bubbles necessary for the plant to grow. These systems usually require more maintenance than the passive systems.

You may be gardening hydroponically now. If so, great. If not, this is the module for you. Regardless what type of elective surgery you plan to have you can garden within days of being released from your hospital or clinic. Shoulder surgery? No problem. Elbow surgery? No problem. Lower body surgery—hips or knees? No problem. Hydroponics is a viable option to consider so you can continue to enjoy gardening at any time of the year. No need to wait until you are fully recovered or even half-recovered. If you can walk with (or without) an assistive device and have the use of at least one arm, you can garden hydroponically within days of discharge. Yes, as in less than a week.

There are two basic systems: active and passive. The focus will be on the passive deep-water culture system (DWC).

Brief History. Hydroponics goes back almost 7000 years. The ancient Egyptians used it. The folks who built the famous Hanging Gardens of Babylon used it. The Aztecs in Mexico used it. The Chinese used it. Some countries in Asia and Europe have used hydroponics extensively,

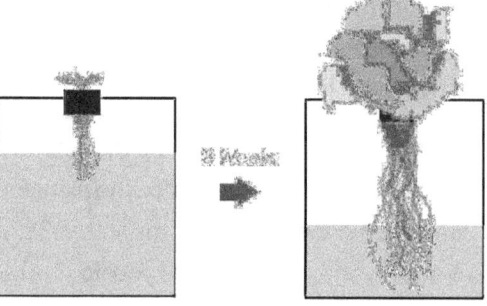

Hydroponics. Passive Systems do not use electricity. You provide aeration to the root system by providing an air space between the container cover and the water level. Passive systems are as close to set-it-and-forget-it systems that you can get.

well before we have here in North America. Angkor Wat, the temple complex in Cambodia, was built in the 12th Century. The moat surrounding this largest of all religious monuments served, in part, as a floating garden. Today, on the island of Sardinia in the Mediterranean Sea, farmers have been able to harvest four crops of tomatoes during their growing season. Very impressive to say the least. Hydroponics can allow homeowners and commercial operations to grow throughout the year and realize multiple harvests, regardless of the weather.

Within the last thirty or so years hydroponics has expanded as a positive, eco-friendly alternative (and complement) to traditional soil-based gardening and, even more recently, as an alternative to small-farm farming. There are many articles and books written about hydroponics. And I have my own book, *Hydroponic Gardening The Very Easy Way* (*Amazon.com* 2018), which is the only book to focus exclusively on the passive DWC system for the homeowner. The word passive means that no electricity or pumps or special tubing is needed when gardening outdoors.

The one system that you will learn about in this module can be especially well suited to you, the home-owner, the single or retired person, the person who lives in a detached home or in an apartment or condo or an assisted-living facility. The Passive Deep-Water Culture System (DWC) has the longest track record, is the easiest to set up and maintain, and is the least expensive and least complicated of all the current systems. You can do this without an advanced degree or any degree.

We all are indebted to Dr. B.A. Kratky who taught at the University of Hawaii and is now retired. He basically set the parameters for the DWC system and eliminated the use of having to use electricity when gardening outdoors.

What is it? Quite simply, hydroponics is a form of container gardening that uses water and specialized hydroponic fertilizer. There is no soil. Plants are suspended in a liquid called the *nutrient solution*. Hydroponic fertilizers provide the essential elements and minerals that allow your plants to grow and thrive. No need to add supplemental fertilizers. The macro and micro elements in hydroponic fertilizers include elements found in nature. People process those elements and package them for you, ready to use. Plants do not care if the nutrients they need to grow and thrive come from a factory or the back end of an animal.

There are six types of hydroponic systems. Four systems are often used by commercial growers—Nutrient Film Technique (NFT), Ebb and Flow or Flood and Drain, Aquaponics and Aeroponics. Two are used by the home-owner—Wick and Deep-Water Culture. There are many variations of these six systems depending on who is marketing which system. Bucket-Bubbler is an example of a DWC system. You may also hear about aquaponics which incorporates fish as the source of nutrients for the plants.

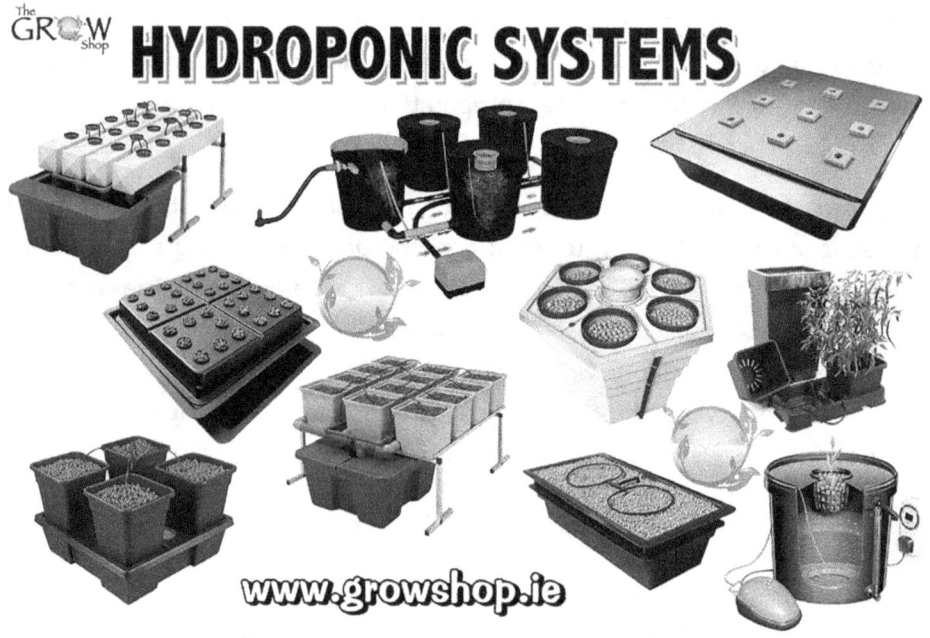

There are many variations to the basic types of systems. Homeowners tend to select the passive DWC system because of its low cost, low maintenance, expandability and sustainability benefits.

NUTRIENT FILM TECHNIQUE

A. NUTRIENT TANK STORES NUTRIENT

B. NUTRIENT PUMP CIRCULATES NUTRIENT

C. NUTRIENT FLOWS INTO GROW CHANNEL

D. NUTRIENT ABSORBED BY PLANT ROOTS

E. UNUSED NUTRIENT FLOWS BACK INTO TANK

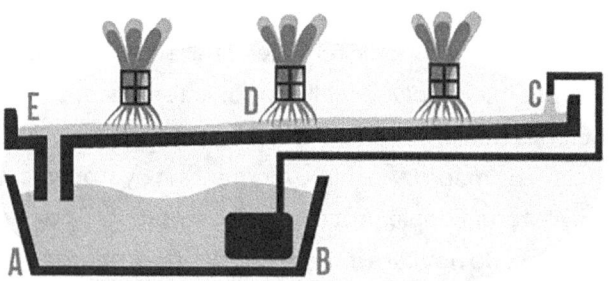

NFT systems are usually seen in commercial or high-production operations. This system does not use a substrate medium. It is an active recovery system. The submersible pump (B) circulates the nutrient solution (A) into a grow tube (C). Plants are suspended by a collar or tube (D), keeping the root system in constant contact with the nutrient solution. The solution (E) is returned to the solution container and the cycle repeats.

PREPARING YOUR WATER WORLD

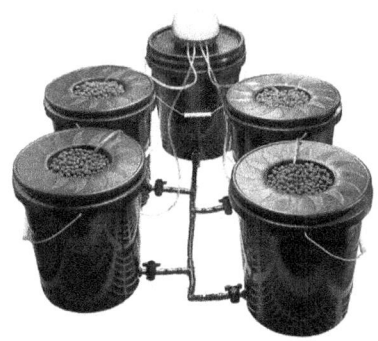

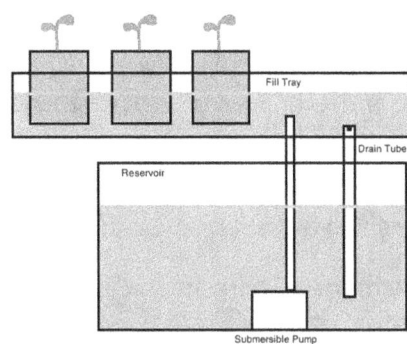

The Bucket and Bubbler system is another version of the DWC system. It is an active system versus a passive one. It uses an air pump, plastic tubing, and an air stone to circulate the nutrient solution and air-oxygen to easc plant set in a line or array of buckets. It is like the wick system without the wicks.

Ebb and Flow is another active recovery system. Sometimes referred to as the flood-and-drain system. There are two containers with this system. The lower reservoir contains the pump and nutrient solution. The pump brings the solution to the upper reservoir. The root system absorbs the solution and an overflow pipe drains the solution back into the lower reservoir and the cycle repeats.

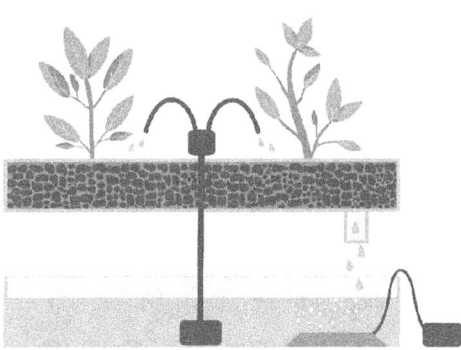

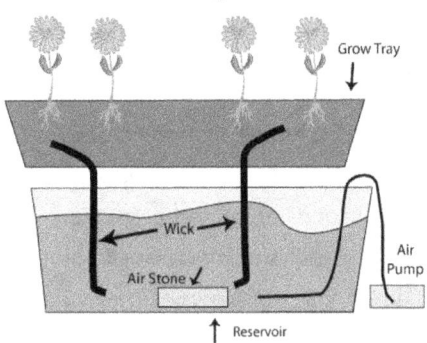

The Drip System, or continuous drip system, is like the drip irrigation system in your soil-based garden. It can be an active recovery or nonrecovery system. A submersible pump connects a tube that goes to each plant. Usually, you can adjust the flow-rate for each plant.

This is a passive, nonrecovery system. There is an air pump and air stone. The nutrient solution is sucked up (wicked up) from the reservoir to the plant grow tray. Sometimes an individual wick is more efficient than another, resulting in different rates of growth for any affected plant.

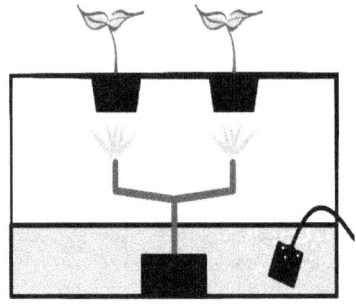

*The aeroponic system uses a pump that **spritzes** the nutrient solution to the root system on a timed-basis. The plant is suspended above the solution. An aerator provides the oxygen. NASA uses a more elaborate and expensive version in the Space Station.*

Low-maintenance DWC System. The deep-water culture system (DWC) is a perfect gardening alternative for sports-folks and anyone else who cannot play with their balls and racquets and clubs and paddles and other toys and tools during the winter. Anyone can learn how to garden the easy way, without the soil and toil and expense. They could even do this after playing their sport. Non-gardeners can now enjoy gardening without the time and toil and expense needed for soil-based gardening.

Advantages. There are many advantages and benefits to the passive hydroponic process. One advantage is to garden during the winter months allowing you to harvest fresh veggies and herbs and grow flowers. You can also garden in those areas that are stifling hot and humid where fungus and mold thrive under those conditions. You can garden during wet and dry seasons, in the desert, and even in Antarctica. NASA uses a sophisticated variation of *aeroponics* to grow potatoes in outer space. NASA's version suspends the food-tuber or potato-eye in the air and spritzes it with hydroponic fertilizer multiple times per hour. Their goal is to find a process to produce food for astronauts who will be sent on extensive journeys. As you read this, they are also experimenting with peppers and other veggies as possible food sources. The Chinese, among other societies around the world, are currently using this system as well.

> *When I started writing this book there were three major E-coli warnings and subsequent directives about not eating Romaine lettuce. The FDA recalled thousands of packages from grocery stores and restaurants. That disease can make you very sick. It can kill you. Good news: you should not have to worry about any E-coli problems when you grow your own veggies hydroponically. The source for most of those incidents came from spreading manure as fertilizer and from people not washing their hands. Bad news: if by some slim chance you do contract E-coli, you will absolutely, positively know the source of the problem (you).*

The DWC system is flexible and highly portable. You will dazzle your friends with your expertise and ability to grow plants in water. Research has shown that plant growth is at least 30 to 50% higher than traditional soil-based gardening, with higher yields. The taste and texture of your produce is as good or in most cases better than what you might purchase at your favorite grocery store. When you incorporate hydroponics, you have more control over what you and your family are eating. There is no waste or spoilage. You harvest what you want to eat that day, just before feeding-time. There is no need for pesticides or herbicides, especially if you garden indoors. There is no run-off or pollution of a waterway. There is no need to be concerned about the quality of your soil, whether it is sandy, clay, rocky, or infested with a toxic menu of construction rubble. You are gardening in water, not soil. You are gardening that is as close to low-maintenance as you can get. Set it and forget it until harvest time.

Yet, in all fairness and to be as forthright as possible, I feel that it is my civic duty and ethical obligation to make you aware of the many downsides to hydroponics. Users beware!

Disadvantages. When compared to soil-based gardening, hydroponic-gardening involves ...

- No weeding and no need to mulch
- No need to use herbicides (a real bummer if you like to spray stuff)
- No need to use insecticides (a real bummer if you like to kill stuff)
- No daily or weekly or monthly spraying of anything
- No need to wait for your soil to dry out so you can start gardening
- No need to hassle your favorite partner or spouse or neighbor to prep your garden
- No soil preparation in the spring (no springerizing)
- No winterizing in the fall
- No need for ergonomic tools or pretty much any other type of tool
- No need for shovels, pitchforks, wheelbarrows, hand tools or roto-tillers
- No heavy lifting and hauling of soil, compost or other amendments
- No need to water an inch or more each week
- No need to wait for rain
- No need to worry about dry spells or dust storms or drought
- No more complaining about a sore back, knees or hips (a real bummer)
- No little or big doggies marking their territory on your salad greens
- No bending down or crawling on your hands and knees
- No garden pets to cuddle and hug—no earwigs, no slugs, no wireworms, no spiders, no creepy crawlers to crawl up your pants or sleeves to freak you out
- No need for gloves or knee pads or back-support belts
- No problems with bunnies or woodchucks
- No problems with snakes or jumping earthworms

Wait. There are more disadvantages ...

- Gardening indoors during the cold, wintry, snowy and icy months means you may have to sell your snow-bird vacation place and stay home
- Your friends will think you gave up gardening because you can now wear those three-inch nails you have always wanted to have (not sure why, but ...)
- No more dirt under your fingernails
- No more chapped and cracked hands (as when you work in soil)
- Your orthopedic surgeon may feel unwanted and lonely
- Kiddies think gardening in water is cool and will get in your way and want to help
- Friends and neighbors will constantly lift the plants out of the container to see if you really are growing plants in water or if you are fibbing a bit
- Your lettuces and salad greens will have a buttery texture, es decir, mantecosa/o
- You will have too much leisure time. You may be compelled to take up a new hobby. Or, you just may chill and get all lazy and become a couch-potato
- You will finally be forced to clean out your cluttered, gadget-filled garage and tool shed and have a garage sale
- And if you live where it is nice and hot and dry where the temperature cooks up into the three-digit mark (even though it is a very dry and nasty hot-heat) you can garden indoors where you have air-conditioning instead of going outdoors to play in the burning sand and have your body-fluids ooze out of your pores and not get all lathered up to ward off flying and crawly, biting-critters that suck up your blood and generally see you as lunch
- And perhaps the biggest disadvantage is that you can garden all year-round, whether it is hot or cold, which means you could raise fresh tomatoes and a wide range of fresh salad greens and herbs in the winter and still be dragged outside and play in the ice and snow and sub-zero temperatures with wind-chill readings of *are-you-kidding-me* and getting frost bite and pretend that you are enjoying that type of forced fun because that is what you did when you were growing up and you want folks to think how tough and rugged you are (that could be a real bummer). Your snow-birding days could be over.

Behavior Change. You read about changing behavior and attitude in **Module One**. How do you feel about *having* to change? How do you feel *thinking* that you may have to change? How do you feel about alternatives to what you are doing now, what you have been doing most of your life? Scary?

Hydroponic gardening requires a behavior change for some people. If you were born and raised on a farm your family probably experienced flooding in a low area at some point. The crop died or was set back because of the flooding. Gardening in water? A bit skeptical? Hydroponic gardening is not a fad. You can do it inside and outside, year-round. You cannot do that with a soil-based garden, especially if you live where there is chilly-cold weather. Did I mention that you do not need any gardening experience? You can do it. Got kiddies hanging around? They could do it.

Why bother changing? You have a soil-based garden now. You have been gardening in soil since your earliest days. Your parents and grandparents may have grown all types of veggies and crops in soil. So why consider hydroponics? There are several reasons, among which there is no need to worry about the composition of your soil, whether it is sandy, clay, or muck or a toxic concoction of whatever someone before you buried there. It is environmentally safe. It is sustainable. No erosion. No leaching of fertilizer into any waterway. No need for herbicides or pesticides. You would use about ninety-percent less water. And once you set it up it maintains itself with very minimal effort by you.

In the second book in this series, *Getting Your ADL Groove Back After Surgery with PAPS: Living Better, Living Longer,* I focus on the different rehabilitation protocols for some of the more common elective orthopedic surgeries that may be on your agenda. If you garden in soil only, you will discover that it will take weeks even months (perhaps the better part of a year) of physical exercise and healing before you can safely and confidently return to the therapeutic and gastronomical joys of gardening and yard-work, with all of its lifting, bending, stooping, crouching, kneeling, squatting, digging, raking and shooing away the bunnies and woodchucks and swatting insects and running scared-to-death from hornets and things that you are sure will sting you. It could take you even longer if you intend to return to your sports activities.

If you garden hydroponically, whether exclusively or as a complement to your soil-based efforts, you can return to gardening as soon as you can stand and walk. You can return to gardening in just a matter of a few days.

Hydroponics is not just for post-surgical procedures. It can be easily integrated into your yard and, best of all, your home. Hydroponics requires less physical work and almost no tools or heavy bags of stuff to haul around. The passive DWC system is easily expandable as your interest (and success) grows. It is a great way to involve the kiddies. Continue gardening in soil if that is what you like to do. Start gardening hydroponically and enjoy what you like to do with a lot less effort, time and energy.

> **NOTE:** I do not sell hydroponic systems. I do not sell hydroponic materials or supplies. I teach young and older folks and all folks in-between how to set up their own passive hydroponic system using standard, low-cost, locally-sourced, ready-to-use materials and supplies.

DWC: The Passive Hydroponic System

Plants do not grow in soil. They grow in the air spaces and channels found in the soil. Nature creates these channels. You create those air spaces when you add composted material and other course materials to your soil. Earthworms and soil-dwelling bugs help the decomposition process and aid in the air-space-structure of your soil. The critical key to having a successful *passive* DWC system is to maintain that air space. The passive system does not require electricity or any moving parts when gardening indoors or outdoors. Yes, you would need artificial lighting when you choose to garden indoors, but the lighting system is an external component of the DWC system. It is not an integral part of a passive DWC system.

Providing that air space is simple. You provide your plants with air by keeping at least an inch of air space between the seedling and the top of the nutrient water line, at

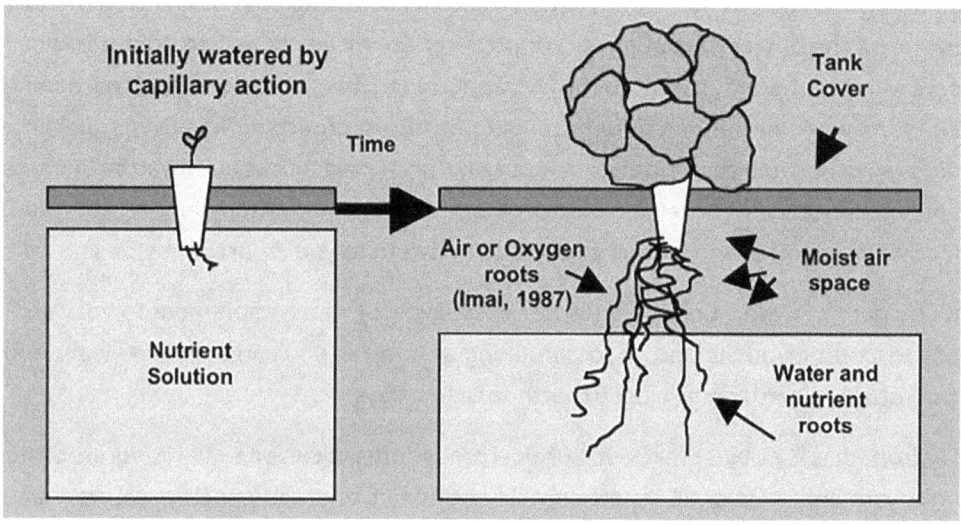

As the seedling develops, the root system expands, the water level drops and the air space increases. The moist air space increases. Illustration used with permission, B.A. Kratky, University of Hawaii.

least initially. As the plant takes up the nutrient solution, the root system develops, the water level drops, and the air space increases. At least a third or half of the root system should stay in constant contact with the nutrient solution. Keeping the air space is why your plants will not die as sometimes besets houseplants or those low-lying areas on your parent's or grandparent's farm with all your fond memories of muck and mud and ruined crops and perhaps a descriptive and colorful word or two.

Basic Materials. The materials and supplies you need are contingent upon the type of container you want to use. You will learn more about each of these materials and supplies in this module. Here is an overview of what you need for a quick-start passive DWC system.

- A food-safe container (select one):
  - Choose a three and one-half or up to a six-gallon **bucket** (with cover)
  - Choose a Wide-Lip Basket (WLB) instead of the cover, which sits or snaps on the bucket and comes in different inside diameters, six- or eight- or ten-inches; or
  - Choose a ten-gallon **tote** (with cover), 24" L x 15" W x 9" H; or
  - Choose a PVC **tube** (4" diameter x 24" long) with end caps
- Hydroponic fertilizer *only*: choose liquid or granular
- A teaspoon, tablespoon and a measuring cup
- Water (choose what you prefer):
  - Use tap or bottled water
  - Use rain-water
  - Use water from a dehumidifier
- A substrate media to support the plants:
  - Use a mix of peat, or coconut coir and perlite; or
  - Use perlite only; or
  - Use LECA (clay pellets) if you use WLBs
- Two-inch net pots to hold the substrate, seed or seedling
- Standard 1020 trays (solid bottom 11"x21") for holding the net pots during seed germination and initial root system development
- A fine-flow watering can
- pH testing kit

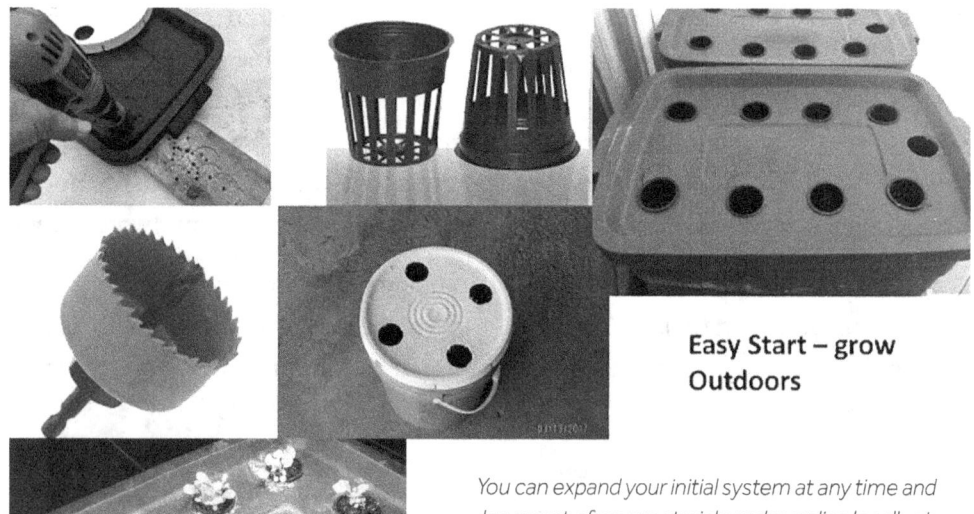

Easy Start – grow Outdoors

You can expand your initial system at any time and buy most of your materials and supplies locally at big-box or hardware stores. You need a drill (or very sharp knife) to cut two-inch holes into the covers of your bucket and tote and PVC tubes. Those holes support the two-inch net pots, which hold your substrate mix and seeds or seedlings. You can mix and match different containers at any time.

Initially, you would decide which container best meets your needs—standard buckets, totes or PVC tubes. As you gain confidence, experience and excitement and become the envy of your less-enlightened neighbors, you may decide to expand your initial system. You can mix and match different types of containers. You are not tied to a single vendor's components. You can create and expand your own system from your local big-box stores, hardware and garden centers. You may need other materials and tools, depending on what you have selected above.

- If you use the two-inch net pots, you will need a drill (12V or 18V), a two-inch hole saw (with a drill-guide), a piece of scrap lumber (so your hole-saw does not cut into your antique table or work-surface).
- To elevate your system, use a pair of resin saw-horses or a spare table to keep the bunnies and other critters away and avoid having to bend down or crawl around on the ground.
- If you plan to garden indoors, you will need an artificial light source, e.g., an LED unit.
- On-going supplies include the seeds or plants you intend to grow.

You can purchase food-safe buckets, totes and PVC tubes from big-box stores, such as Lowe's, Home Depot, Menard's, ACE Hardware and others in your area. The cover for

PREPARING YOUR WATER WORLD

each bucket should be included in the price of the bucket so make sure you grab up the cover. You can also pick up free buckets from your favorite grocery store bakery department or from smaller, mom and pop bakeries in your area. Most (all?) states prohibit stores from re-selling these buckets. Make friends with the bakery manager and ask for a bucket or two (or more). They are happy to have you get them out of their way. Usually, a bakery has buckets of different sizes. Monday is often the best day to grab your buckets. Free is good.

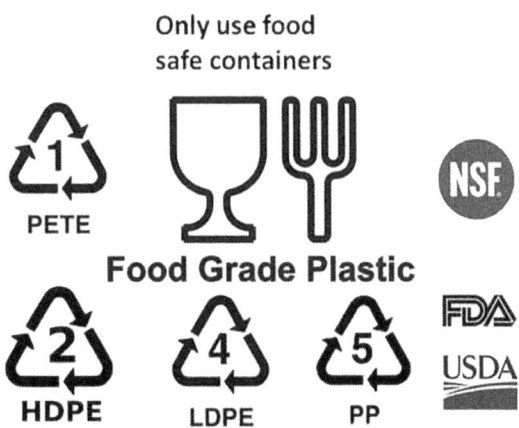

Only use food safe containers. You can use any color bucket, though white buckets work best outside. PVC tubes (PP5) that are marked as Schedule 40 (SCH 40) are food safe as are other containers with these numbers and/or symbols.

Food Safe Containers. Got a handy bucket that once was home to some pesticide or paint or a chemical other than plain water? Don't use it with any veggie or herb you plan to eat. Your containers should be food-safe. You will see the food-safe symbol or number on the bottom of standard buckets or totes. The illustration listed above identifies those food-safe numbers. Number two is considered the best of these because it handles extreme heat and cold very well (among other qualities). PVC tubes (white) are usually made of PP (polypropylene) or Number Five, but all of those listed above are considered food safe. Your government would not lie to you.

Tool-free Easy Start. Not too excited about working with a drill and any other tools? Not to worry. Once you have the materials you can set up a passive DWC system in minutes. Most of these materials will be one-time costs and should last several years. Here is a list of materials to get you started with an outdoor passive DWC system using a standard five-gallon **bucket** *without* tools ...

- One 5-gallon food-safe **bucket**- $4.00 (or get a freebie)
- One 10-inch **WLB** that snaps on to your bucket (no tools needed)- $7.00
- One bag each (8-quart size) of **perlite** and **peat** (or **coconut coir**)- $10.00
- Five 2-inch **net pots**- $1.00/5
- Blend the perlite (80%) and peat or coconut coir (20%) to create a substrate mix; dampen it and fill each net pot then add 2-3 seeds per net pot (eventually, you would cull the weakest and keep one seedling per net pot)

- Add only **hydroponic fertilizer** at **one teaspoon** per gallon of water or not more than two-tablespoons (or six teaspoons) per 5-gallon bucket-$20/14 ounces*

- Fill your container with **water** (tap water, rain-water, dehumidifier water) up to the *bottom* of your WLB, maintaining your air space. Do **not** fill the bucket up to the tippy-top of the WLB

- Add about two-inches of your damp substrate mix to the bottom of the WLB, set your net pots on the mix and fill in the spaces with perlite only, or additional substrate mix or LECA (clay pellets; more on this substrate later)

- Initially, top water your seeds until the root system grows through the slots of the WLB

- No tools. No drilling. Relax and watch your plants grow. Sports-folks will have hydro-envy. **Done!**

> **NOTE:** It is almost always better to use slightly less fertilizer when your plants are young, then increase the dosage to the recommendations provided on the brand-type of fertilizer you buy. You can start with two or two and one-half tablespoons per ten-gallon tote initially, then increase it a bit as your plants develop. Just for fun, read the directions (even if you are a male-person).

Cheating with Store-Bought Plants. Want even less work to get you started? You may not have the time, place, willingness or patience for starting your seedlings from seed. And if you are in the early stages of your rehab protocol after surgery you may

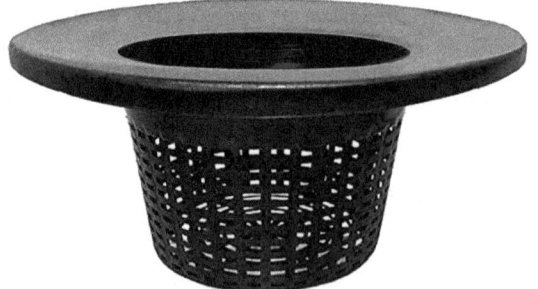 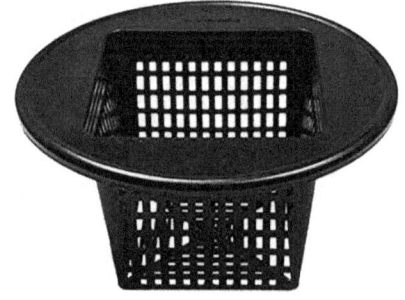

Wide-lip baskets designed to fit over standard 3.5 to 6-gallon buckets. You can set or snap them on to a bucket. No tools needed. Some have rounded bottoms, others square. Regardless, they work the same—very well thank you. The outer dimensions (OD) of WLBs are the same. The inner dimensions (ID) come in six- eight- and ten-inch sizes. You can plant one tomato plant or one pepper or one eggplant directly in the six-inch size and up to five Romaine lettuce or Asian green plants with their net pots in the ten-inch size.

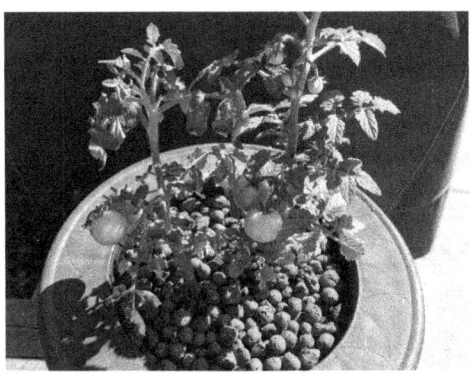

This is an eight-inch (ID) wide-lip basket (WLB) that sets or snaps on standard buckets. WLBs are an easy way to grow larger varieties or multiple plants of smaller varieties, such as salad greens and herbs such as Arugula. In this photo I have a cherry tomato, patio-variety, that was started in a net pot. Both the net pot and plant are set on a layer of perlite-peat and filled in with LECA.

decide that you do not want to spend the time or energy planting and nursing them. If so, buy your plants from your favorite garden center. Buy plants that are about four to six inches tall with deep green leaves and sturdy stems. Using smaller and healthier plants will reduce the shock of transplanting and make the transition from soil to water easier.

Remove the plant from its container and remove the potting soil by gently dipping the plant in water. Hold the plant by its leaves, not the stem. It is not critical that you remove all the soil. Once done, add an inch or two of the substrate-mix to the bottom of your WLB then place your plant(s) in the WLB with the root system extending down into the WLB. Fill in the space with perlite, with more substrate mix or LECA. You would not need net pots when using store-bought plants. No tools needed. **Done.**

Buying plants is instant gratification without the anxiety of *will-they-germinate*. The root system is established. The garden center treated the plant as a soil-based item. When you place it in a hydroponic container you are growing it hydroponically, unless you are a purist. Regardless, I consider it as being grown hydroponically from that point forward.

Many hydroponic gardeners consider growing plants in water as being organic. All (most) organic gardeners tend to disagree. Your federal government cannot decide either way. They leave it up to each state. The plant doesn't care one way or the other, but people-folks do.

Start small and easy. You can always expand your initial set-up using additional buckets or by adding different containers—totes and PVC tubes—if you want. In this section, you will learn

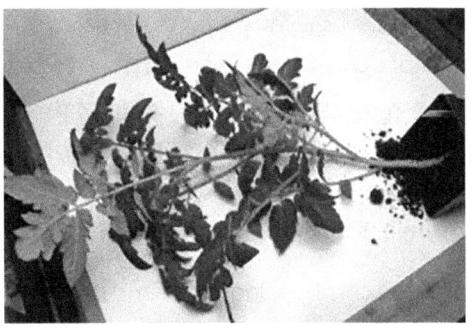

You can use store-bought plants for your hydroponic system. Buy shorter, healthy-looking plants, remove as much of the soil as you can and transfer them into your or a wide-lip basket. Fill in the space with your substrate-mix and LECA. Instant gratification.

more about the materials and supplies, the net pots, substrates, fertilizers, how to build a low-cost PVC light-frame and what you will need when you choose to garden indoors.

Net Pots come in different sizes—two-, three- four- and six-inch units. I use the two-inch size because they are readily available and inexpensive, about $.20 each and are re-usable. The larger sizes would require a larger hole-saw or special holding trays. A two-inch net pot will support almost any salad green, Asian greens, such as Bok choy or Tsoi-sim or Kailaan, as well as some varieties of collards, mustard greens, kales, beets, turnips, arugula, basil and rosemary.

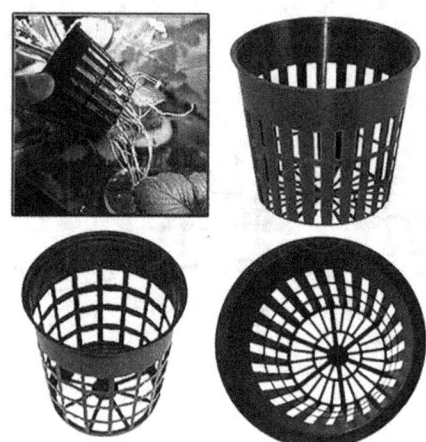

You can use net pots with totes, bucket covers/WLB and with PVC tubes. Identify the number of plants you want to grow in your container cover. Before you drill the holes, place a two-inch thick piece of scrap lumber under the cover so you do not gouge

You can use two-inch net pots to grow a very wide variety of veggies and herbs. Note the root system growing through the slots in the net pot (upper left-hand corner). The substrate material (peat and perlite) supports the seedling shown in the upper left-hand corner.

your antique dining-room table. Mark out where and how many holes you want for the cover. Drill a hole and use a screwdriver to push out the cut-out piece from the hole-saw. Repeat the process. **Done.**

You can cut in eight to twelve holes per 10-gallon tote cover and four to seven holes per bucket cover. If you prefer to eat salad greens as *micro-greens,* then cut twelve holes in the tote cover. If you want to grow tomatoes or cucumbers in a tote, drill two holes in the cover, one hole at each end. For peppers, eggplants, collards or kale drill four holes with one hole at each corner of the tote, keeping the center area open. Or, if you prefer, cut in three holes: cut one at each end of the far corners and the third between them on the near side of the tote. For bush squash, drill one hole in the center of the tote cover.

Still not comfy using a drill and hole-saw or don't want to spend the money to buy them? You could cut out each two-inch hole with an Exacto-knife or sharpen the open end of an empty tomato paste can. These are just options to consider. However, you may want to update your medical and life-insurance policies before you use these weapon-like devices. And again, if you are not crazy about using a drill go with the WLB. Easy and **done.**

I use the two-inch net pots because drilling the holes is easy with a drill and the net pots are inexpensive at less than twenty-cents per pot and they are reusable. And I can fit up to twelve net pots in a standard ten-gallon tote. You can purchase larger net pots. You could find them in three- to six inch sizes. Cutting holds that large will be a challenge. Many of these larger size net pots come with special trays-or support grids, so you would not have to drill anything.

Ten-Gallon Totes. Using totes will allow you to use the cover to grow up to twelve plants. Two of the food-safe totes you may want to consider are a Rubbermaid product, 'Roughneck', and a Husky product, their 'Heavy-Duty Tote'. Mark out the number of holes you want and drill, again placing a piece of scrap lumber under the tote cover.

Each of these totes are approximately 24" L x 15" W x 9" H and two will fit under one 48" LED shop light if you are growing your plants indoors. You could place them on a table or bench or on resin saw-horses to keep them up and away from critters.

PVC Pipes and Tubes. Is your space limited? Grow vertical. Build a low-cost and easy to assemble PVC frame with one-inch diameter thick-walled pipe. You could use the frame indoors to hang your lighting unit or outdoors to hang the PVC tubes. The tubes can be four-inches in diameter and whatever length you want. The pipe and tube are usually sold in ten-foot lengths. Once you cut the pipe fit the pieces together and suspend the four-inch diameter PVC

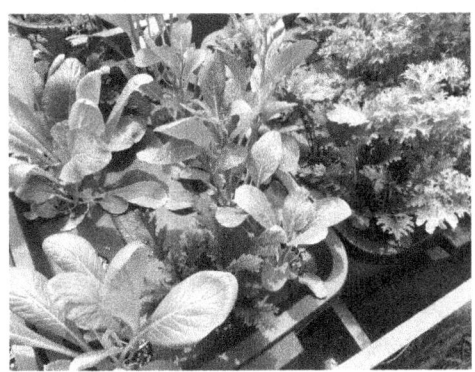

A mix of Asian greens and lettuces growing in ten-gallon totes. Harvest as micro-greens then let them grow to a mature size for a continuous harvest throughout your growing season. You can grow up to twelve plants in each tote. Grow plants that have a similar growth habit, e.g., vertical Romaine lettuce varieties, and mature about the same time. Keep each hole about two- to three-inches apart to allow for plant growth. Consider growing more of the vertical-growth varieties so you can maximize your yield in a small amount of space.

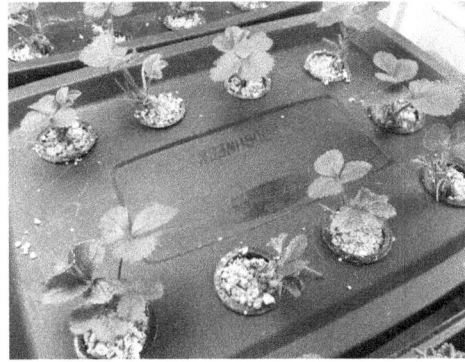

Do you like strawberries? The variety, 'Seascape', after nine-days in a ten-gallon tote, from bare root to three-inches high. Fifty plants growing in totes for a K-12 school project. Ever-bearing or day-neutral varieties are typically recommended for indoor and/or container gardening. Grow them indoors under artificial LED shop-lights.

tubes with bungee cords (or wire) from the top, horizontal pipe. You will need to buy one-inch elbows (two) to assemble the vertical and horizontal pipe. Set two 48" x ½" rebar pieces about 12" into the ground and slip the PVC pipe (legs) over the rebar. The rebar will support the PVC frame and prevent it from tipping over. **Done.**

> **TIP:** Some big-box and hardware stores will cut the PVC pipes for you at no or very little cost. Otherwise you will need a cutter or saw to cut the pipe to the dimensions you want. Identify the lengths you need. The nice helper-person will cut them for you.

My hydroponic containers are set above ground, high enough so the bunny-rabbits and woodchucks cannot reach them for their daily snack. Five-gallon buckets set on the ground or your deck or patio should deter the smaller bunnies. However, I place my totes and buckets on resin saw-horses that are about 30" high to keep both the bunnies and the wild-turkeys from chomping on my produce. I place my PVC tubes on a half-inch rebar frame that I designed so that I can include three to four 60"-inch PVC tubes, each supporting eleven net pots with plants, on a footprint that is only 36" wide by 12" deep. I can easily garden standing up with no kneeling and minimal bending. I can dramatically increase my yield in this small space by growing vertically. I have different lengths of PVC tubes. My 24" tube holds five plants; my 48" tube, nine plants and in my 60" tub I can grow eleven plants.

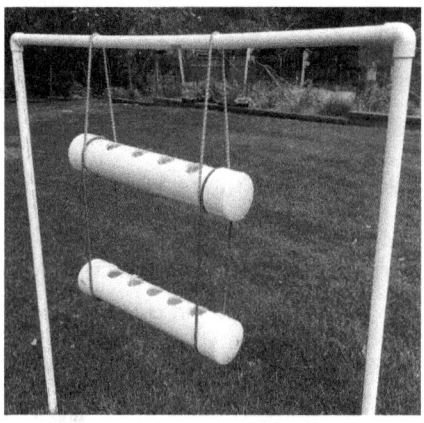

A portable PVC frame is great for outdoor use if you have limited space. Each 24" PVC tube will support five plants or a total of ten plants as shown in this photograph. High yields within a small footprint. This PVC frame is 36-inches wide by one-inch deep. I use one-inch diameter PVC pipe, but if you prefer more stability use the one- and one-half inch pipes. You could use six-inch diameter PVC tubes, but I have found the smaller size works great.

PVC, or **polyvinyl chloride**, is one of the most widely used thermoplastic polymers in the world. Contractors use the rigid variety for siding and plumbing in homes and office buildings. When you use PVC, look for the *codes NSF-PW* or *NSF-61* or *Schedule 40* stamped on the pipe. These are newer plumbing components and comply with the American National Standards Institute (ANSI) which sets the standards for our potable or drinking water. As of this writing, about 70% of homes in the United States

PREPARING YOUR WATER WORLD

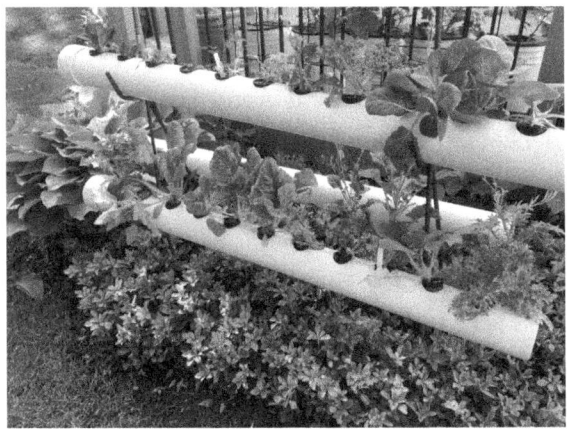

I have several rebar frames in my yard. Growing vertically allows me to grow more product within a smaller foot-print. In this photo, the 60" tubes are supported within a foot-print of 12" deep x 36" long. Each tube holds eleven plants for a total of forty-four plants in this narrow and vertical space. This is one example of a vertical gardening set-up that can dramatically increase your yield in a small foot-print. I sealed one end of the tubes with clear caps cut from a sheet of acrylic. In this way I can easily check the water level without having to lift a net pot. The other end has PVC caps. In 2019, I planted two sets of strawberries—'Seascape' and 'Honeoye'—and a variety of salad greens and herbs in these PVC tubes with very good results.

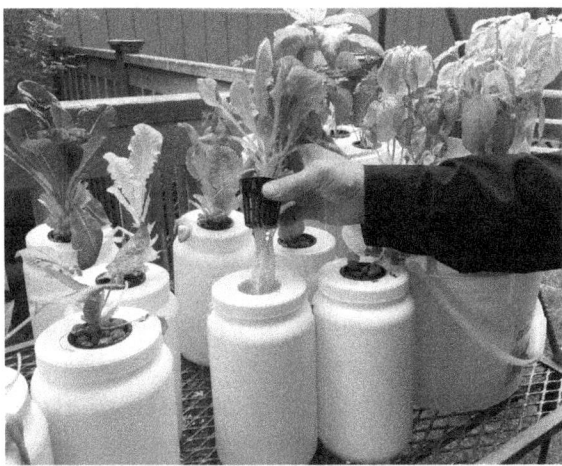

Buckets work well and so do smaller containers. Here you see sixty-four-ounce containers with salad greens and basil. Note the root structure on the lettuce plant. Use your drill and two-inch hole saw to make the holes in each cover.

have (or should have) this type of PVC for cold water outlets. Copper is expensive. PVC pipes are cheap and these are food-safe. Builders are using PVC.

Rebar and PVC tubes. Can you weld? Do you want to weld? Do you live near a vocational school? Is there a welding company near you? If you are a bit handy or know someone who is handy working with rebar and a welding-torch, consider creating a vertical frame from half-inch rebar. Rebar is often sold in twenty-foot lengths and like PVC pipe and tubes is inexpensive. Either material should last you close to forever.

Smaller containers and buckets. If space is an issue for you, consider containers as small as thirty-two or 128- ounces. You can grow salad greens and herbs in these containers. Larger plants, such as peppers, maybe not so much. Regardless, these containers can easily fit on a kitchen counter, table or bench. They are great for the kiddies (K-6) and seniors and folks who live in apartments or condos or assisted living facilities.

The two-gallon bucket and thirty-two-ounce container size is great for kiddies who may want to help you during your rehab process. If you are a bit older than a kiddie, keep in mind that water weighs eight pounds per gallon. The smaller buckets are easier to move and haul around than the larger buckets and will go easier on your joints, such as knees and hips. They can be convenient with almost no maintenance and provide salad greens to seniors and other folks who just need a small quantity of fresh greens each week.

> *I have had success growing heirloom tomatoes in five-gallon buckets and ten-gallon totes. Cherry and patio-type varieties seem to be easier to grow and bear fruit quicker. The space allows the plant to develop an extensive root system. Tomatoes take up a lot of nutrient solution. Best to check the water level on a weekly basis, especially during hot, dry days and when the ambient temperature remains above 85-degrees for several days (and the nights remain above 70-degrees during that period).*

Indoor Lighting. The passive DWC system does not use electricity when you grow your plants outside. The sun provides the energy source. You will need to provide a light-source if you plan to grow veggies and herbs indoors. Buy a four-foot LED lighting unit, with bulbs, which will allow you to place two 10-gallon totes with up to twenty-four plants or three buckets with larger plants under that unit.

Gardening indoors is an absolute treat. Enjoy fresh veggies and herbs during the winter, while everyone else is buying their greens grown from who-knows-where and sprayed with who-knows-what. It is not necessary to buy *grow lights* or units marked specifically for hydroponics, unless you want to spend more money than you need to. Many lights listed on the Internet are for commercial operations. Some give off high levels of heat which can burn plants if the lighting unit is too close to the plants. The ceilings in commercial operations are normally higher than twelve-feet. In addition, some communities may have a restriction on high-energy, high-heat units because they could be a fire hazard if there is not adequate ventilation. Shop smart. Save your money. Check out those lights at COSTCO, Home Depot, Menards, Lowes, ACE Hardware and other outlets that are in your area.

> *TIP:* You can purchase an LED lighting unit, aka a *shop light*, from the electrical department in your favorite big-box or hardware store. Some units include non-removable bulbs that are rated at 50,000 hours (COSTCO). That converts to about ten- or fifteen-years of use, all for about thirty dollars for the unit, with bulbs. No need to change bulbs. Cost effective.

The LED or fluorescent bulbs should have a Kelvin rating (K) of at least 4000K. Bulbs that emit a white or bluish light (5100 to 6500K) are best for vegetative growth (when you want to eat the leaves) while those emitting a yellowish light (3000 to 4100K) are better for flower and fruit production, such as tomatoes, peppers, cucumbers, eggplants and so on.

You can still find the old-fashion fluorescent T12 bulbs that are now quasi-LED-types and they work just fine with older lighting units. Check the packaging. Not all LED bulbs will work with those older units unless they specifically indicate that they do. These newer T12 fluorescent bulbs are not as energy efficient as the newer LED units, especially when compared to the T5 or T8 LED bulbs, but your plants will do well under them.

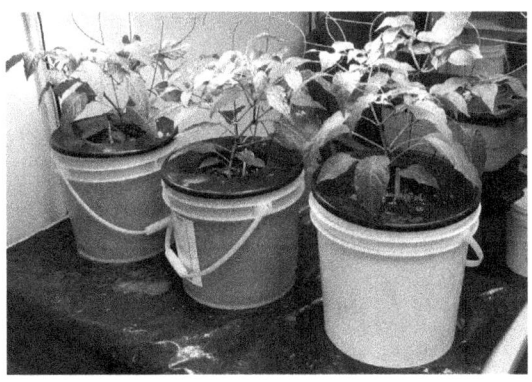

Six-inch (ID) WLBs support these hot pepper plants. A shelving unit made from metal or resin is an efficient way to grow a wide range of veggies and herbs indoors. Some units have adjustable shelves allowing you to grow taller plants, such as peppers and patio-type tomatoes, as well as shorter plants, such as lettuces and Asian greens. Most of the newer metal and resin shelving units are easy to assemble and do not require the use of any tools. The buckets are freebies from a local bakery.

Substrates. Think of substrates as a soil substitute. Your soil contains some elements and minerals and supports the plant and root structure. The hydroponic substrate supports the plant but does not contain elements or minerals. That is the job of the hydroponic fertilizer. You can use a variety of substrates to start your plants from seeds. Now that you have an idea about the types of containers you can use, you can easily start your seeds with different types of substrates. If you are comfy starting plants from seeds, go for it. If not, there are plenty of garden centers and plant sales to consider as I mentioned earlier.

Perlite and Peat and Coir. You read about using net pots. Now let's focus more on what you fill the net pot with. You may recall that you can start by creating a substrate mix that includes perlite, peat and/or coconut coir. Mix and fill each net pot with perlite (80%) and peat or coconut coir (20%) or in perlite only (100%). Dampen the mix before you place it in your net pots or WLBs to avoid having it fall through the slots. All these materials are natural.

Perlite. This is a form of *volcanic glass* and is typically formed from the hydration of obsidian, a volcanic rock that is usually black. In its natural state it is like *rock glass* and if chipped in a certain way was used as a knife or cutting tool by our ancestors and maybe even some modern folks as well. Perlite for hydroponic gardening is not sharp, but white and light. You will see it included in many potting soils. They are those little white things. They are not Styrofoam. You can reuse 100% perlite with a 1:10 ratio of bleach to water. Very sustainable and reusable.

Some perlite creates a dust when you open the bag and work with it. You may be allergic to the dust. Wear a mask and moisten the perlite before you mix it with peat or coir. Wetting the perlite will prevent dust.

Peat. This is another natural material usually found in bogs and fens. Scotland comes to mind. It comes from vegetative matter and over time decomposes. The peat acts as a wick, bringing the nutrient solution up into the root system. Perhaps its most famous use is in the making and mellowing of Scotch whiskey, just in case you wanted to know.

Coconut Coir. It is a newer product from a gardening point of view. It is made from recycled coconut husks which are shredded and sold as *coconut coir*. Coir is sold as solid bricks and needs to be soaked in water before you can use it. Like peat, it wicks the solution into the root system. It is also sold loose in bags that you can use immediately. No soaking required.

> *I first learned about gardening from my father when I was about seven or eight years old. He started many plants from seed and though he always started too many, he did not like to toss any of them. He always found a space for his extra tomato and pepper plants, "just to see what would happen." His garden was crowded but produced a whole lot of food for our family.*

Starting Seeds. You can start your seeds directly in your substrate mix and germinate them in your net pots. Remember to moisten the substrate mix with water to prevent it from falling through the slots of the net pots. Fill the net pots with the mix and add two or three seeds in each net pot. Top water and when the seeds germinate and have their second set of leaves, keep the best seedling, one per net pot, and discard the rest. Cut, do not pull, the seedlings you want to cull. If you pull them out of the net pot, you will damage the roots of the plant you want to keep.

You can place thirty-six net pots in a solid 1020 tray (11"x21"). Top or bottom water the seedlings and when the root system has grown through the slots of the net pot you can transfer the entire unit—seedling and net pot—to a container of your choice. You can also start your seeds in potting soil (maybe you already do that) and when the seedlings develop a reasonable set of roots, remove some of the soil and transfer them to your net pots, add your substrate mix (or just perlite) and set them into your container—totes, buckets or PVC tubes.

TIP: If you have a problem *killing-culling* a seedling, gently tap out all the seedlings from the net pot, carefully separate them and replant them in separate net pots—one plant per net pot. You can do this after the plant has its second set of leaves and before the root system extends too far out from the net pots.

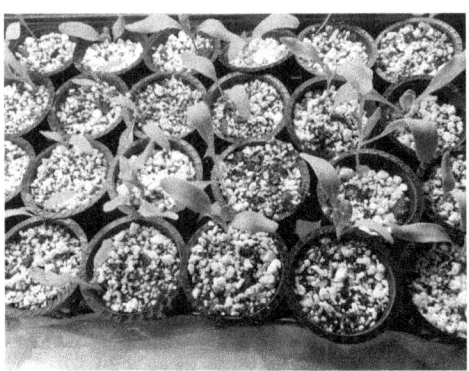

You can add your seeds directly into each two-inch net pot, using a mix of perlite and peat, perlite and coir or use only perlite. Place your net pots in Standard (1020) trays. Only keep one seedling per net pot and cull or transplant the rest in their own net pot. These are chard seedlings-red, orange, yellow and green.

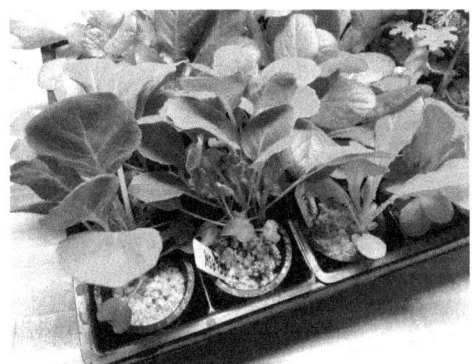

You can keep your seedlings in the 1020 tray to allow the plant and root system to develop before you transfer them to your containers—buckets, totes, tubes. Do not remove the seedling from the net pot. These plants are about six weeks old and are ready for transplanting. Note the size of the plants. You could start harvesting the larger outer leaves of these plants as micro-greens at this point in their development. Harvesting some of the leaves at this size, then allowing the plant to grow to maturity or to the size you want, allows you to realize multiple harvests from the same plant.

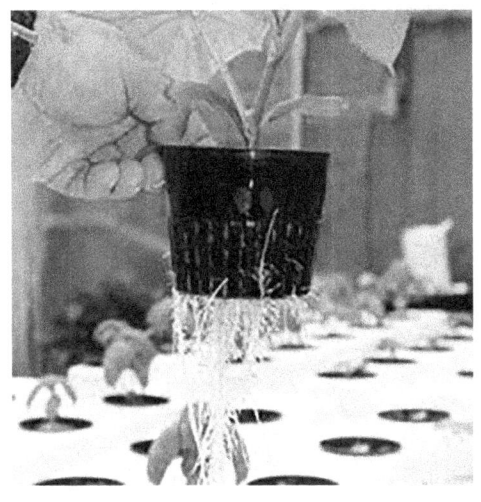

Note the root system growing through the slots in the net pot. The plants can now be transferred to your container of choice. Do not remove the seedling from the net pot, otherwise you will rip some of the roots and shock the plant. Your seedlings should thrive so long as a third to one-half of the roots are in contact with the nutrient solution. Do not fill your container with nutrient solution all the way to the top of the container. Always keep an air space. As the plant develops the water level drops and the air space increases.

> **TIP:** After top watering to help the seeds germinate, add about a quarter- to a half-inch of water to the bottom of your 1020 solid tray. The peat/coir will wick-up the water to the root system. You do not need any fertilizer at this point. Why? *Cotyledons* are the first leaves produced by plants. Cotyledons are not considered true leaves and are sometimes referred to as *seed leaves,* because they are part of the seed or embryo of the plant. The seed leaves serve to access the stored nutrients in the seed, feeding it until the true leaves develop and begin photosynthesizing.

Rockwool Cubes. This is another substrate option to consider. You can direct seed into rockwool cubes. Rock wool is often associated with insulation. The rock wool used for hydroponic gardening is not the same product, nor does it include asbestos or other nasties. Rock wool is made from spinning *molten basaltic (volcanic) rock* into fine fibers which are then formed into cubes and blocks.

Rockwool is a brand name. The generic term is rock wool. The more commonly available hydroponic rock wool cubes are between one- and two-inches wide and one and one-half-inches deep and are used for germinating seeds that are then transplanted directly into soil (yes, soil) or your hydroponic container once the root system emerges from the cube. When you use these cubes, you avoid having to create a substrate mix of perlite and peat/coir. Some folks find the cubes to be more convenient with less work. The results should be comparable to a substrate mix of perlite and peat or coir. You can only use the cubes once. Toss them into your compost bin.

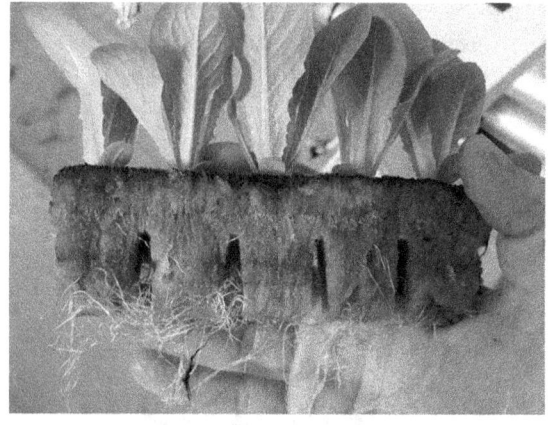

Once the root system has grown through the rock wool cubes, you can transfer your seedlings to the container of your choice. Note the roots extending through the substrate (rock wool cubes). You can use this substrate with net pots and buckets with WLBs. Do not remove the seedling from the rock wool cube. Doing so will rip out the roots and shock (or kill) the plant. Plant the entire cube in the WLB or net pot. Plant the entire cube in your soil-based containers.

The cubes are usually sold in sheets of ninety-six, depending on the size you order and the vendor's packaging. There is an indentation in each cube. Place a sheet in a standard seed starting tray; soak the cubes, following the directions of course, then add one or two seeds per cube in the indentation. If both seeds germinate, cull the weakest one.

> **TIP:** Only use hydroponic rock wool. Buy it online or from your local hydroponic store. Do not buy rock wool if you see it stacked in the building products department along with insulation products. That version of rock wool is for insulation, not for growing food.

Once the root system has penetrated the cube you can transfer the entire cube—seedling and all—into a net pot or a WLB. The cubes fit into a two-inch net pot. When you use the cubes (or net pots) with a WLB, add a mix of perlite and peat to the bottom of the WLB, say about one-inch deep. Place and space multiple rockwool cubes in the WLB depending what you are growing, then fill in the remaining spaces with perlite or **LECA** (clay pellets). The root system has already developed and should not have a problem passing through the slots in the WLB and into the nutrient solution.

> **NOTE:** You can transfer hydroponically grown plants, along with their net pot or rock wool cube, directly into your soil-based garden and containers. The reverse is not always successful. That is, transferring a mature or semi-mature plant from soil to a hydroponic system may fail because you will probably rip out too many roots in the process. This can shock the plant and either kill it or inhibit its growth.

LECA. This is a natural aggregate that you can use to support your net pots and rock wool cubes in WLBs. This is an expanded clay aggregate pebble that is made from *100% natural clay.* It works better in WLBs and with transplanted seedlings. It is pH neutral, clean and can be re-used multiple times by soaking it in a bleach solution (10%) for a few hours, rinsed, dried and ready to act again as a support for your plants. Sustainable. Reusable. Cost effective.

The name LECA means *lightweight expanded clay aggregate.* Use it straight out of the bag. Rinse it to remove any dust. Typically used in hydroponic systems you can also add it to your soil-based garden, especially if your soil is a bit heavy (clay). LECA can prevent compaction and enhance aeration by creating more air-spaces in your soil. Just remove it from your WLBs when you want and spread it on your soil-based garden.

Household bleach is a strong and effective disinfectant. You can buy it almost anywhere. The active ingredient, *sodium hypochlorite*, effectively kills bacteria, fungi and viruses (including flu and COVID-19 viruses). Use it to clean and disinfect your net pots, WLBs, PVC tubes and other materials when you are done harvesting and before you start a new batch of plants. You may not have any bad stuff growing-living in or on your materials but disinfect them anyway. First, dump your nutrient solution; rinse out your containers; create the bleach and water solution (one teaspoon to one gallon) and soak the materials for about ten to sixty-minutes. Rinse until the bleach odor is gone.

> *Confession: I soak my materials overnight. I do not measure the amount of bleach. I just pour. I know what the ratio is and how long to soak the things that I want to disinfect. I want to make sure I have killed what needs to be killed, dead. Perhaps a tad over the top and overkill, but that is what I do. You may want to read the directions.*

You know that plants do not grow in soil. They grow in air. Most of these substrates, except LECA, can also be used to start your seeds. LECA is the only substrate that is not suitable for starting seeds because the seeds will fall through the spaces between the round clay balls and, therefore, may not germinate.

How to Use Different Substrates

Substrate	Net Pots	WLBs	Container Type	Comments
Perlite alone	Yes	Yes	Totes, Buckets, PVC Tubes	Use to start seeds in net pots
Peat-Coir and Perlite Mix	Yes	Yes	Totes, Buckets, PVC Tubes	Ratio: 80% Perlite, 20% Peat or Coconut Coir Use to start seeds in net pots Use at bottom of WLBs
Rock wool Cubes	Yes	Yes	Totes, Buckets, PVC Tubes	Insert the cubes in two-inch net pots to start seeds
Clay Pellets	No	Yes	Buckets Larger net pots: 3, 4, 5 and 6-inch sizes	Use to support your plants growing in net pots or rock wool cubes

Fertilizers. What fertilizer do you use and how much should you use? Use hydroponic fertilizer only. It is more complete and almost every brand includes the thirteen or so essential minerals and elements for plant growth and viability. The fertilizer will be labelled as hydroponic or aqua. It is more concentrated than almost all the soil-based fertilizers you may be familiar with. Read the directions please. In most cases you will be using only a *teaspoon* per gallon versus a tablespoon per gallon for traditional soil-based fertilizers, such as Miracle-Gro and Fertilome and other brands. A ten-gallon tote requires two-to three-tablespoons, compared to ten-tablespoons for soil-based fertilizers. Using only hydroponic fertilizer is easy. You can purchase powder or granular and ready-to-use liquid types. Mix with water. **Done.**

When your goal is to eat the leaves of a variety, select a fertilizer when the first number is high or higher than the others. That first number on a fertilizer bag, box or container is the level of nitrogen (**N**) in that bag, box or container. If your goal is to produce bigger or more flowers or fruit, the second number, or phosphorous (**P**), should be higher than the nitrogen number. The third number is potassium (**K**), which is a beneficial element for plants.

These numbers represent the percentage or total weight ratio within that bag, box or container. For example, a fertilizer labelled as 16-4-17 means the fertilizer has 16 pounds of nitrogen per 100 pounds of total mass or is 16 percent of the contents. The number 4 indicates there is 4-percent or 4-pounds of phosphorous and 17 percent or 17 pounds of potassium. All bags of fertilizer list these three primary or macro elements in this order. All these elements are natural. They are found in the ground, the air or once living animals. Phosphorous is a rock and bone meal comes from animal bones. Nitrogen is a gas and extracted from the air. Your lawn looks a lot greener after a thunder-storm. Why? Free Nitrogen. No need to add additional fertilizer to your lawn after a thunder-boomer storm.

There is at least one added benefit with hydroponic fertilizer. You can use it with your soil-based plants as well. You should not, however, use soil-based fertilizers with a hydroponic system. They are not as complete with respect to providing the plant with the macro and micro elements they need to develop fully. If you do, you will need to add supplemental fertilizers to compensate for what nutrients are missing. As a result, you can get double usage from hydroponic fertilizers. If you grow flowers or veggies that produce a fruit, such as tomatoes, peppers, cucumbers, use a hydroponic fertilizer labelled as *bloom or flora*. Those types of products will (should) enable your plants to produce more and larger flowers or fruit.

Scientists can create fertilizers comprised of N-P-K and any of the other macro and micro elements. There is consistency with the product. If you are an organic gardener of the purist variety, these *lab-produced fertilizers* are on your naughty list. If you are not an organic gardener purist, then these fertilizers will work just fine. Plants do not know, nor care, whether their N-P-K and other elements come from a test tube or the back end of a moo-cow or seaweed scooped up from the ocean. Only people care, but they are not plants. You could also combine different fertilizer products from different companies. Read the directions. Do not over-fertilize.

> *I have used both liquid and granular fertilizers. I also have combined dry with wet, granular with liquid. For example, I have combined Jack's 16-4-17 with General Hydroponics Flora Micro 5-0-1. The results were the same-very good with respect to growth rates and yields. You may choose to experiment (that is okay and legal) in order to find what works best for you, based on what you are planning to grow. Start with Jack's granular 16-4-17 and add Flora Micro liquid at the prescribed dosage, about 2.5 to 3-tablespoons per ten gallons as a starting point. You could increase the dosage as the plants mature. Follow the directions. And, if you are growing tomatoes or peppers or flowers, you could experiment and add a third product called Hula Bloom. This granular baby is a 0-50-30 mix. You ONLY use one teaspoon for five-gallons. Follow the directions. Apply this tri-product mix on one plant. How is it doing? How did it do? Let that be your guide as to whether you want to experiment with multiple products or just keep to one—simple and done.*

Water Options. The beauty of a passive DWC system is that you do not need to change the water as often as you do with an active hydroponic system. Nor, do you need to water as frequently as you do with a soil-based garden. The water reservoir in your bucket or tote should suffice for at least three weeks. Less maintenance. Less work. Less expense. You can use two watering methods, which I mentioned earlier: top and bottom watering.

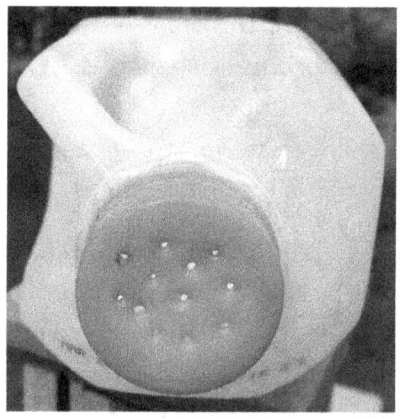

You can create your own fancy-fine watering can from a half- or full-gallon milk carton. Use an awl or heavy-duty needle to punch some fine holes in the cover. Test out the flow. Is the flow fine enough? If so, you are done. If the spray is too wimpy, make each hole a little bit bigger and test again. You can always make the holes bigger, but you cannot return them to the smaller size.

Top Watering. Initially, you will need to top water your seeds and very young seedlings, just as you would when you start seeds in potting soil. Use a fine spray, otherwise the flow of water will bury your seeds and could disrupt or inhibit germination. You can make your own fancy fine-watering cans by using empty half-gallon milk containers. Drink or dump the contents. Punch several small holes in the cap with an awl or a heavy-duty needle to create the holes for the fine spray. Make the holes small at first, then test what you did. If the spray is what you want, you are done. If not, make the holes slightly larger. Test it. You can always make a small hole larger, but you cannot make that larger hole smaller.

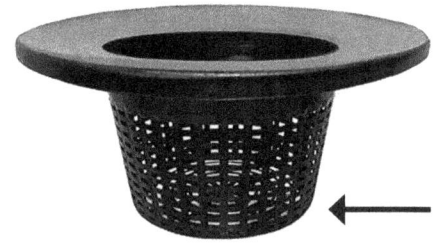

After you fill your net pot or WLB with a mix of perlite and peat and have added your seed, fill your container with the nutrient solution and set the initial water level so that it just touches the bottom of your net pot or WLB. You need to maintain an air space with a passive deep-water culture system. You do not need a pump or bubbler. As the plant matures, make certain that at least a third of the root system maintains contact with the solution.

Bottom Watering. One option after top-watering is to add about one-half inch of water to your seed starting tray. Adding water to the bottom of the tray allows the peat to wick-up the nutrient solution into the developing root system. Add your fertilizer after the secondary leaves appear. Start with a weaker solution first, then use the dosage recommended on the fertilizer package. Keep that air space! Once the seeds germinate, you can stop watering from the top. Maintain bottom watering until you are ready to transfer the net pots to your container.

> *TIP:* Always use cold water, which has a higher oxygen level than warmer water. When growing leafy greens indoors in totes you may not have to add any additional water or fertilizer for about one month (or more). Depending on the temperature outdoors, you should not have to add any additional water for at least three weeks (or more), though you can certainly check the level each week if you want. Go away on vacation. Your plants will be fine.

Water changes. You may have read or been told to change out your water-nutrient solution on a weekly or bi-weekly basis. That recommendation applies to active systems, such as NFT, Wick, Flow and Drain, etc. Active systems have tubes and filters and bubblers that can clog, especially if you are using a granular fertilizer. Generally, that frequency is not applicable to a passive deep-water culture system.

It is not necessary to add additional fertilizer every time you add water to your system. I often change out my nutrient solution about once a month, then add the appropriate amount of fertilizer for the gallons of water added. It is not necessary to fill your container up to the bottom of your WLBs or net pots when you change out the water after that first month or so. How extensive is the root system? As a rule of thumb, so long as at least half or a third of the roots are in the nutrient solution you should be fine. The remaining space will provide the necessary air space for you passive DWC system.

> How often do I check the level of my nutrient solution? That depends on the type of container I use and whether I am growing indoors during the winter or outdoors in summer. Indoors (from September-October to April), I check my totes and buckets about every two weeks and usually do not have to add additional cold water for at least a month and sometimes not until the sixth week. Tomatoes will take up more nutrient solution during that period than salad greens and herbs, such as basil. Outdoors (from May to September-October), I need to check plants growing in totes or buckets every week and, depending on the heat, may need to add additional water by the second week. Totes seem to hold the water level better, but PVC tubes need checking every week and I usually have to add water, and sometimes fertilizer, within a two week period, again all of this depends on the ambient temperature, especially if days stay in the upper 80s to mid- 90s for an extended period of time. A two-foot long PVC tube holds about two-gallons of solution and a five-foot tube holds about five-gallons.

Floating Gardens. Here is fun idea to consider. It is almost free. Do you live by a lake or pond? Buy a piece of two-inch thick Styrofoam. Set your net pots and plants in the Styrofoam sheet, keep it moored to your dock or the bank. Next, pull up a comfy chair and relax while you wait for the plants to mature. The pond or lake provides the water; the fish provide the fertilizer.

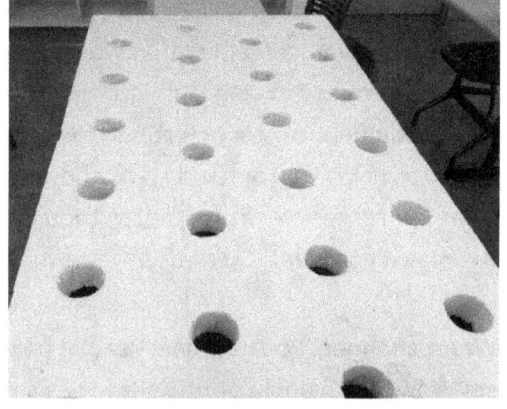

Drill holes in a section of one or two-inch thick Styrofoam for your net pots. The overall size will depend upon your pond or water feature. For a passive DWC system, use a smaller hole-saw size, one and five-eighths. Set the net pot so just the bottom touches the nutrient solution and the bottom of the Styrofoam board. The rest of the net pot is above the surface of the Styrofoam and provides the necessary air for the plants.

Don't live by a water pond or lake? Buy a kiddie pool or a stock tank. Cut the Styrofoam board so there is space on all four sides so it can move around freely and allow the fishies to check out the sunlight. If you include fish, such as goldfish, in the kiddie-pool, you do not need to add fertilizer. The fish will provide the manure, aka fertilizer. **Done**. Sports-folks will have envy.

Use a one and five-eighths-inch hole saw (not the two-inch size) to cut out as many holes as you want for the piece of Styrofoam. Though the size of your hole is smaller, you can still use the two-inch net pots. Your two-inch net pots should fit in these holes so just the very bottom of the net pot touches the water. *The air space is basically above and on top of the Styrofoam.* Do not push your net pot all the way into the hole. Cut holes about four-inches apart, add your plants and perlite/peat mix and set the Styrofoam in your water feature, pre-formed unit or stock tank. **Done**.

Aquaponics. Aquaponics is a variation of hydroponics. When you add fish to a water container you have aquaponics. Aquaponics is more complicated to set up and maintain, but you could do this. You do not need any hydroponic fertilizer. The fish provide the poop, the fertilizer.

There is at least one drawback with aquaponics if you include the fish and the plants in the same tank-container. Fish, especially Koi and Tilapia, will chomp on the root system. Eating the roots will impede the growth of the plant. You can avoid this problem when you use two tanks: one for the fish and a separate tank for the plants.

Some folks advocate including a filter unit to the fish tank. The filter will remove all or most of any solid waste matter from the fish before it reaches the plants. Some folks may get a tad squeamish thinking about the fish-manure-plant cycle. Some folks raise certain species of fish (Tilapia) for food consumption.

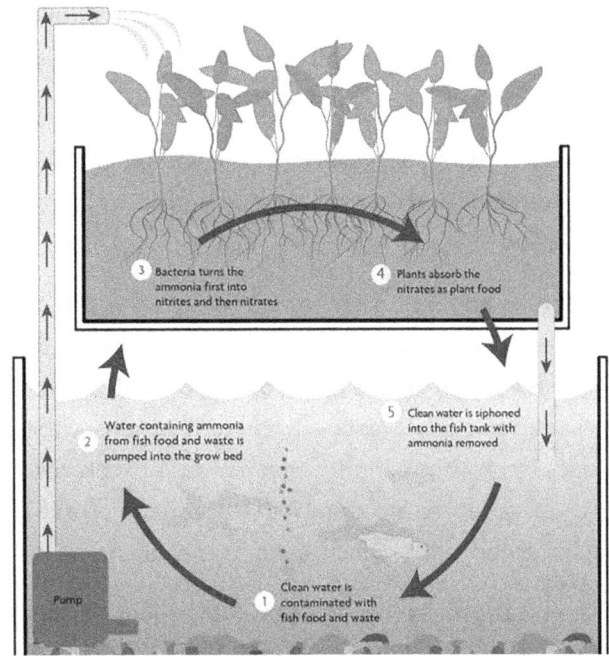

This two-tank illustration includes a pump and a filter system, both requiring electricity. You add fish food to the fish tank. The fish take in the food at one end and push out the waste at the other end, which is carried by the pump to the hydroponic tank or tube system. The plants extract the fish waste (fertilizer-poop) and in the process clean the water which then returns to the fish tank. The cycle will take a few months to set up properly, but once established the fish and plants should be happy (University of Michigan, aquaponics).

You could set up a seasonal aquaponic system on your deck or patio by adding a few fish to your kiddie-pool or stock tank. Aquaponics on the cheap. When you add fish, elevate your water feature to keep the racoons, cats, dogs and other fish-loving or water-loving critters away or use fencing if that is easier. Use a pair of inexpensive resin sawhorses to elevate your system. You will need to use electricity to run a small bubbler to provide extra oxygen to the fish.

Plant Options

You can grow anything (almost) hydroponically. In **Module Three**, you read about a few cool-weather plants that you could grow in your soil-based garden. You can grow those same varieties hydroponically. Whether you want to garden in soil or water or a combination of both is up to you. You may not be able to grow everything you would like to grow during those first months (or the first year) after surgery. You need to focus on your rehab protocol. With hydroponic gardening you will be able to return to gardening quicker and grow what you want with less effort and less maintenance.

Start easy with salad greens and Asian greens and other varieties that require less maintenance and that will provide you with a continuous harvest. Here are a few to consider.

Lettuces and Asian greens. There are a wide range of varieties and colors, from shades of green to shades of reds and varieties that include both reds and greens. Likewise, Asian greens can provide you with a choice of shapes, colors, textures and flavors. You can harvest both as micro-greens within four to six weeks. Maximize your space by growing varieties that have a vertical growing-habit. Romaine lettuce is one lettuce variety as are many Asian greens, such as bok choi, bo pak, mustards such as 'spicy green', and spinach, such as the Japanese variety, 'komatsuna'.

Harvest these leafy veggies by cutting just the outer leaves. Do not cut the central stem or the whole plant. Harvesting this way allows you to extend your harvest period. You could expect to harvest a single plant over a two- to three-month period. You can eat young micro-greens raw or sauté them, then let the plant mature. You can also cook-sauté mature lettuce leaves and eat them as you would spinach or combine them with a pasta dish.

Kales and Broccoli Raab. You can eat almost any veggie leaf raw when the leaves are young and tender and that includes the leaves of beets, collards, mustards, kohlrabi, broccoli, broccoli raab and cabbage leaves. You are getting dual usage and enjoyment—eating the young leaves, then the mature veggie. Consider the smaller varieties of kale, such as 'Prism' and collards, such as 'Flash'. Grow the beet, 'Bull's Blood', for its colorful, deep red-maroon leaves. Does anyone eat turnips anymore? Try the Japanese variety, 'Hakurei'. They are white and very tender when you harvest it about the size of a large golf-ball.

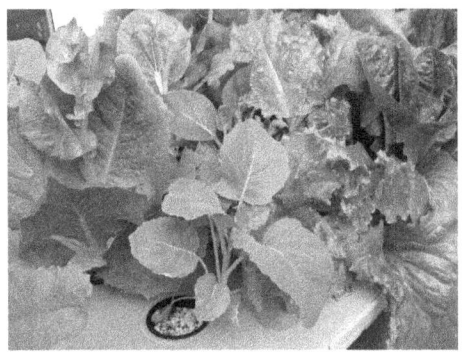

Grow varieties of broccoli raab, mustards, collards and cucumbers and more in ten-gallon totes.

TIP: Do you raise rabbits or gerbils or Guinea Pigs? Grow some veggies for the critters. Rabbits will eat basil, carrot tops, cilantro, dill, parsley and lettuces, such as the Romaine varieties.

Cucumbers and Squash

Lots of folks want to grow tomatoes and rightly so. Fresh tomatoes from your system should taste a whole-lot better than the cardboard varieties often found in grocery stores during the winter months. Tomatoes, peppers, eggplants, bush cucumbers and bush summer squash require a bit more maintenance as they mature. If you grow tomatoes, grow the patio varieties that mature quickly and can easily be grown in a container. Gain confidence with these smaller varieties, then move on to the larger determinant and indeterminant varieties. Determinant varieties produce their fruit over a short period of time. Indeterminant varieties will produce over a longer period of time and, often, up until the first frost.

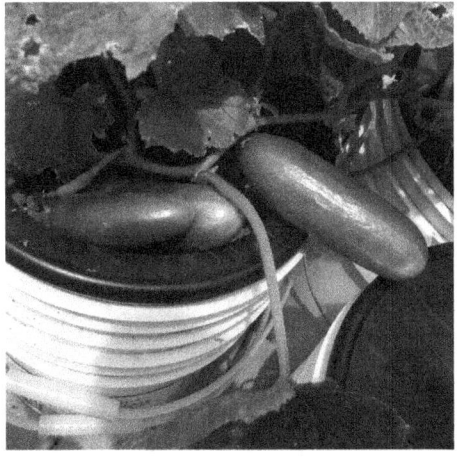

*Grow cucumbers and bush-varieties of squash in buckets and totes. Use a trellis to support the cucumber vines, though they may be listed as a **bush** variety. I use two white buckets, one inside the other, to help keep the water a bit cooler during the hottest days of summer. The variety shown here is 'Diva'. A patio variety of summer squash can grow in a bucket or a tote.*

TIP: As a rule of thumb plant one plant per one gallon of water. You can squeeze in an extra plant or two if you intend to harvest the leaves as *micro-greens*. Start with salad greens and build your confidence and prove that the process works for you. Then, move on and include those crops that take a longer time to mature, such as tomatoes, peppers, cucumbers, and eggplants.

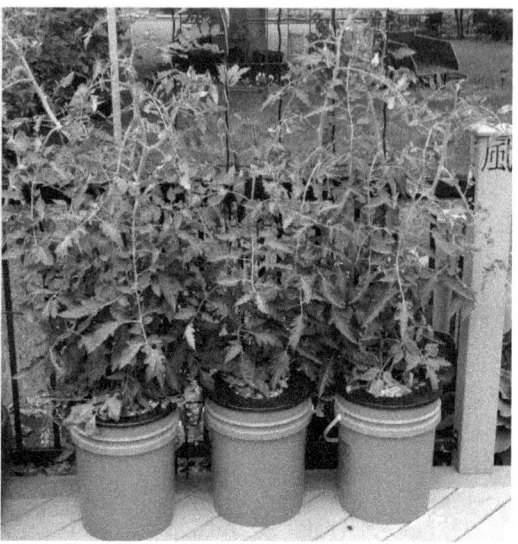

Eat the Rainbow. What you eat and how much you eat can affect how quickly you recover from surgery. There are other varieties to include on those shown on the next page. Select those that are relatively easy to grow, or are readily available where you shop, while you are in your rehabilitation period. Build your confidence level. Eat the rainbow. Grow it. Buy it. Get well.

Want minimal maintenance? Got a bucket? You can grow tomatoes hydroponically in standard five-gallon buckets that take up residence in your yard and garden or on a deck or patio. Make better use of your railing by using it to support your tomatoes as they grow. Here I am growing 'Cipolla's Pride' set in eight- and ten-inch WLBs. These are indeterminant heirlooms and produce fruit over an extended period of time. Darker bucket colors will tend to warm the water, so you may need to check the volume and temperature if you are experiencing hot weather over an several days (or weeks).

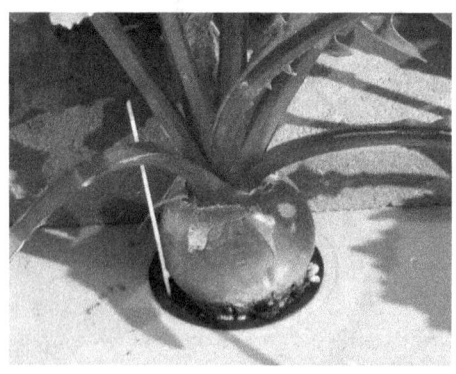

Japanese Red Turnip. Harvest some of the young, tender leaves, then harvest the entire bulb. Grow kohlrabi and beets in two-inch net pots. The product grows above the surface, on the cover.

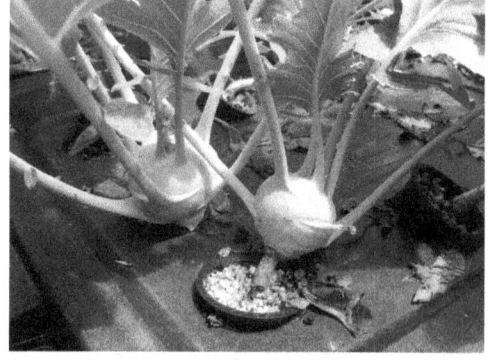

Kohlrabi grown in 10-gallon totes are ready to harvest. You can eat the leaves of different Cole-family varieties, such as kohlrabi, cabbage, broccoli, when they are small and tender. Note how the entire bulb is exposed.

This Color	And these Foods	Will provide you with these Benefits
RED	Strawberries, raspberries, tomatoes, tomato juice, red peppers, watermelon, cherries, guava, pomegranate	Lycopene: antioxidants, heart health, memory
ORANGE	Carrots, pumpkins, orange peppers, sweet potatoes, apricots, squash, cantaloupe (muskmelons)	Beta-carotene: immune system, healthy eyes
YELLOW-GREEN	Oranges, lemons, papayas, peaches, bananas, yellow peppers, pineapple, corn, yellow apples, yellow pears	Vitamin C: detoxify harmful substances in your body
GREEN	Spinach, kale, collards, lettuces, green apples, kiwi, pears, celery, cucumbers, peas, zucchini, green peppers, honeydew, green beans, limes	Folates: builds healthy cells, bones, teeth, eyes
GREEN-WHITE	Broccoli, Brussels sprouts, cabbage, jicama, mushrooms	Indoles, Lutein: helps to eliminate carcinogens
WHITE-GREEN	Garlic, garlic chives, onions, chives, asparagus, ginger	Allyl methyl sulfides: anti-oxidants help to destroy cancer cells
BLUE	Blueberries, plums, black currants, black grapes, prunes, blackberries	Anthocyanins: helps to destroy free radicals
RED-PURPLE	Grapes, purple cabbage, raisins, figs, eggplant, purple carrots, purple cauliflower, berries	Resveratrol: decrease estrogen, improve memory, healthy aging
BROWN	Whole grains, legumes	Fiber: carcinogen removal

Red Onions. If you grow onions, the small, red onion varieties have the highest level of anti-oxidants. Use onion sets or plants rather than seeds. Onions are the most popular and most consumed veggie in the world. Red onions are healthier than yellow or white onions. The smaller red onion-sets are healthier than the larger red varieties. The biggest potential health benefit of a red onion comes from its organosulfur compounds — a family of nutrients that are also present in garlic, leeks and other Alliums. *Organosulfur compounds* are powerful antioxidants, which means they help scrub your cells clean of cancer-causing free radicals. While research continues, the Linus Pauling Institute has found that organosulfur compounds might have anti-cancer properties and benefit heart health by helping to control cholesterol levels

And just for all of you folks out there who happen to cook, the *flavonoids* in onions are more concentrated in the outer layers of the flesh. Therefore, peel off as little of the fleshy portion of the onion as possible. If you remove more than the outer-most layers, a red onion could lose up to seventy-five percent of its *anthocyanins* and twenty-percent of its *quercetin*, which is an antioxidant that fights against free radicals, – chemically reactive compounds that damage cell membranes and DNA and also cause cell death. Trim sparingly. Your body may love you for that.

Vernalization. Berries and other fruit varieties, which include blueberries, raspberries, blackberries, and strawberries to name a few, need a dormant or cold period before they can produce flowers and a crop for the next season. The process is called *vernalization*. The plant is exposed to the cold of winter or by artificial means, such as being stored in a refrigerated area for a few months. Once exposed to this cold period, the plant typically will flower, though some varieties may need additional cues before they start to flower. You can grow any of these in the northern climes in your soil-based garden. Treat them as annuals if you want to grow them hydroponically, or trot down to your grocery store and buy them.

> *I am always asked whether folks can grow strawberries hydroponically. The short answer is yes. The longer answer is that many varieties require a cold period-vernalization. You can certainly grow the plants hydroponically during that first year and may get a small harvest, depending on the variety you have selected. However, most varieties produce in their second year, after their cold or dormant period. I have planted 'Seascape' and 'Honeoye' and 'Albion' with good results. I treat them as annuals. And for you folks who live in the colder Zones, you can order your strawberries from Nourse Farms, located in Massachusetts. They ship throughout the winter. Start your plants indoors o/a Labor Day and prepare to harvest before Thanksgiving.*

You can grow strawberries hydroponically, inside or outside. Grow varieties called *everbearing* or *day-neutral*. If you live in the colder Zones and want to grow them indoors, you may need to toss them into your compost bin and do it all over again the following spring because they will not have that period of vernalization. No problem. Treat them as annuals and purchase new plants each year. Eating your own pesticide-free berries during the winter is a fantastic treat. Use this checklist as a starting point:

☐ First, buy bare-root plants. Seeds take about three or so years to do much of anything. An everbearing variety, such as '*Seascape',* (and there are others) is everbearing, producing a crop on or about June (depending on your Zone) and then with lighter yields until frost.

☐ Second, do not use coconut coir or peat moss in your net pots. They will retain too much moisture and could suffocate the root system, which needs air. Perlite is a good substrate to use. You could support the plant and its root system with straight (100%) perlite. Use a courser perlite versus one that looks a bit powdery.

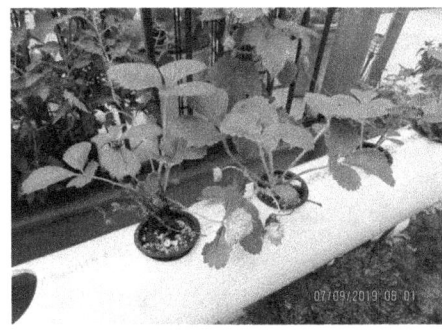

- [ ] Third, set your plant inside the two-inch net pot making sure some of the roots stick out through the slots in the net pot. Remove any dead or dry leaves. You could grow them in PVC tubes, totes or smaller buckets (3.5-gallon size). And like any berry, if you grow them outside critters will eat them before you do, so you may need to elevate them off the ground and/or cover them with netting or a floating row cover just as you would if you were growing them in soil in your garden.

'Seascape' strawberries growing in four-inch food-safe SCH40 PVC tubes. You can get reasonable results in tubes. You may need to check the nutrient level every week and plan on adding water about every two weeks. This two-foot tube holds about 2.5 gallons of water. You will need to check the water level every week, especially during hot summer days.

- [ ] Fourth, fill the remaining space in your net pot with perlite, but do not cover the crown of the plant. They need to be above water, above the perlite, for them to grow and produce fruit. Add your water and fertilizer. Consider two fertilizer products from General Hydroponics: Flora Gro and Flora Micro initially, then add

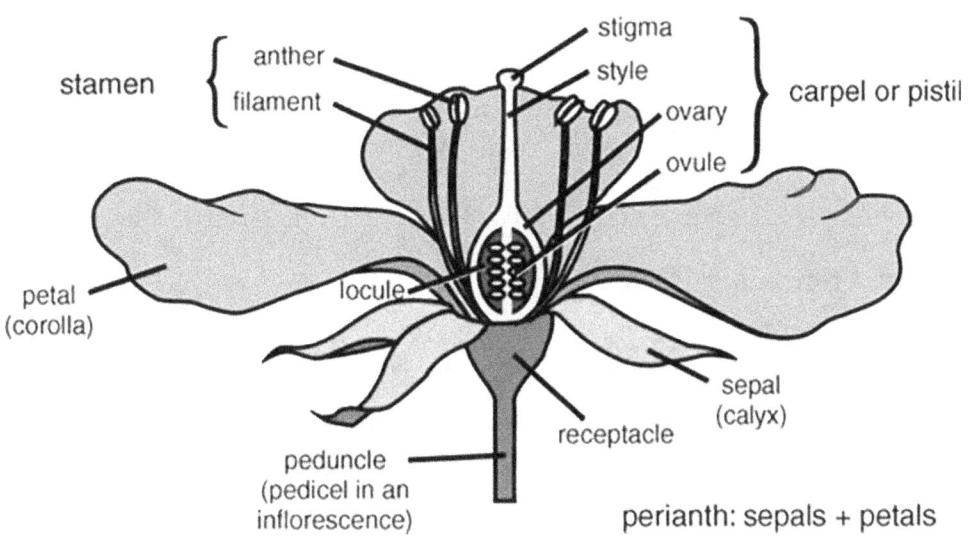

Flora Bloom as the blossoms develop. You could experiment with Bloom and Micro initially, if your store-bought plants have already started to form buds.

☐ Harvest your strawberries full-ripe. Unlike other berries they do not continue to ripen once picked.

Strawberries need pollinators. Bees and birds help when you grow them outside. Inside, you will have to be the bee and hand pollinate them. Use a small, natural-bristle soft brush (or cue-tip) to brush the pollen from the stamen (the boy-part, which can be brownish in color) to the pistil (the girl-part), which is a yellow-greenish color and looks like an un-ripened berry that you eat. Pollinate the entire pistil, otherwise the plant will not produce fruit.

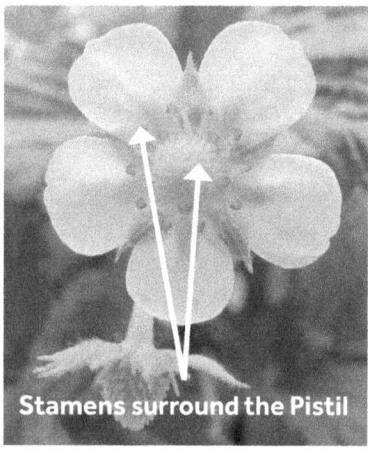

Stamens, the male-part, surrounds the Pistil (top arrow) the female-part (bottom arrow). When you hand pollinate, remove the pollen from the Stamen with a soft brush and apply it to the entire Pistil area (the part that looks like the berry that you will eventually eat).

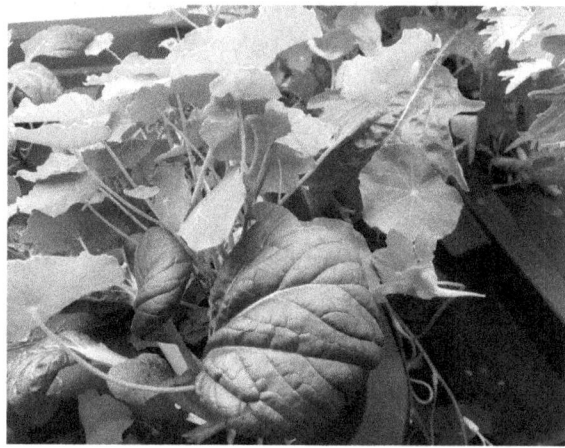

Mix and match. Grow edible flowers (nasturtiums) with vegetables (mustards, chards) and herbs. Plant plants that have about the same growing habit, e.g., vertical growth and mature within the same time frame, e.g., within two weeks. Taller, early maturing varieties could shade and stunt the growth of smaller, late maturing varieties. Nasturtiums are just one variety of edible flowers that does well hydroponically.

Module Summary

You can expect to return to soil-based gardening, depending on what procedure you are having, your physical situation, how much lifting you are allowed to do, the nature or protocol required of your surgical procedure and clearance from your surgeon and/or physician, anywhere from one-to-seven months after discharge. Always check with your medical care-team about what you can and cannot do and when you can do it safely.

Given these same parameters, you can expect to return to hydroponic or soilless-gardening, approximately three days after discharge from the hospital or recovery facility. If you can walk and support your weight reasonably well with a walker, cane, or crutches and have full use of at least one arm, you should be able to garden hydroponically within a week, tops.

Grow almost anything you want in water. No soil is needed. No gardening experience is needed. Set up your system and forget it (almost). The passive deep-water culture system uses no electricity. No pump. No tubing. No bubbler. No weeding.

Hydroponic containers can include food-safe totes, buckets, and PVC tubes. Food-safe containers should include one of these numbers: 1, 2, 4, or 5 on the bottom and PVC tubes should have SCH40 or Schedule 40 stamped on the side.

Substrates are readily available at most garden centers and, of course, hydroponic stores. Use a mix of perlite (80%) with peat or coconut coir (20%) to start your seeds and to support your plant throughout its life in your net pots and wide-lip baskets.

There are a wide range of hydroponic fertilizers to choose from, liquid and granular. Most are complete and include thirteen to sixteen macro- and micro-elements. You can use hydroponic fertilizers on your soil-based plants as well. Hydroponics has its advantages and disadvantages.

Advantages. flexibility and portability; expandable; low cost, low maintenance; garden the year-round and enjoy eating fresh, pesticide-free food. Sustainable. Environmentally safe.

Disadvantages. You will not have to prepare the soil; no digging, raking, chopping, roto-tilling, hauling in compost or fertilizer; no need for shovels or hand-tools or other such implements and be forced to have a garage sale to get rid of all that stuff; you will not have any weeds to pull; no creepy-crawly critters up your pant legs or down your neck; no crawling around on your hands and knees. No worrying about rain making your garden muddy—no soil composition issues.

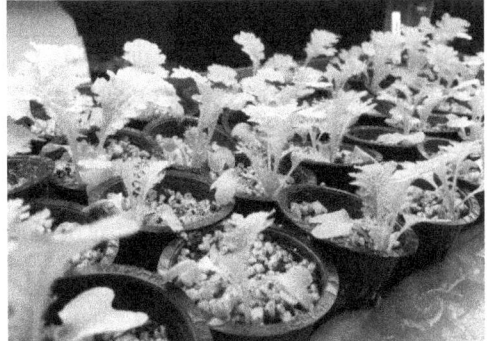

Keep your seedlings in the 1020 tray until they have developed their secondary leaves and the roots have grown through the slots on the net pots. You can then transplant the net pot and its seedling into the container of your choice—totes, tubes, buckets, Styrofoam.

Low-Maintenance Hydroponics

Soil-Based Gardening	Soilless (Hydroponic) Gardening
Winter: Planning what you want to grow and where; start seeds in potting soil and 1020 trays/plastic pots/ Jiffy-7; wait for warm weather and spring; then transfer seedlings to your garden/containers; add fertilizer of your choice as needed; use artificial lighting indoors	Basically, the same, except you can direct seed into a mix of perlite/peat in your net pots; no transfer needed; add hydroponic fertilizer after seeds germinate and form their secondary leaves; garden the year-round, no need to wait for warmer weather; use artificial lighting indoors.
Spring: Prepare your garden for the growing season-dig, rake, rototill; spread fertilizer before planting; mark out rows/square foot grid; plant seedlings in soil or containers.	No soil preparation; no spreading of fertilizer; no marking out of rows or need for square foot grids; transfer seedlings (growing in net pots) to your containers—buckets, totes, PVC tubes, floating garden.
Summer: Weed, water, fertilize, mulch, harvest; scare away the four-legged critters; wash-clean produce before eating; add non-diseased plant material to your compost bins.	No weeding; check water nutrient level weekly; change out water once a month; no supplement fertilizer needed; no mulching needed; no need to wash-clean produce before eating or scare away critters when your containers are elevated above ground; add non-diseased plant material to your compost bins.
Fall: Prepare to winterize your garden-clean up weeds and plant residue, add any remaining non-diseased plant material to your compost bins, dump and turn under any excess fertilizer or soil amendments by hand or with a rototiller; snow-bird to someplace warm and toasty and wait until spring before you can garden again; buy your produce and be careful about E-coli or other nasty diseases.	Harvest last of your produce; clean, drain and move hydroponic containers inside for year-round gardening, grow and harvest regardless of the weather outside; dump plant material in your compost bins; snow-bird to someplace warm while your plants keep growing while you are grabbing some Vitamin D; return and continue harvesting your disease-free veggies and herbs and keep gardening throughout the winter and spring and summer and fall with minimal effort.

You may or may not live in Asia or South-East Asia, nor care to grow Aloe or Potatoes. Regardless, hydroponics is not a fad. There are many residential and commercial applications.

There is no try only do.

—YODA

PREPARING YOUR WATER WORLD

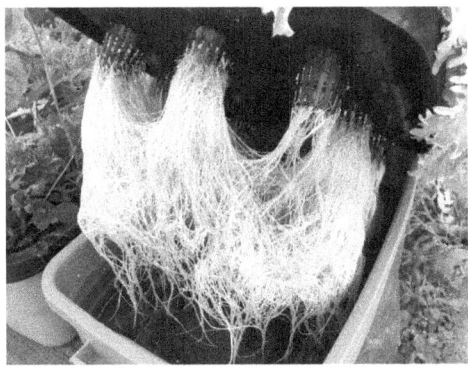

The vibrant root system from lettuce grown in a ten-gallon tote. From an educational perspective, displaying the root structure can be quite astonishing to K-12 students and adults. Very difficult to display the complete root development process with soil-based plants.

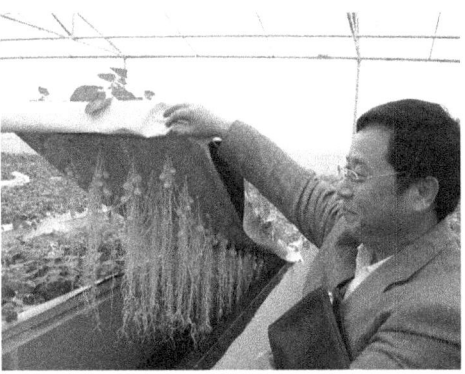

Potatoes growing hydroponically in China. Hydroponics can be used in any country, in any environment, including outer space and (now) in Antarctica.

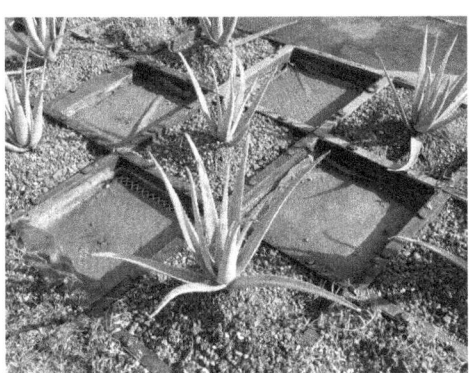

Aloe Vera growing hydroponically on the top floor of a car park (parking ramp), Singapore. Hydroponic systems can exist in or on almost any building, anywhere.

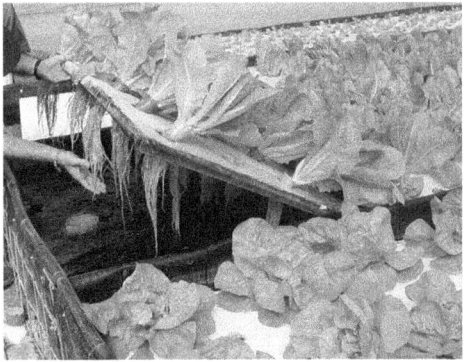

Got room? Want to start a small business and provide fresh produce to your local schools, restaurants or grocery stores? Easy to do. Easy to expand. High sustainable yields, year-round.

Your Notes

MODULE 5

COLLABORATING WITH YOUR MEDICAL CARE-TEAM

The focus and outcomes of this module include ...

- Living your life after surgery
- Trusting your medical-care team
- Asking better questions to get better answers
- Self-directed action plans

Overview

Let's assume that you have completed your pre-surgery physical. And hopefully your hospital had a mandatory educational session that included an illustrated guide of exercises and information about what you can expect during and after your procedure. That session and guide established some organization and protocol for your recovery period. Your primary physician made some suggestions about what to expect and what your responsibilities will be both before and after surgery. You may have already met with others on your medical care-team—physician's assistant,

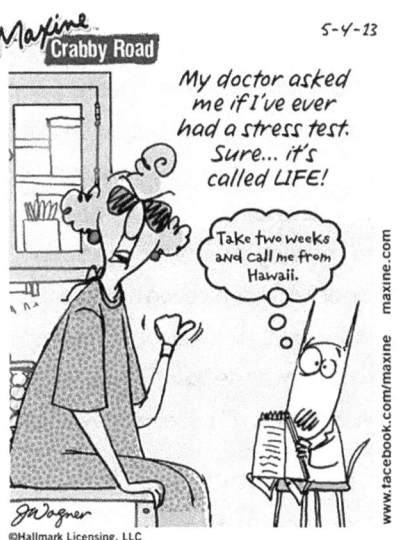

physical therapist, nurses and the folks who will be an integral part of your procedure. On the day of your surgery, you will again meet with some of those folks as well as your surgeon and the person(s) responsible for injecting you with a dose of happy juice so you can nap while the other folks do whatever it is that they do when they hang out and hover over you in the operating room chatting about this and that but you won't care because you will be out like a light. You know what to expect. Or, maybe not. If not, then this module will help you establish a clearer line of communication with the happy medical folks you should be meeting with prior to your surgery.

Doubtless, during chats with your medical team you heard at least three recommendations that may or may not be what you want to hear (or may not apply to you at all, of course)—stop smoking, lose some weight, stop drinking before and after surgery and especially when you are taking opioids for pain control. Sometimes, those recommendations can be fightin' words. You may have wondered why on earth you ever agreed to go with *this* surgeon. Too late.

Change is difficult for most people. For others, it is very difficult. We are creatures of habit. We drive to work or to school or to the grocery store or mall on the same roads. It is much easier to suggest that others change, rather than hear that you are the one who may need to change.

Butts, Binging, Boozing and You

Stop Smoking. Okay, you don't smoke and no one in your home smokes. No one you know smokes. And no one you work with or associate or socializes with smokes. Fantastic! Then feel free to skip this section.

If you smoke, you have heard people telling you (I assume) to quit smoking a thousand times. But you know better and you can quit anytime you want. At least that is what you say to folks. Or maybe you just didn't say that. You like to smoke. You aren't giving it up. Okay. Just for fun, do you realize that tobacco products, such as cigarettes, cigars, pipes and chewing tobacco contain almost 7,000 chemicals and at least fifty of those can cause cancer? And don't even think that e-cigs or those vapy-thingies are safe. Have you listened to the news? E-cigs contain some nasty ingredients, such as ultrafine particles that will find their way deep into your lungs. The flavorants, such as *diacetyl*, is a chemical already linked to lung disease. Happy inhale. Okay, so it is not going to happen to you. Got it.

Forget the health part. Think about the financial part that you are tossing away. What do you pay for a pack now? What do you spend each week? In a month? In a year? You may not be a financial-wizard but add it up. How much do you puff away in a year? Stop smoking and stash the cash into your retirement account.

> *For the record, I stopped smoking on 6 January 1966. I started when I was ten. During summer, I worked on tobacco farms in Connecticut from age eleven to my sophomore year in high school. It was the highest paying summer job. One or two ciggies a day evolved into a pack a day by the time I joined the Air Force. I was in the US Military in the 60s and a pack of cigarettes cost ten-cents a pack, one dollar per carton. We could only buy five cartons a month. The Military did not cause me to smoke. They just made it easy for me to expand and enjoy my habit. By the time I left the service, I was smoking four packs a day. I quit several times over the years, sometimes for up to a month, then returned to smoking but always increased the amount that I was doing before quitting. At one point I quit and smoked Dutch Master Panatela cigars. Fifty cigars to a box. One and one-half boxes per week. Back to cigarettes, mostly unfiltered Camels and Pall Malls. I quit cold turkey for good and never looked back or regretted it. No gum chewing. No sucking on candies. No jamming down junk or comfy food. No finger-nail chewing. Within the month I could taste food, without drowning it in salt. The yellow stain on my fingers disappeared. No more tiny fire-holes in my clothes. No more morning hack. No more afternoon cough.*

Back to the health-thing. Well, you don't have cancer and don't intend to have cancer so what's the big deal? Tobacco products do great things to your body. One of the great things it does is to delay your body's ability to heal from your surgical procedure. Of course, if you don't care about how long it takes you to get back to playing golf or tennis or any of your other ADLs, then maybe the delay is no biggie for you. But, cheer up, there are more great things it does. It…

- Constricts your blood vessels which reduces the amount of oxygen-rich blood in your bloodstream;
- Causes your blood to clot faster, which can lead to heart problems;
- Causes your blood pressure and heart rate to rise;
- Causes strokes and heart disease;
- Makes asthma symptoms worse;
- Dulls the taste of your food (which is why you tend to add a lot of salt to your food);
- Turns your fingers yellow and makes you and your clothes smell (stink?); and
- Best of all, it keeps you coughing and hacking throughout the day.

Give us a break here. Why should you quit? None of those bad things will happen to you, right? Right?

> *Quitting can be difficult. Very difficult. I am a bit skeptical about the gene-thing where you smoke because of a wayward gene or two. Folks smoke for lots of reasons. I was so good at (chain) smoking that I could smoke while taking a shower and not get that wicked-witch-white- stick wet. What a great accomplishment. I quit cold-turkey. No patches (they didn't have those patchy-thingies back then). Quitting was (is) a great accomplishment. I got to walk up a flight of stairs without doing any heavy-breathing. Amazing.*

There are multiple options that allow you to quit smoking if you are willing to do so. You can gradually decrease your dependency. You can wear one of those patchy-things on your arm. Or, you can quit cold-turkey. You may have found it very difficult to quit. You may have tried to quit several times only to return to your habit with increased dedication and probably smoked more than before you attempted to quit. Congratulations! You are a member of the club.

Going through the process of quitting will increase your overall health. There are few, if any, disadvantages to quitting. Well, maybe at least one. You will have to decide what to do with all the money you will save. Save it for your retirement? Take a vacation? Buy a boat? Donate it to your favorite charity? Stuff it under your bed?

The key to quitting is simple. It comes down to just two words—able and willing. You are able to quit, whether that means going cold-turkey or gradually reducing the amount you smoke each day until finally you stop for good. The barrier to quitting is your willingness, or unwillingness, to stop. You can stop. You can do it. You have the ability to do it. But are you willing to do it? Are you unwilling to change? Of course, you say, you can quit at any time. Great. You have conviction. You convinced me. Now prove it.

Rationalization is the key to your mental health. If you are not willing to stop, you will rationalize and come up with some dandy excuses for why you do not need to quit. Make a list of all the excuses you have used over the years. I'll bet you could come up with some real dandies. Able and willing. What's in your head?

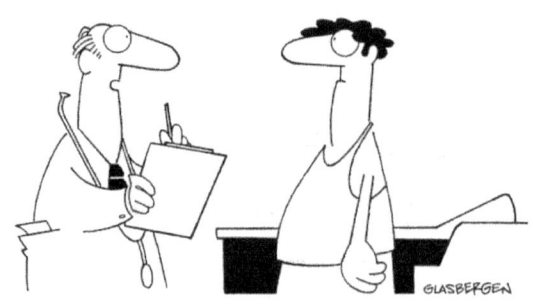

"If smoking relaxes you, then don't quit. Being dead is very relaxing."

Smoking is smoking. If you are filling your lungs with smoke, whether from a cigarette or cigar or pipe or e-cigs or vaping or marijuana or snorting or a shisha pipe (aka hookah or nargile) you will experience health problems. Guaranteed. You are betting the life of your lungs on it.

Lose the Weight. You learned about exercising and what types of exercise you could be doing to treat arthritic pain in **Module One.** Those same exercises, and others (re: **Module Six** and **Appendix Six)**, could help you lose some weight. Sometimes losing just five pounds can take pressure off that bad knee or hip or arthritic ankle and reduce your pain level. Check with your primary doctor about whether losing a few pounds will benefit you. I am talking about a few pounds, maybe ten or twenty tops, at least for the short term. And if you really need to lose a lot of tonnage, check with your doctor for the best way to do that. Change your behavior. Change your attitude. Make weight-loss an integral part of your ADLs. It is not just a campy thing to say on New Year's Day.

Do not go on a crash diet or a program that promises that you can lose thirty or forty or fifty pounds in a short period of time. Marketing propaganda aside, a sudden and significant loss of weight is not good for your body at any time. It is certainly not good for your surgical procedure. It could leave you weaker and impact your recovery process. Better to lose a couple of pounds each week over several weeks or a few months, than trying to lose five or more pounds per week and more than thirty pounds per month. Losing one or two pounds per week may seem a bit slow, and you may decide that that little amount of weight-loss comes under the category of why bother? Do it anyway.

The point of weight loss is to lose weight. Got it? The other and more critical point is to modify your behavior so that eating sensibly is your way of life. It is not something you start and stop. It does not mean that now you are stuck eating leaves and twigs and foods with exotic-sounding names that you have never heard of.

And if you are able (yes, you are) and willing (maybe) losing weight and changing your eating behavior can help you keep your weight off for the longer term. Eat when you are hungry, not when you are bored or lonely or feeling sorry for yourself. And just because it is feeding-time, breakfast or lunch or dinner, does not mean that you automatically eat. Pavlov lives. Eat when you are hungry. Forget the clock. Your stomach will tell you when. Your eyes and nose can deceive you.

Losing a lot of weight quickly may be more water loss or lean tissue loss than fat loss. There are programs that can help you lose more weight more quickly. These

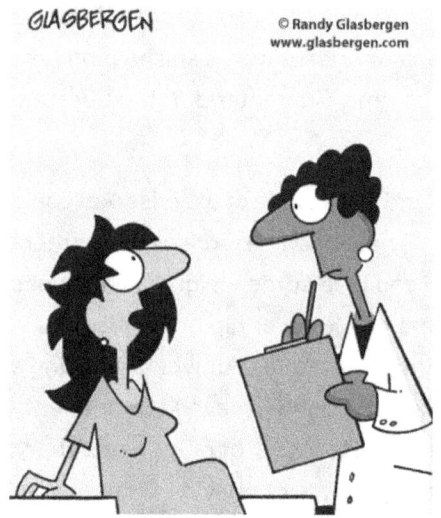

"I stay healthy by following a strict vegetarian diet — nothing but coffee and cigarettes!"

programs are almost always under medical supervision and include low-calorie diets for obesity coupled with an exercise component. These are not extreme diet programs (*Hensrud,* Mayo Clinic). Best to start sooner, well ahead of your scheduled surgery date. You can thank me later.

Any weight loss or any weight loss program should not weaken your system and cause problems during your post-surgery rehab process. Losing weight can be as simple as eating less per meal, eating less chubby-food and exercising more. Less in, more out. Less calories in, burn more calories out. There are many health benefits to you when you quit smoking and lose some weight. The advantages outweigh any excuses you may have if you continue to smoke and choose not to lose weight. Not concerned? Okay.

Stop smoking. Lose some weight. A pound or two a week is healthier. Your ability to modify your behavior is doable. Your willingness to do so is the hard part.

Booze and Surgery. Maybe your medical care-team recommended a third tidbit: quit drinking, at least before surgery and while you are on brain-pain-numbing narcotics. You may not want or need to quit drinking alcohol all together, but you may want to consider shutting it down prior to and after your surgical procedure. Why? Studies (and probably your care-team) has shown that having even moderate amounts before and after a surgical procedure can weaken your immune system and slow down your rate of recovery. Give it up for a while, then if you insist on going back to having a drink after your surgeon says your rehab is done, then that is your decision. Besides, how much damage can stopping do to your internal organs? Ask your care-team for their feedback.

Your medical-team may not have just been talking about excessive drinking. Even that occasional drink during the week and especially drinking just prior to surgery can be detrimental to your health as you prepare for and engage in your post-op rehabilitation program. What does your team have to gain if they tell you to stop? Maybe not much. What do you have to gain if you stop? Maybe your health.

What does excessive mean?

- For men, that means drinking five or more drinks in two-hours. Or, fifteen or more drinks in a week.

- For women, that means four or more drinks in two-hours. Or, twelve or more drinks in a week.

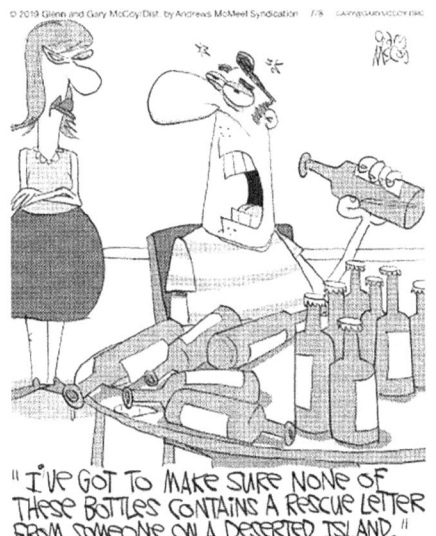

Rationalization can be your key to mental-health. At least, that is what you think.

Okay, so you say you drink just under those amounts in a two-hour period. What? Continue drinking at that pace? Maybe not. Granted, alcohol affects individuals differently. Regardless, just as with smoking, drinking prior to surgery can present you with a problem that you may not want to have. Some folks will say there is a family or a genetic issue. Fine. Still are you willing to stop (even for a short time) prior to surgery? You are able to stop, but are you willing to stop (Jha, 2008)?

Drinking, like smoking, is a habit. You learned to do that. You smoke before (during) and after you eat. You drink before (during) and after you eat. You have a drink and have a smoke. Your habit could become compulsive if you look forward to having that drink or two (or more) when you come home from work or are just hanging around your home thinking about having that next drink. Pavlov lives.

You cannot hide if you are overweight. There are visual clues. And wearing dark colored clothes will not make you thinner. You cannot hide or fib about whether you smoke. Your fingers may be stained a pretty yellow. Your clothes may have a distinct odor (or stink). You may be able to hide how much you drink, unless you have those cute ruddy checks with lots of little red blood lines running up and down your face. That could be one tip-off. But you could be good at hiding your habit.

My suggestion is that you fess-up and be honest with your care-team regarding your eating, smoking and/or drinking habits. The more information you share prior to surgery, the better your anesthetist and surgeon can take proper precautions and, if necessary, modify some aspects of your pre-op preparation.

What could you do if you were willing to stop? First, if you don't drink, don't start. Second, just stop if you do drink. Okay, you want more options or ideas?

- Refrain or limit consumption two- to eight-weeks prior to surgery to reduce your risk of complications. The sooner you stop or cut back, the better.
- Do not drink any alcohol while you are on narcotics or other brain-pain-reducing medications. The drugs tend to slow your reaction time down and adding the alcohol component just makes things worse for you (and others).
- After surgery if you choose to have that drink, do so based on the recommended amounts by your care-team. Generally, those amounts should not exceed one or two drinks a day, whether you are prone to enjoy beer, wine, or hard liquor.

Some of the complications from drinking before-during-and too soon after surgery include, but are not limited to the following:

- Longer bleeding times
- Higher risk of infections
- Delayed incision healing
- Often a longer stay in the hospital
- Sepsis and shock (when your blood becomes poisoned)
- More stress on your body
- Weakened immune system

Whether you choose to lose some weight or stop smoking or reduce your alcohol consumption is totally up to you. It is your body. It is your recovery time. But just in case something nasty happens and your recovery is a bit longer than you expected you may want to look in the mirror, rather than looking to blame your surgeon or care-team. Just a thought.

> *Always go to other people's funerals,*
> *otherwise they won't come to yours.*
>
> —YOGI BERRA

Whom to Trust

Which brings me to another potentially sensitive topic—your relationship with your surgeon. How did you select your surgeon? Did your primary physician recommend your surgeon? Did you use darts? A recommendation by a friend (or enemy)? You now have a surgeon. You have established rapport. The surgeon can engage in a conversation with you. Informative. Answers your questions clearly so you understand what to expect during and after surgery. (S)he makes you feel comfy. Good bedside manner. Maybe buys your book. Maybe encourages you to write another book. So, what's not to like?

The pre-surgery protocol has been explained to you and you understand what you need to do. Here I go again. Perhaps one of the recommendations by your physician was that you lose a bit of weight, before you undergo your surgery. Well, maybe lose a lot of weight. You think you don't need to lose any weight, okay, maybe a couple of pounds. You can handle that. But (s)he recommended that you lose forty pounds. Sixty pounds. Now you have a problem. And maybe a concern. You may become defensive. You may even question his or her heritage or lack thereof. Who is this stranger telling you to lose weight? Why doesn't (s)he lose weight? Did you have thoughts about finding another surgeon after hearing that breaking-news?

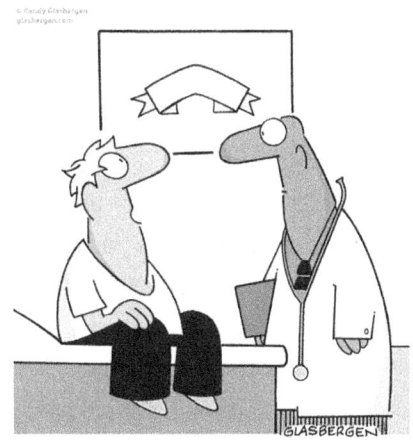

"I already diagnosed myself on the Internet. I'm only here for a second opinion."

Does this surgeon know what (s)he is doing? What is (s)he recommending and why? What's the big deal. You have been on a diet. You even enrolled in one of those weight-reducing programs that you saw on TV or that was recommended to you. You lost a couple of pounds. Maybe even fifteen. Okay, six for sure. What's the next step anorexia? *Kwashiorkor*? And would a surgeon refuse to operate on you until you did lose the recommended weight? What? S(he) doesn't want to buy a larger boat?

There are some surgeons who will refuse to operate. They know from experience that folks who are over-weight, by a lot, will not be keen to do the post-surgery exercises. And if they start the exercises they will stop shortly after discharge. They will not modify their eating habits. Their recovery will be longer than expected. They will complain to their surgeon and probably others that the operation was not successful, that it was not done properly, that the physical therapist caused too much pain. They will not blame themselves or acknowledge that their behavior had anything to do with any post-surgical issues. Some surgeons will refuse to operate.

Who wants to be told to do something differently? Who wants to be told, congratulations, you are a mess? Who wants to be told your lifestyle needs to be changed if you want to realize a speedy and healthy recovery? Your ego and vanity and feelings are hurt. To protect yourself emotionally you have decided that your surgeon is a border-line village idiot. You decide to change surgeons. Well, you will show 'em who's the boss. You will find another surgeon who really understands you and has a better bed-side manner, is more empathetic to your situation and is not so direct and abrupt and so inconsiderate of your feelings.

God gave us the gift of life;
it is up to us to give ourselves the gift of living well.

—VOLTAIRE

Surprise! If someone, such as your surgeon, recommends that you lose weight, then lose it. Your surgeon has your health and recovery in mind. Changing surgeons is not the path you should be taking. Changing surgeons is not going to alleviate your weight problem. Losing the recommended weight could. Stop smoking could help your lungs and allow you to walk up a flight of stairs without huffing and puffing. Stop (or cutting down) on your drinking could help your liver, kidneys and heart perform better.

The ball is in your court. Take the recommendations and put your ego or vanity or emotional block aside. Maybe you are your worst enemy. Maybe it is time to go with the recommendations of your care-team.

There are multiple reasons why you may have the urge to change surgeons. Whatever you come up with will seem logical to you. Again, rationalization is the key to mental health. Changing surgeons or physical therapists or hospitals because they want you to change your behavior—stop smoking, lose weight, whatever—is not going to earn you *The Smartest Move of the Year Award*. Sometimes when folks ignore recommendations and their recovery is not as positive as they want or expect, whom do they point a finger at—themselves or their surgical team? Guess.

Getting a second opinion on these basic issues may be an option for you. Yet if your surgeon is competent, why consider going to someone else? Take responsibility for your decision. Who knows, maybe you will have a much more positive and enjoyable lifestyle. And, just for fun, how will you respond if your new (second) surgeon also says you should lose weight? Would you look for yet another (third) surgeon? Don't do that. Whom do you trust and believe—your physician or your ego?

We are what we know.
And when the body of knowledge changes, so do we.

—JAMES BURKE, CONNECTIONS

Joint replacement procedures. What type of elective orthopedic surgery are you having? You may already be familiar with your procedure. You may be preparing for what lies ahead. If not, here is some other information that you may want to know and clarify with your surgeon. Communicate with your care-team.

If you need to have a body-part replaced, it will most likely be either a partial or total procedure. There are different types of joint diseases and both surgical and non-surgical treatments may be prescribed, depending on your situation. When surgery is prescribed, joint replacement is recommended and can take one of two avenues to correct the pain and problems you may be experiencing: partial or total replacement. Hips and knees typically come to mind, but other joints can involve partial or total replacement, such as neck and spine, shoulders, elbows and hands or wrists.

Partial Joint Replacements (PJPs). As the term implies, half or a section of a joint may need replacement. Partial knee replacement surgery is one example. The surgeon removes that part of your knee that is diseased or damaged and replaced with a prosthesis or artificial part. In the case of a knee, you may be released the day immediately following your surgery. Short hospital stay-arrive, get doped up and cut up on Day One; get released on Day Two. And who knows, the way procedures are going maybe more joint procedures, such as hips, will be an in-out, same day procedure.

Total Joint Replacements (TJRs). Total joint replacement means the entire joint, knee, hip, shoulder, elbow, and so on are replaced, usually with a prosthesis composed of plastic and metal. TJRs are more involved and generally require that you remain in the hospital for an extra day or two. The rehabilitation process is a bit longer.

The type of procedure you have will be a result of the conversations you have with your surgeon. Sometimes the final decision is made on the operating table. Regardless, the goal is to resolve your problem, alleviate your pre-surgery pain and get you back to a normal lifestyle.

Types of Surgery. First, there is no such thing as non-invasive surgery. Getting a flu shot or having your blood drawn or getting a mosquito bite is an invasive process. Your skin, which is the largest organ in your body, has been pierced and invaded. *Minimally invasive* is the term to remember and keep in your mind.

Generally, elective surgery on and around the area of your joints involves one or two primary procedures—arthroscopy or arthroplasty (or open-surgery).

Arthroscopy Surgery. Arthroscopy is minimally invasive surgery that uses a tiny camera called an arthroscope. The camera helps the surgeon examine and repair the tissues inside or around your shoulder joint (or knee joint, for example). The arthroscope is inserted through a small cut (incision) in your skin. This type of surgery is generally performed within an hour or so allowing you to arrive and depart for home within a few hours. In and out. **Done.**

You may be familiar with the term arthroscopy in connection with knees and hips. Yet surgeons use it with shoulders, elbows, wrists, feet and ankles. Probably the most common are repairing cartilage and meniscus problems in knees and repairing rotator cuff tears in shoulders. One advantage is limited damage to the tissues—muscles, tendons, ligaments—surrounding the affected joint. Typically, there is less surgical trauma to the joint; less bleeding, swelling, and inflammation. Opioid pain meds are not needed for as long as they could be for other surgical procedures.

Perhaps the one downside to this type of procedure is a false sense of confidence on the part of the patient (you). That is, you may consider the procedure to be less complicated than, say, open shoulder replacement surgery or rotator cuff surgery, and therefore not take your rehabilitation as seriously as you should. You may be too quick to garden after surgery or engage in golf or tennis or higher-impact activities sooner than you should. Not good. Be patient.

Arthroplasty or Open Surgery. The word arthroplasty (or orthroplasty) may sound similar to arthroscopy but the difference is as distinct as a knight is to night or as a lighting bug is to lightning. The term arthroplasty is an all-encompassing word that refers to joint diseases. Some doctors will use the term interchangeably with arthritis, which means joint inflammation. Yet there are some forms of open-surgery that are distinct from arthritis such as *neuropathic arthropathy*, which is nerve damage from diabetes, or *hypertrophic pulmonary osteoarthropathy*, where the ends of bones in your ankles, knees, wrists, and elbows grow abnormally and *hemarthrosis*, which is bleeding in the joint and is often common in people who are hemophiliacs.

Arthroplasty is a more invasive and involved procedure. You could expect surgery to last a couple of hours or so, depending on your situation. But not to worry because you will be zoned-out during that time and won't feel a thing. You probably will be required to remain in the hospital over-night and perhaps for a couple of days, again depending on your situation.

Debridement. Debridement is the medical removal of dead, damaged, or infected tissue to improve the healing potential of the remaining healthy tissue. Surgeons can remove that material by surgical means, mechanical, chemical, autolytic, or by maggot therapy (which was very common in times past, just in case you wanted to know and would like to consider that as an alternative form of treatment, or not).

Anesthesia options. You may not want to be fully awake while your surgeon is invading your body. Enter anesthesia. This is a process of inducing a pain-free, tranquil, sleep-like state while you are undergoing the procedure. Gone are the days when it was suggested that you bite hard on a piece of leather or wood. Your anesthesiologist has several ways to make your experience as comfy as possible. (S)he will, no doubt, meet you before your scheduled surgery time to ask you a few questions and identify the technique (s)he intends to use to make your experience as painless and tranquil as possible.

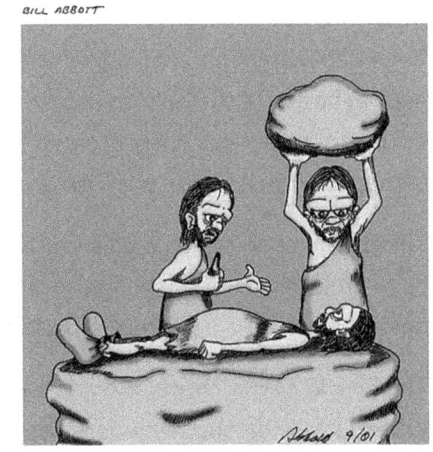

This is Ralph, your anesthesiologist.

General Anesthesia. Typically, you will receive medication to induce a sleep-like state, followed by a gas anesthetic agent that is administered to you via a mask into your lungs. During your procedure you will be attached to monitors that display information about your heart rhythm and rate, oxygen level in your bloodstream, body temperature and blood pressure. Your anesthesiologist continually checks these monitors throughout your procedure.

Regional Anesthesia. You may believe that this type of anesthesia will keep you awake during your procedure and therefore you may reject this technique. Not true. You will receive medications that allow you to nap peacefully throughout the operation. Unlike the general anesthesia technique, when regional anesthesia is stopped you will awaken almost immediately in the operating room, without pain. The anesthesia is still working to control your pain, though you are wide-awake (pretty much) and can hear and carry on a conversation with those attending you as you wish. Depending on your situation and the procedure, you may be given an *intrascalene block* used in conjunction with light sedation, especially if you are having surgery of the shoulder or upper body. You will be monitored and watched over as with the general anesthesia technique.

Are you a tad nervous about having anesthesia? You could ask to bite on a bullet or piece of leather or wood if you prefer.

Communication and You

Questions for Your Care Team. Lots of folks have surgery each year. Millions? Some are well informed about certain aspects of their procedure and have a good idea about what the rehabilitation process will entail, how long it will take, and what precautions they need to be aware of. These folks have asked questions. They got answers. On the other hand, others feel intimidated, embarrassed or feel that asking their surgeon questions is impolite. Whose body is it? Yours or theirs? Ask questions. Ask better questions.

There is no need to make your conversation into an inquisition. Yet, you may want to be aware of some of the basics so you can better prepare for what is going to happen before and after your procedure. At the very least here are five basic themes to consider.

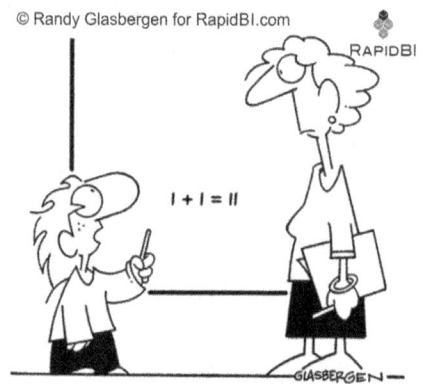

The Five W's Plus Three: Who, What, Where, When, and **Why** are key words that will help you create your own set of questions so you can feel more comfy with what will happen to your body. You can also add the words **How** and **May I** or **Can I** to the mix if you like. Again, you are not a trial-lawyer nor a member of a federal investigative team, but these basic **Five W's Plus Three** words can help you frame the types of questions you want (need) to ask your team, which includes your primary physician, surgeon, physician's assistant, physical therapist, and the helpful folks you will meet in the hospital or care-unit. You decide in what order or sequence you want to ask your questions. Prepare and plan ahead. Here are a few examples to use as a starting point. Select those that are most important and relevant to you.

> *I do not have a specific order but tend to ask further clarifying questions as I interact with my medical team. That is, one comment leads to one question and if I need to understand the answer better, I ask another question. I consider my body a temple, a bit bionic and perhaps abused and bruised and very used, but I need to know certain things about what others are going to do to that temple. And besides, I am the one who will be paying the bill. I ask questions.*

Who? For example, rather than say, **Who** will assist you in the operating room? consider saying, In addition to yourself, **Who** will assist you in the operating room? or **Who** should I contact at the hospital/physical-therapist facility/extended-care facility if I have some more questions?

What (and What if). What will happen before my procedure? **What** tests will I be having prior to surgery? **What** should I be doing to prepare myself or to get in better shape before my procedure? **What if** I do *that* this way instead of doing it *your* way? Or, **What** will happen if I do it this way? **What** will my recovery process be like? **What** are the risks with this type of surgery? **What if** I decide to put the procedure off until next year or two-years from now? **What if** I want to have non-surgical treatment options? **What** supplies, equipment and help will I need when I return home? **What** restrictions in my daily routine should I be aware of? **What** type of anesthesia will be used and **What** effect will that have on me after the procedure?

Where. Where do I go for surgery? **Where** will you perform the surgery? **Where** can I get a second opinion?

When. When will I have to take further tests? **When** should I arrive at the hospital-surgical facility? **When** will I know the outcome (the results) of my surgery or **When** will you visit me in my hospital room to update me about the results? **When** should I start my exercise program? **When** can I return to work? **When** can I return to gardening after surgery? **When** can I return to my golf game, tennis, racquet ball, hand-ball, pickle-ball or my other contact sports?

Why. Why are you recommending this procedure versus another procedure? **Why** do you think this is the best time for me to have surgery? **Why** do you think I need this surgery now?

How. How long will the surgery take? **How** long will I be in the hospital? **How** long will I need to stay overnight at the hospital or extended-care facility? **How** much pain will I have after surgery? **How** long will my recovery take? **How** much improvement can I expect after surgery and how will that affect my lifestyle? **How** long will I need to take my pain medications (opioids)? **How** long before I can play golf or tennis or baseball or run a marathon?

May I. May I ask you some questions about my procedure? **May I** follow-up with you if I have more questions (before or after surgery)? **May I** follow up with your assistant if you are not available? **May I** get a second opinion please? **Can I** do those exercises on my own or do I need a therapist? **Can I** schedule any physical therapy through you, or should I contact your PA?

Use these questions. Create your own. The purpose is to make you feel comfy about what you will be going through, from the initial meetings to the end of your rehabilitation process. The purpose is to help you prepare and organize what you want and need to say in as clear and succinct way possible. You are preparing for a surgical procedure. Prepare yourself.

Questions from your care-team. On the other hand, your surgeon and even your primary physician will want to know more about your situation before any tests are scheduled. They will be asking you questions. I do not have a clue who your doctor(s) is or what types of questions (s)he will ask you, but it would be wise to prepare to answer at least these basic questions.

- **When** did you first experience pain (in your shoulder/hip/knee/ankle, etc.)?
- **What** were you doing when you first experienced this pain?
- **What** movements or activities aggravate your pain?
- **Have you** experienced any other symptoms in addition to this pain?
- **Does the pain** seem to be localized or does it travel below your neck/shoulder/elbow/hip/knee?
- **Does your work** or hobby or sports activity aggravate your pain?
- **What** have you done to cope with your pain?
- **How** would you rate your pain over the last few days?
- **Are you** experiencing this pain right now?
- **On a scale of one to ten**, what is your pain level now, with ten being extreme pain?
- **What** questions do you have for me and your upcoming procedure?

There will be other questions, no doubt, but at least be prepared to describe the *what* and *where* and *how long* your situation has been going on. Be as specific as possible. At the very least, your doctor(s) will want to know **when** your pain started, **what** were you doing at that time, and **what** is your situation now, with respect to pain levels and mobility or movement restrictions. Communication between you and your care-team is critical. Communication among your care team members is also very critical.

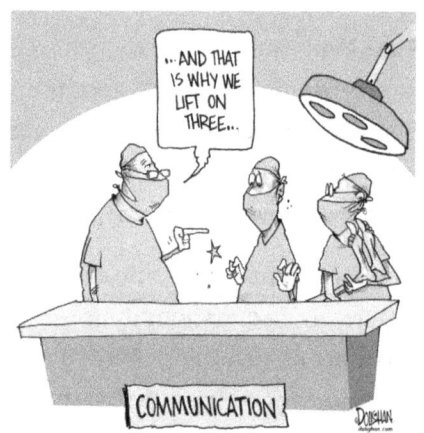

Setting Appointment Times. Before you come face-to-face with your surgeon, you will need to chat with the reception-folks to make an appointment. Getting through to a receptionist can be easy and quick or it can seem like a short-term career while you wait on the phone listening to the same music over and over again.

Has it been difficult for you to get an appointment? How long have you had to wait in the waiting room? Physicians or the appointment-person book patients back-to-back and generally allow you only about fifteen-minutes. And if your surgeon is running late for whatever reason, your wait time can feel like a short-term career. Here are a couple of suggestions that may make your day.

- Avoid Mondays and Fridays, which tend to be the busiest. Tuesday, Wednesday or Thursday is better.

- Schedule for the first appointment of the day. Your physician should not be backed up at 08:00 or for that first time slot, unless of course there is a weather or traffic delay.

Okay, so now you have your appointment. Your wait-time is over, right? Maybe not. You may be waiting in the waiting room waiting for the PA to call your name and lead you to the examination room. Sometimes that wait seems like a very long time. And sometimes it is.

- Generally, the receptionist will indicate your expected wait time if the doctor is running late. At some point you think that your wait-time is getting long. And maybe you think waiting is becoming a short-term career. Ask the reception (politely) how long it will be? If the wait seems too long, ask if you should re-schedule. The receptionist will probably suggest you keep this appointment and that the doctor will be able to see you any minute now and may check that out just to make sure. Don't be pushy. When you bring this matter up to the folks behind the counter, they should realize that everyone's time is valuable, including your time. Be nice. And don't get mad and all huffy at the receptionist. (S)he is not the one who is running late.

- Finally, the PA calls your name and together you go to the examination room. S(he) asks you several questions, takes your blood pressure, maybe even has you get on the scale, which almost always seems to be at least ten-pounds off. S(he) will tell you that your doctor will see you shortly and leave and there you wait, again.

- Finally, the physician enters. Plan on a quickie meeting. You may only have about fifteen minutes. When you ask a question, some physicians will simply tell you the time in as few words as possible; others will build you a watch and expand upon the topic and flood you with detail until your eyes glaze-over, whether you want those details or not. And, as a result, you may become confused or over-whelmed with the details.

- Prepare for your appointment by writing down your questions and be able to answer the physician's questions clearly and succinctly. Remember the Five Ws Plus Three. If the surgeon wants to know more, (s)he will ask you for more information.

- Be prepared to discuss your situation with respect to your symptoms. For example, **When** did your situation start to appear? **What** has changed about your situation over time? **What** is your situation today?

- Clarify what the doctor is telling you. Ask to have terms or procedures defined or explained more fully. At times when information is dumped on us (you) there is a tendency to get that glazed and spaced-out look in our eyes. You may even decide that is a good time for a short nap. You may want to summarize what you believe you heard and understood. Do not parrot back exactly what the doctor said but frame your comments as you believe you understood what was said. For example, "You were explaining some techniques that I would like try. Does that mean I can do those exercises on my own without needing a therapist or a steroid injection and can continue eating my favorite chubby-food?"

Surgery: Go or No Go

When do you decide that joint replacement or another elective procedure is something that should be high on your wish-list? When your spouse or partner or friends keep nagging you to do it? When you cannot handle the pain or inconvenience any longer? When you decide eating hospital food and having folks wait on you would be a good experience? When you and your physician decide that surgery is the best option for you? How extensive a procedure will you undergo? Total? Partial replacement? Minimally invasive?

You may be a candidate for total (or partial) shoulder, elbow, hip, knee or foot replacement when you experience all or most of the following. Check all that apply.

- ☐ Your pain has increased and limits your everyday activities, such as playing golf or tennis, walking or climbing stairs, even getting in and out of cars or your favorite chair.

- ☐ Your normal walking gait has changed and you rock and sway when you walk on a flat surface.

- ☐ Your knees are bowing in or out.

- ☐ You experience pain even while resting, which keeps you up at night (and makes you a bit cranky in the morning).
- ☐ When you blame the weather.
- ☐ Any swelling or inflammation does not subside with over-the-counter medicine.
- ☐ Your joints feel stiff when you swing a racquet or golf club or even when you are just sitting there, watching television clicking the remote.
- ☐ You feel very little relief from steroid injections, physical therapy, acupuncture or other remedies that you have tried.
- ☐ Your spouse-partner hassles you about why you are complaining, when you should be doing something about it (aside from complaining).

Trusting your surgeon and others on your care-team can relieve some of the stress or concerns you have about your upcoming procedure. No doubt your hospital or surgeon should have a complete checklist for you that identifies what you need to do before, during, and after your surgical procedure. No? Ask for one.

Pre-Surgery Checklist. Review this common-sense checklist before you step into the medical facility and before you take that exciting, fun-filled ride to the operating room. What hasn't happened that you believe should have happened? Check with your care-team about that. Be prepared. Get prepared.

- ☐ What is your scheduled surgery date?
- ☐ Where is your hospital or surgical facility located?
- ☐ Where can your coach or helper-person park while you go to the Admissions office?
- ☐ What door should you enter and how early in the morning can you check in?
- ☐ What identifications and insurance information do you need?
- ☐ Who is a key contact for you at the hospital?
- ☐ How to contact your surgeon and who is the PA (physician's assistant)?
- ☐ When is your pre-op physical scheduled with your primary doctor?
- ☐ When is your pre-op meeting scheduled with your medical facility?
- ☐ Does the hospital (or another organization) offer free pre-surgery educational classes?

- ☐ Have you registered for this free educational class?
- ☐ Have you started your pre-surgery exercises?
- ☐ Have you received your pre-surgery antiseptic cloths (if those are required)?
- ☐ Are you planning to come home right after your surgery?
- ☐ Are you planning to go to rehab facility instead? Who will take you there? Where is it?
- ☐ Did you contact your insurance company about your procedure and whether your policy covers everything? Some things? What is not covered?
- ☐ What medications can you take and stop taking before surgery?
- ☐ Should you stop taking vitamins or supplements before surgery?
- ☐ Do you have a coach? Who can help you during the group therapy sessions at the health-care facility? At home?
- ☐ Have you washed and set aside the clothes you will wear in the hospital? Pack sparingly. Remember, you are going in for surgery, not a fashion show.
- ☐ Keep your computer and cell phone and jewelry home. You don't need it. There should be a phone in your room. Your goal is to recover, not to report your minute by minute status to the world.
- ☐ Don't even think about letting social media know that you are in the hospital for X-number of days, unless of course you want to invite some not so friendly folks to come over and break into your house.
- ☐ Are you easily bored? Do you feel the need to fill the air with your voice? Chill. Go quiet for a bit. Read a book. Watch television. Take a nap. Take another nap. Twiddle your thumbs. Think nice thoughts. Give your vocal cords a rest. Enjoy the sound of silence.
- ☐ Bring and wear loose fitting sweat-pants or shorts and tops. Trust me, no one cares if you are wearing designer-somebody clothes. Wear comfy clothes. Have a nice set for discharge if you must, just in case you want to stop by a friend's house to show off your cast or splint or scar.
- ☐ Have you decided, before surgery, that you want to be released as soon as possible after surgery? That staying an extra hour or day in the facility is not high on your wish-list.

> **NOTE:** Medical insurance policies change. Federal and state policies change. Laws and regulations change. You may have decided to leave the hospital as quickly as possible, maybe even on the next day or two, regardless what your surgeon says. Fine. You are going home. If something unforeseen happens after an early discharge, your insurance policy (or Medicare) may not cover all your expenses. For that expense to be covered (your policy-Medicare says) you had to remain in the hospital for three days or more. Maybe your policy covers some procedures and tests, but not others. Maybe you have to go to another facility for that test. What is covered? What is not? Talk to your insurance agent. Talk with the hospital administrator (or billing department). Find out what is covered and how long do you have to remain in the hospital to have that expense covered. Financial surprises may be not fun.

What else can you expect? Your primary physician or surgeon will want you to have a few tests. Maybe you already had them. Blood samples would be a given to check on your *hemoglobin* and *iron* levels. Knowing the level of both is important. Hemoglobin carries oxygen from your lungs to tissues within your body. Iron helps your cells make energy. If your blood level is low, you will have less energy and tend to feel tired most of the time. And you may become grumpy and crabby. Got a short temper? It could get more explosive. Got zip patience? It could become shorter.

Having a normal blood level before surgery will help you tolerate the procedure better and lower your risk of needing a blood transfusion. Regardless of your blood level prior to surgery, it will drop a bit as a result of the surgery. Depending how low that level is after surgery you may be wise to increase your level of protein by eating more red meat or liver or chicken or turkey or fish all of which have higher levels of iron. Raising your *hemo* level and increasing your iron level can make for a quicker recovery.

Your diet is important both before and after surgery. Folks tend to complain about hospital food. They often make the same complaints about airline food. Call me silly, but are you going to the hospital because you expect fine five-star dining or are you going there to get something fixed? Ditto with an airplane ride: You go there to get from point A to point B, safely and quickly. Which is nice. Hospital food is okay. It keeps you alive, which is a handy thing. You can increase your strength and stamina after surgery by eating specific foods (re: **Appendix Four**). So rather than get all worked up about the food, get worked up about what you are eating *before* you go to the hospital. And then continue to pay attention to what you eat and why you are eating what you are eating *after* surgery.

You can also start eating (or not eating) certain foods before surgery. Generally, folks who get in better shape prior to surgery need less supervised physical therapy. Check with your surgeon or the hospital staff responsible for surgical patients for their recommendations. Better yet, chat with a nutritionist-person. They should know. That is what they went to school for. They can help you create a dietary program specific to your situation.

What if eating lots of nice red meat is not high on your wish list? Eating the Mediterranean diet, with its focus on fish, nuts, fruits, vegetables, beans, whole grains and using olive oil are all great for keeping your body healthy. There are non-meat alternatives made from plant protein. And if the recommendation is that you eat certain foods, rather than what you are eating now, not to worry. The earth is not flat. The sun will rise in the morning. You will survive.

Here are a few examples of foods to eat and foods to avoid before (and after) surgery.

- Do not eat trans and saturated fats, usually found in processed foods, because they can contribute to inflammation, which in turn can increase your pain level.
- Eat leaner cuts of meats, low-fat cheese and low-fat milk.
- Do you have problems eating veggies from the Solanaceae family, that is, tomatoes, peppers, eggplants, and potatoes? These veggies contain a chemical called *solanine*, which can increase pain levels in some folks, especially after surgery. Avoid these if they affect you in a negative way.
- Cut down (cut out) high-sugar chubby-foods, such as soda, candy, pastries, honey, and certain cereals (by the way, sugar is sugar to your body, regardless of its name or what the marketing folks say).
- Eat more Omega-3 foods, such as walnuts, pumpkin seeds, cold-water oily fish, can reduce inflammation.
- Protein is good for building body tissue so consider poultry, fish, seafood, nuts such as pecans, legumes (beans, peas), soybeans and tofu.
- Dark green veggies, such as kale, romaine lettuce, Asian greens, and collard greens are jam-packed with anti-inflammatory phytochemicals and antioxidants and their fiber will help alleviate constipation, which is common from anesthesia.

Over the Lips and over the Gums.
Look out Tummy, here it Comes.

—RED SKELTON

Your Surgery Day. The important day will arrive as scheduled. What can you expect when you walk through the door of your health-care facility? Granted, your procedure may not be scheduled for a few weeks or months yet, but you may be curious about what your day will be like when you step inside your health-care facility. Your hospital or clinic will have their own protocol to prepare you for your surgery.

Generally, you can expect to arrive at least two hours prior to your scheduled procedure. This time is needed by the administration and nursing staff to prepare you for your procedure. They will ask you questions. Your surgeon probably asked you some of these same questions. Didn't someone take notes or something? Anyway, expect questions. There will be periods of waiting filled with periods of activities and more questions and then some more waiting. And maybe even some more waiting. Chill and relax. You will be in good hands. So, what if you wait a bit longer than you want. Where are you going anyway? You are having surgery in a couple of hours or so. Chill. Relax.

If the person who brought you to the hospital or clinic is going to wait there and chat with the surgeon after the procedure and before you see your spouse-partner-friend-relative-neighbor in the waiting room, suggest that they bring a book or magazine or entertain themselves because they will probably be waiting until your procedure is done. How long did your surgeon say the procedure will take—an hour, two-hours, more? And what about the time you will be in the recovery room? How long will that be (approximately)?

Some of the activities you could experience on the big-day could include the following.

- Wait in a reception room.
- Walk to another room where you will fill out some administration forms.
- Go to another room to chat with a pharmacist in order to clarify the types of medications, non-prescription vitamins and herbal supplements you are taking and when the last time you took them and when was the last time you had something to eat and drink? Can I have my cup of coffee now? No.
- Return to one of the earlier rooms and wait for a nurse or assistant to take you to the actual surgical-preparation room.
- A wrist band will be strapped on you and you will be asked a thousand times to verify your name and date of birth to verify if you are the person listed on the form and at times, I assume for sheer entertainment, you will be asked what type of surgery you are having and what side of your body will be operated on. Some medical folks sure have a sense of humor when they ask you that. Well, maybe they are bored.

- Depending on your procedure, you will get buck-naked and asked to wipe down your body or the areas around the surgical area to guard against infection and then inserted into one of those style-challenged gowns designed to expose your back-side and bum and make you self-conscious while you wait or walk down the hall to go to you-know-where to do you-know-what.

- An IV inserted in your arm or hand with a hanging saline bag will disgorge its liquid contents in your vein, which may feel cool (cold?) to you, but no big deal. When was the last time you ate or drank something? You were already asked that but humor them anyway. Respond politely and accurately. Now can I have my coffee? No.

- A procession of other nurses, anesthesiologists, assistants, and eventually your happy-face surgeon will appear and ask what do you think you are you here for. What? (S)he doesn't know? More humor. (S)he will mark the body part with an "X" or his or her initials to make sure there is no mistaken body part fixed that did not need fixing, then you will wait some more.

- You probably will see medical folks walking back and forth going somewhere and at times just sort of hanging around the nursing station, chatting while you wait and wonder why you have to wait so long (clearly, more medical humor here).

- Finally, one or two folks will arrive with a cart or wheel-chair or some sort of transportation vehicle. A final (final?) kiss to someone you live with or know and you will be wheeled into the operating room and gently tossed on the operating table and covered with a toasty blanket. You will be given a spinal or other anesthetic needed for your surgery, exchange pleasantries with part of the surgical team and at some point your lights will go out, the procedure will take place, and you will awaken an hour or so later, and taken to the recovery area awake, maybe a tad goofy and mildly foggy perhaps and there wait until you can be transported to your room.

- You will be asked if you want something to drink (they will not have what you really want) and do you want something to eat (dry crackers probably).

- You will be given more pain meds every so often and asked to rate your pain level on a scale from zero to a gazillion.

- Once your pain level seems comfy for you and your room is ready, you will be wheeled to your room where you will spend the next day or so having folks wait on you hand and foot every two hours or so, especially throughout the night while you are trying to sleep.

- Relax. Enjoy the gurney rides. Be patient. Do your exercises. Eat some food. Get well.

- Of course, if you had an out-patient procedure you will return home later that day. No need to fret about the food or inattentiveness from the health-care folks or noise from the other patients and their hoard of visitors who crowd into the room next to you and decide that it is party time. You can be in your own quiet little space in your home.

- Or, you may have elected to go to an extended care-facility if you live alone or if the person you live with may not be able to provide you with the recommended post-surgical care or has a problem boiling water.

- Did I mention to do your exercises? Don't overdo it. Don't baby yourself. Listen to the experts who are waiting on you hand and foot and you should have a great recovery.

The prelims are over. You have done all the preparations that were recommended to you. You are on your way to the first day of getting relief from the pain you have been experiencing. That will be the first day that you can start living your life after surgery. Congratulations. You did it.

> *I had my second hip operation. All went well. I created a pre-surgery exercise program to condition my lower and upper body. I thought I was in okay condition. Surgery done. Recovery room done. On my way to my room. The gurney driver stopped at the door to my room and soon I was surrounded by four other people. I assumed they were there to gently drag me off the gurney and drop me on to my bed. I was prepared. A nurse was among the group and asked if I wanted to walk to my bed. Walk? I just had surgery. Yes, walk. Can I do that? Absolutely. Do you want to? Sure but... Not to worry. We are here if you need any help. Okay. I got off the gurney and stood for a few seconds, then took my first step, then more until I got to my bed. Turned around without hanging on to anything or anyone and backed by butt against the bed, swung my good leg over, then the surgical leg and that was that. I think I smiled and said something dopey. Some laughs. Tucked in. Everyone left. I knew then that what I had done to prepare and lessons learned from my other ortho surgeries paid off. I felt pretty good about that.*

Module Summary

Listen to your surgeon. (S)he is the person whose goal is to make you feel all better. Listen to the other folks on your care-team. They are the ones who make your pre- and post-op process go well so you can return to your ADL groove and go on

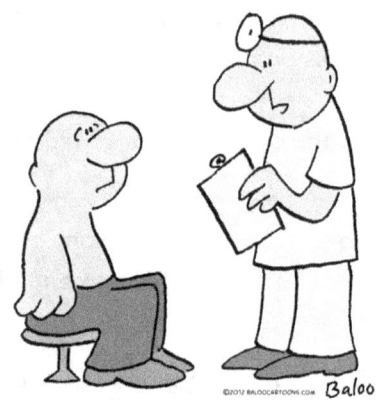

"I'll give it to you straight — This disease is almost *impossible* to pronounce."

to living your life after surgery. If you think you know better than your team, then why are you still having pain? Why are you not doing all of the things that you would like to do? Why are you less active?

Medical folks make mistakes. Medical folks are human. Humans make mistakes. It is part of our DNA. Regardless, your medical team has made suggestions. Implement them. Exercise. Lose weight. Quit smoking. Lay off the alcohol for the recommended time, especially if you are on pain-medication. Follow their recommendations. Get your surgery. Complete your rehabilitation process. Get back to your ADLs and, if you feel the need to re-assert control over your favorite body, then go back to your old unhealthy habits and deal with the consequences. Take responsibility for how you choose to go about your waking hours.

Make a list of questions (the **Five W's Plus Three**) for your surgeon and others on your medical care team. Your questions and their answers should help you feel more comfy. This is not an inquisition. It is a way to establish a collaborative communication link. And be prepared to respond to the questions they will ask you.

Take a few minutes to create a self-directed action plan (SDAP) that identifies what you plan to do and how you plan to do what you plan to do prior to and after your surgical date.

Self-Directed Action Plans (SDAPS)

It's over (right?). You got your ADL groove in gear before surgery with some pro-active preparations. You have organized your home and yard. You have cleaned and stored all your big-boy or big-girl toys and tools. Your sports equipment and clothing is nice and clean and stored for the next few weeks or until the weather allows you to go out and play. You talked with your medical team and you were more than thrilled about seeing the inside of the operating room. You had your procedure, which you don't remember because you were taking a nap. Regardless, you are out of the facility and home and recuperating. **Done.**

COLLABORATING WITH YOUR MEDICAL CARE-TEAM

This may be your first or last procedure. But just in case you are a candidate for another procedure (who knows), you may want to evaluate what you went through, what worked and what you would do differently that next time. There are some questions on the next page to get you started and thinking about what you did not do, and the support you received from your medical team. You can start to complete this form before surgery or after your procedure. Feel free to make copies.

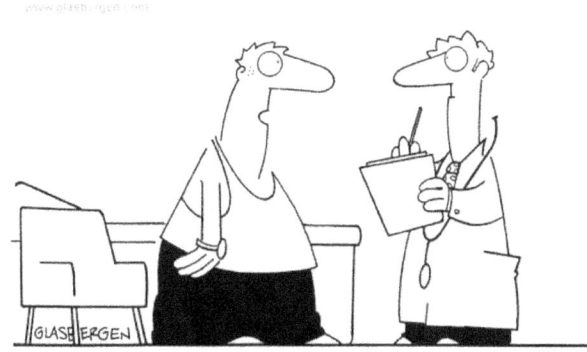

Your Notes

My Self-Directed Action Plan

Before Surgery

What procedure are you scheduled to have? _____

When is the procedure scheduled? _____

Have you prioritized any changes you decided to make, either with yourself personally, within your home, outside in your yard and garden? _____

What is your goal as a result of this surgery? _____

Priorities After Surgery

What did you decide would be nice to do? _____

What were you able to do yourself? _____

What help did you need to complete any other activities you decided to do?
_____

What did you do to relax and reduce any stress you had before your procedure? And how well did that work for you?
_____
_____

What modifications, if any, did you make to your home, e.g., bathroom or other rooms, and did they help? _____
_____
_____

Are you making those changes permanent or were they temporary just for your surgery?
_____

What types of changes did you make, if any, in your yard and garden and did they help?
_____
_____
_____

Who, if anyone, helped you make those changes and were you satisfied with their help?

Did you start your recommended pre-surgery exercises? _____ If so, how many weeks prior to your procedure did you start? _____ If you did not start your exercise program, why not? _____

How helpful was your medical team, e.g., surgeon, assistants, physical therapists, to prepare you for your procedure and who, especially, was the most helpful?

What would you do differently the next time if you just happen to need another surgical procedure?

Additional Notes or Comments:

> *We don't stop playing because we grow old;*
> *we grow old because we stop playing.*
>
> —GEORGE BERNARD SHAW

MODULE 6

EXERCISING FOR YOUR PRE- POST-CONDITIONING

This module contains graphic photographs, illustrations and suggestions that may be disturbing to some people. Caution is advised.

The Focus and Outcomes of this module include ...

- Low-impact exercises to relieve pain for different body parts
- Exercises to build and maintain your strength, flexibility, mobility
- Exercises for living your life after surgery

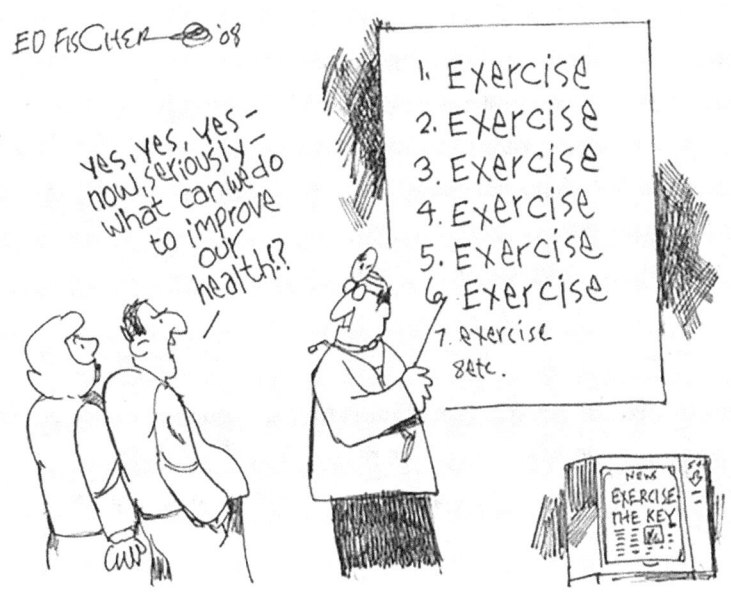

> **NOTE:** This author (that would be me) does not endorse any treatments, procedures, products, physicians or organizations mentioned in this or any of the other modules in this book. The information is provided as an educational service by the author and is not intended to serve as medical advice. Use them as a starting point to learn how to integrate them into your ADLs, whether you garden, play sports or sit and play cards or board games. Anyone seeking specific medical advice, whether associated with a planned or past surgical procedure, should consult his or her surgeon and primary physician.

You can use the exercises in this module to serve your needs in at least four ways:

1. Pre-surgery toning, flexibility and strength-building
2. Post-surgery rehab protocol to get your ADL groove in gear, quickly and safely
3. Integrate them within your current exercise program
4. Establish a longer-term preventive maintenance program (PMX) to help you keep in shape while you enjoy living your life after surgery

Overview

In addition to providing you with lifestyle advice, your medical care-team will talk medical to you. In that occasionally mind-numbing process, they will use terms for different exercises and movements that you may or may not be familiar with. You may call it jargon. All professions use jargon. People who work in a profession do not use the term jargon. The abbreviations and code-words and collections of letters they use are their way of communicating in a quicker and more efficient way. To you, they could be confusing. Jargon. You may not want to be embarrassed by asking *huh questions*.

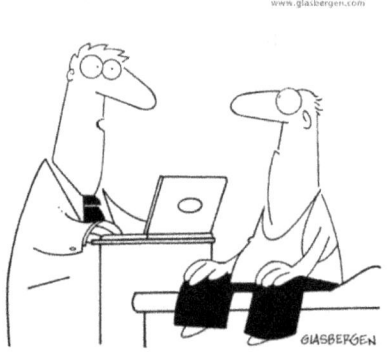

"Doctor and physician are outdated terms. I'm your biological tech support specialist."

Use the questioning suggestions in **Module Five** as a guide. This module should help you have a better understanding of the names and abbreviations for exercises that you may need before and after surgery and for establishing a better dialog when you communicate with your care-team.

EXERCISING FOR YOUR PRE- POST-CONDITIONING

Prepare yourself for your surgery by using the exercises for that procedure. The better conditioned you are before surgery, the easier it will be for you to recover and return to your ADLs sooner.

Terms of Movement: Range of Motion

Your care-team will use many of the terms in this module. Most of the terms and exercises could apply to both your pre- and post-surgical procedure.

Passive Range of Motion (PROMs). This is level one. PROMs mean that someone else, such as your physical therapist, is moving a body part without your help. You just sit around or stand or lie down and they do all the work. Your role is to pay attention and at times just scream out in agonizing pain every now and then to let the therapist know that that movement caused you a teensy-bit of pain. Don't be upset if they smile a bit.

After shoulder surgery, for example, the therapist will move your shoulder for you in a controlled manner. Initially, you would only be allowed to have someone else move a body part for you. If you are the impatient type, you may find this process a tad boring because you will not be in control. You may only meet with your therapist

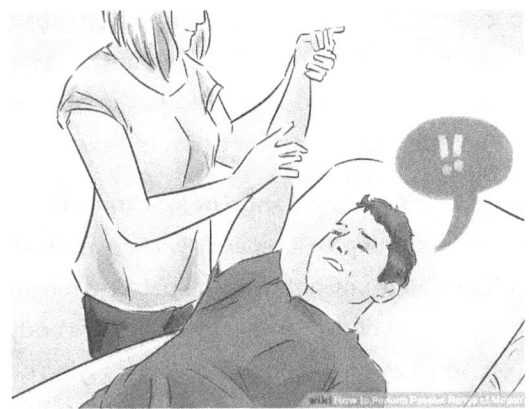

Passive ROM where you just sit or lie there and scream every now and then while your therapist moves the surgical body-part.

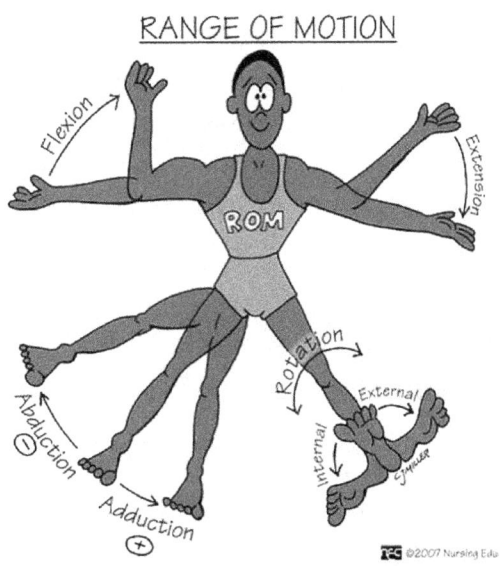

*Movements away from your **body core** include the terms: extensions, abductions and external rotation. Movements returning to or moving back towards your core include flexion, adduction and internal rotation. Flexion is a motion in which the angle of the joint involved decreases. Bending your elbow towards your upper arm is one example. Extension is a movement that increases the angle of the joint. Straightening your elbow is one example. Flexion and extension can be performed at different joints and are controlled by your body's muscles.*

once or twice a week. You want to get on with it. Not to worry. You will get more involved as you progress. Use these PROMs and the time you spend with your therapist or physical trainer to get the proper form down so later you can do them yourself. It would be good to pay attention to what and how the exercise needs to be executed effectively.

Active or Assisted Range of Motion (AROMs). Once you have gained some movement and your pain level and swelling reduced, you are ready to graduate to this level, AROMs. Here you get to participate in a more active way with your rehabilitation. Your therapist is still in charge and will move a body part with some active assistance from you. You may be sitting or standing or lying on your back, stomach, or side and as the therapist moves a body part, an arm or a leg, you may be asked to provide a bit of resistance. You cannot take the therapist home with you, but you may be given a substitute therapist-helper, such as a set of elastic bands or pulleys or other devices to provide that resistance. You may be instructed to tie the elastic band to a door-knob and as you pull on the band with your surgical hand your good arm pulls on the band as well. Your good arm (therapist) is assisting your surgical arm. You now have some control. You will experience a bit more pain but stick with it because as you progress your pain will lessen and you will achieve more ROM and be able to move to the next level.

Active Range of Motion (ARMs). At this level, your physician (or therapist) may include a set of exercises that do not require assistance, either from a therapist or with the help of another body part. ARMs are completed with only your surgical body part—arm, shoulder, elbow, hip, knee, foot and so on. You are making great progress when you are cleared to do ARM exercises.

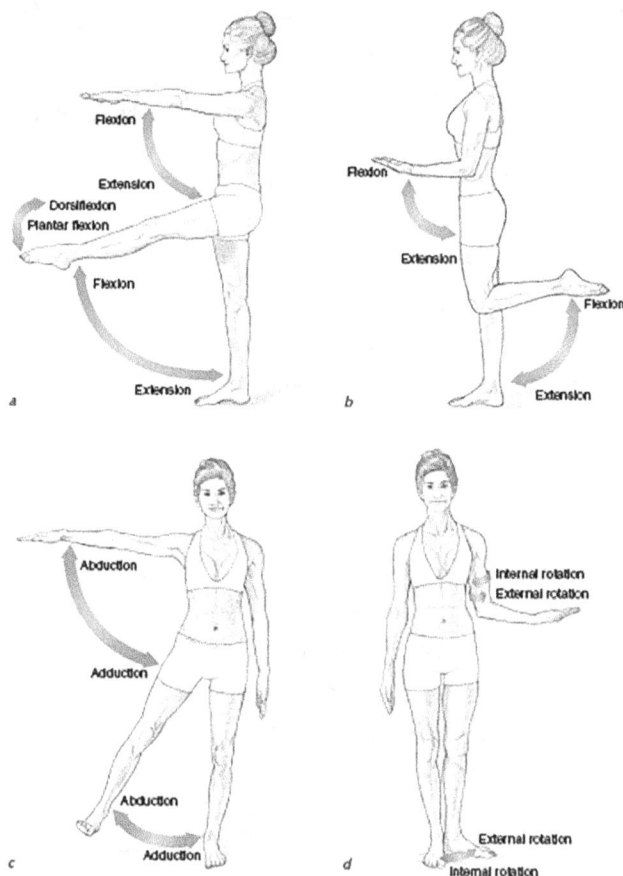

Light Resistance Exercises (LREs). At the LRE level, you will be allowed to use light resistance exercises, with or without weights, as you progress through your rehabilitation process. Usually this will be at least one month after discharge, again depending on your progress and the type and extent of your surgical procedure. If you belong to a club, start with one-pound weights. If you are at home, start with an eight-ounce can of tomato paste, for example. If you were involved in sports or lifting weights or engaged in higher impact activities, start with the lightest weight available.

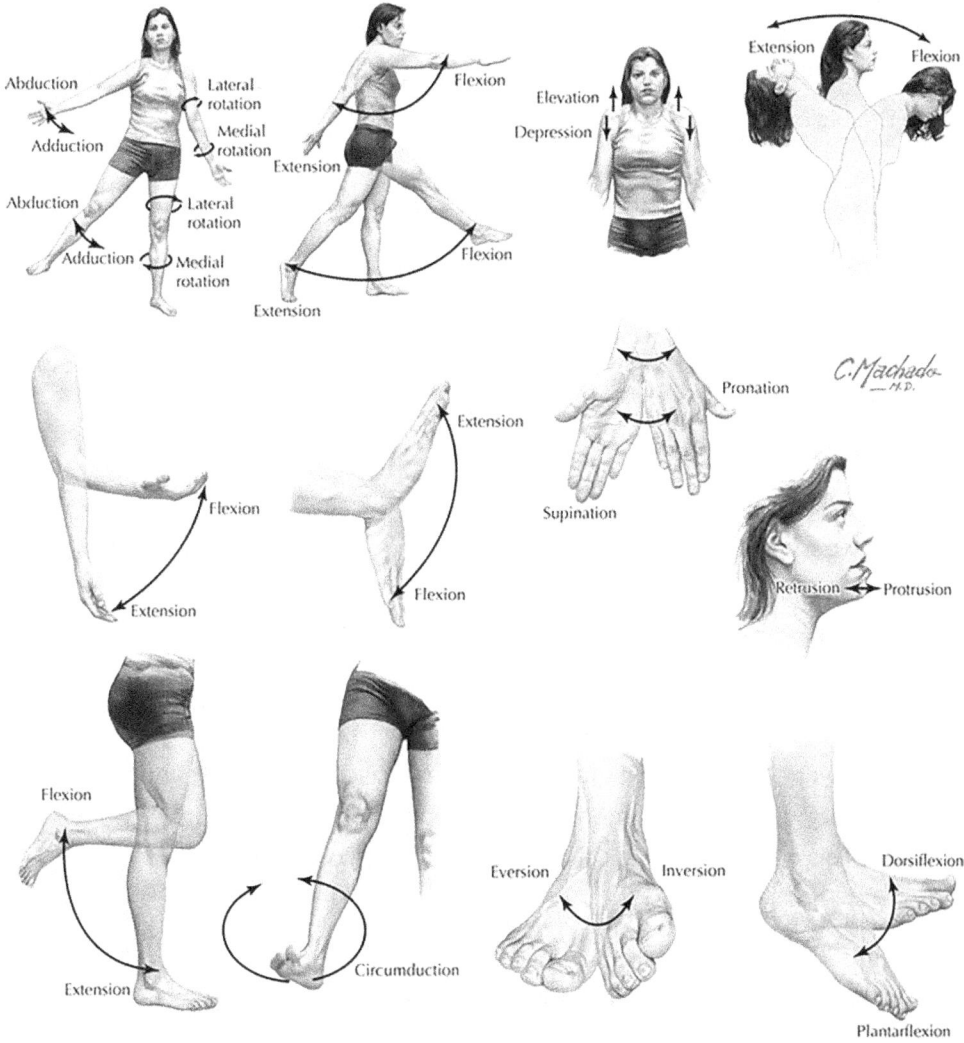

*Moving your foot and toes down, away from your body is called a **plantarflexion** exercise (or movement), while moving your foot and toes up and towards your body is called a **dorsiflexion movement**. Dorsiflexion is movement that lifts the front part of your foot (or your wrist) away from the floor. When you stand on your tippy-toes you are engaging in a plantar flexion movement. Note the other terms of movement, e.g., supination, protrusion, medial rotation and elevation-depression (**Oercommons**, anatomy).*

A common mistake folks make is to start with too much weight and do too many repetitions during a set and doing the exercise rapidly. If you think lifting a one-pound weight is for sissies, then extend the number of repetitions to twenty or forty or sixty for each set. Start light and work up to what you can do without experiencing any pain or swelling. Pain is not part of the program.

Flexion and Extension: front to back motion. Flexion is movement toward your body, in front of your body. Extension is movement that extends that body-part away from your body. Specific tendons and muscles allow your body-parts to move your arm or leg out in front of your body while other tendons and muscles allow those body-parts to come back. Is that all confusing? Well, that is why medical folks make the big bucks.

Abduction and Adduction: side-to-side motion. These are movements side-to-side, left-to-right of your body. As you see from the illustrations, abduction is movement away from your torso and adduction moves your arms or legs back in towards your body.

External and Internal Rotation Motion: away from-back towards. External rotation movement, e.g., your feet, is movement away from your body, to the outside. Internal rotation is movement back towards your body, toward the inside.

Exercise. Why bother? Simple: conditioning. Your successful rehabilitation protocol process depends on it. Proper exercise it is an integral part that should enable you to return to gardening and playing golf and tennis and walking around the Mall without a cane or walker or a knee walker or crutches and doing all of your other favorite ADLs quickly and safely.

And, as always with suggestions in this book, contact your primary physician or member of your care-team to ascertain what exercises should be in your daily exercise routine. Most elective surgeries are scheduled two to three months (or more) in advance. This gives you at least sixty-days to start an exercise program.

Start your exercise program at an easy level, say doing five to ten repetitions a couple of times each day, then work your way up to more reps and with more resistance or weights. As always, stop any exercise if you feel dizzy or experience pain in your joints or if you are having chest pains. Your commitment to complete the exercises recommended by your medical team is up to you. You will probably receive a more extensive set of exercises from your medical team. Confirm that with your care-team to make sure you are doing what you should be doing in the proper manner.

EXERCISING FOR YOUR PRE- POST-CONDITIONING

TIP: Your ADLs may already include an active exercise program. Fantastic. If so, check with your personal trainer or physical therapist to identify what you are doing—the types of exercises, duration, use of weights, and so on. Is it okay to continue with that program? Do they have any other suggestions that you should include, e.g., exercises, duration and using heavier weights?

Exercises for Body Parts

General Assistive-Device Exercises. You may be using an assistive device now. If so, to get you started with an exercise program consider these three easy and effective exercises. Each can help you if you need to use a walker or crutches or a wheel-chair during your post (or pre) protocol. These exercises will help you get in and out of bed or a chair or vehicle. You can do each of these standing or sitting down. Consider these as a starting point.

- **Bicep Curls.** You can stand or sit. You probably have done these or certainly have seen folks do them. With dumbbells at your side, slowly curl your arms up towards your shoulder (flexion). Then slowly return to your starting position (extension). Start with one-pound weights and work up to eight or ten pounds if possible. If the most you can lift is five pounds, then simply increase the number of reps you do during each set. If one-pound is too heavy (sixteen-ounces), grab a six-ounce tomato paste can instead and work up from there.

- **Triceps Curls.** You can stand or sit and follow the same procedure as for biceps curls. You can also lean over a table or bench, using one arm to support yourself. With the other arm, hold a light weight and dangle it towards the floor. Keep your arm straight, do not bend your elbow, raise your arm back and up so it is parallel with your body or floor.

- **Seated Lift-Ups.** Sit in a chair with sturdy arms. Press down with your arms and lift your butt from the chair, then slowly lower yourself on the chair. If you do these in a wheel-chair make certain your wheels are locked.

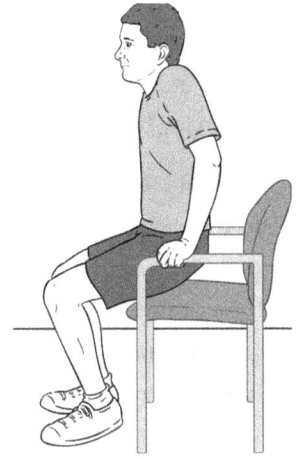

*Seated Lift-Ups. Use your arms to lift your butt off the chair. Raise yourself a few inches, then lower yourself and repeat. Note the difference between this exercise and the seated quad lift shown later in this module. Here you use **only** your arms; with the seated quad exercise you **only** use your legs.*

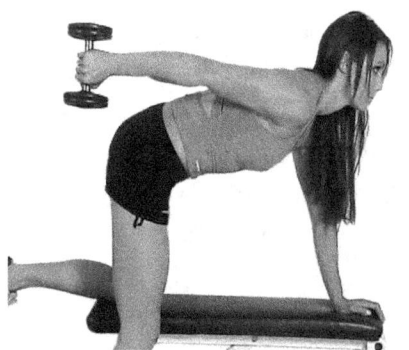
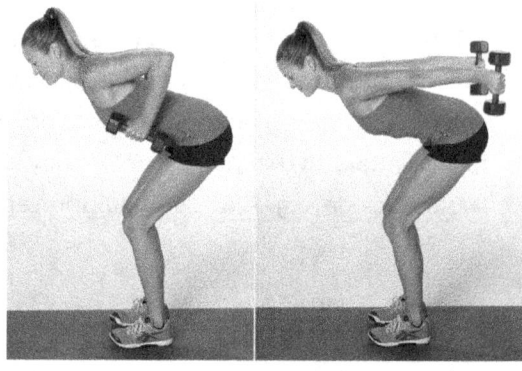

You can do the triceps kickback exercises as shown in these three photos—bending, standing or using a bench or table or your bed for support.

The following exercises apply to specific body parts and selected ailments. These exercises are from multiple medical sources. Some exercises could easily apply to multiple body parts, such as those for your hips and knees. As a result, you will see some redundancy. Not to worry. Note each example and ask your physician or personal trainer or physical therapist which of these exercises could apply to you. We'll start at the top with neck and shoulder exercises and travel down to the bottom of your body with foot and ankle exercises. Enjoy the ride.

Upper Body Parts: Neck to Hands. You can use these exercises before and after your surgery. Long-term, use them for continuous toning and physical well-being as you pursue the various sports and other ADLs that you have been involved in or that you now want to start. As always, rely on your care-team to provide you with a protocol that is specific to your situation. Follow their recommendations and instructions. Ideally, your care-team will demonstrate an exercise that is specific to you and provide you with illustrations and feedback about your form and technique.

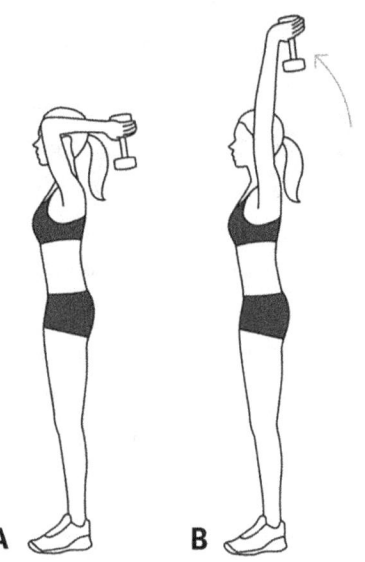

And remember that if doing any exercise causes you pain, nausea, dizziness, swelling or discomfort, stop immediately and contact your physician. Got an oweee-ouch? Did you overdo something? Think **RICE** – **R**est, **I**ce, **C**ompression and **E**levation to reduce any pain and swelling that you might experience.

Necks. Having any pain can be a pain. These exercises could resolve or at least minimize the pain in your neck. Maintain good posture by keeping your shoulders back and relaxed

EXERCISING FOR YOUR PRE- POST-CONDITIONING

and your head back so it aligns over your shoulders. This is called the *neutral position*. If you are having neck surgery, lie on your back as much as possible when sleeping. Do not lift anything heavier than three-pounds until cleared to do so. What is a three-pound object? A steam iron weighs about that much. A half-gallon of milk weighs four-pounds. A gallon of water weighs eight-pounds. A can of beans weighs about one pound.

When doing your neck exercises breathe normally and do not hold your breath. Do not hold your breath for any exercise. Breathe. Avoid fast or jerky movements. Plan to complete them twice a day. You can do these neck exercises at home, without any special equipment and most can be done sitting or standing. Your eventual goal will be to do these exercises at least ten-times per set. Two excellent online sources for exercises and illustrations are from The Memorial Sloan Kettering Cancer Center and *WebMD* 2019.

- **Neck Stretch.** Turn your head so you are looking to the right. Place your right hand on your left cheek and jaw and apply light pressure. Turn your head back to look down and to your left. Place your left hand on top of your head and gently apply pressure. Repeat in the other direction.

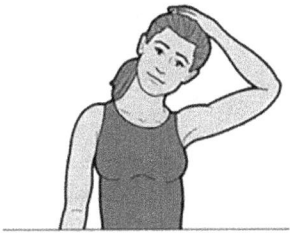

Side Bend
Sit down, bring head into neck-retraction position, then gently guide right ear toward right shoulder with right hand. Stop when you feel a stretch on left side of neck. Return to neutral. Repeat 5 times on each side.

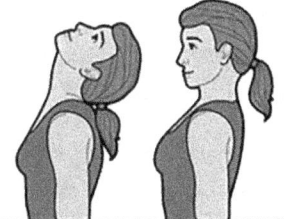

Head Drop
Starting in a seated position, retract neck (as above). Slowly move head up and backward as far as you can comfortably go. Return to neutral. Repeat 10 times. Do this exercise again at the end of each session (so you do it twice each session).

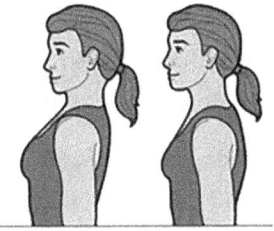

Neck Retraction
While lying faceup or sitting down, bring head straight back, keeping your eyes on the horizon. Then return to neutral. Repeat 10 times.

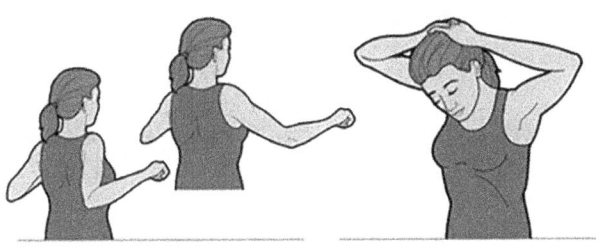

Shoulder Blade Pull
While sitting, bend raised arms at 90-degree angles. Relax shoulders and neck. Keeping arms and neck still, squeeze the muscles between shoulder blades, drawing shoulder blades closer together. Return to neutral. Repeat 5 times.

Flexion
Sitting down, bring head into neck-retraction position. Clasp hands behind head and gently guide head down, bringing chin toward chest. Stop when you feel a stretch in the back of your neck. Return to neutral. Repeat 5 times.

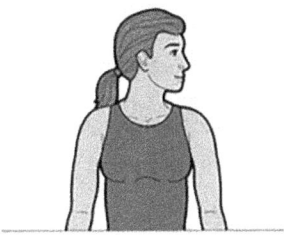

Rotation
While sitting, bring head into neck-retraction position, then gently turn head diagonally to the right so your nose is over your shoulder. Return to neutral. Repeat 5 times in each direction (left and right).

Neck pain exercises could apply to some shoulder issues. Check with your therapist and surgeon.

- **Neck Tilt.** Sit or stand, tilt your head down so your chin touches your chest. Hold for five seconds, return to starting the position. Repeat.

- **Chin Tuck.** This exercise is like the neck tilt. Sit or stand with your back and head leaning against a flat surface (a wall) to maintain good posture. Tuck your chin in with your hand and flatten the back of your neck against the wall. Repeat.

- **Side Neck Stretch.** Sit or stand and point your right arm down and out a bit from your body. Place your left hand on the top of your head and gently pull down your head to the left to stretch the muscles on the right side of your neck. Hold for ten- to thirty-seconds. Repeat on the other side.

- **Side-to-Side Neck Tilt.** Sit or stand and tilt your neck towards one shoulder, keeping your ear in line with your shoulder. Hold for five seconds, return to starting position, repeat.

- **Shoulder Shrugs.** Shrug, move, your shoulders up toward your ears. Drop them back down. Repeat.

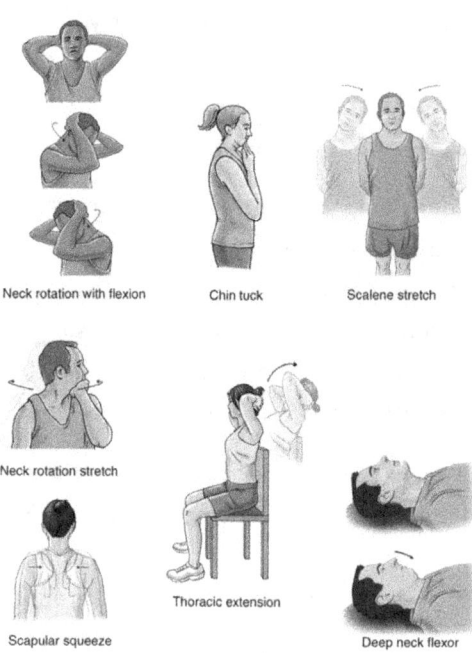

These neck exercises can help relieve neck spasms and general tightness. Always, always check with your personal trainer or physician or physical therapist about any exercises you read or hear about. Do they apply to you? If so, learn the proper way to integrate them into your ADLs.

Pinched Nerve Exercises

Many exercises can be completed in your bed or sturdy bench or table. The guidebook you received (hopefully) from your medical-team should indicate the best or the different alternatives for completing a particular exercise. For example, there is at least one alternative to performing exercises 1, 2 and 3 on the illustration shown on the next page. You could sit on your bed or bench and place your arms behind you. Lean back on your hands-arms and push out with your chest. Your arms will support you as you push your chest up-out. You should feel a stretch in your chest and shoulder area.

EXERCISING FOR YOUR PRE- POST-CONDITIONING

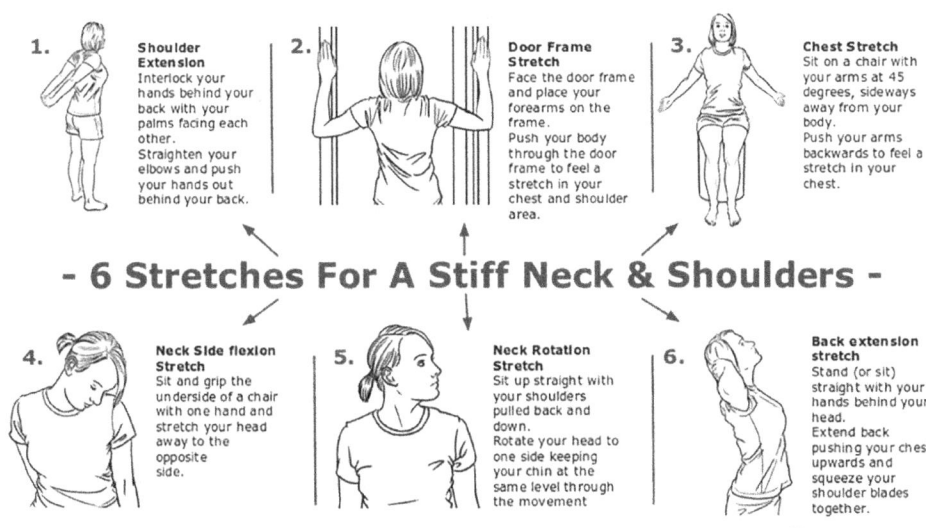

Do you drive? Do you tend to turn your head around to look for other cars or people when you back out from a parking space? Does that cause you any pain? You can reduce your neck pain before and after surgery with some of these simple ROM exercises.

- **Rotations.** Sit or stand with your back and head directly over your shoulders. Turn your head as far as you can to one side, without causing pain. Hold for thirty-seconds, turn your head to the other side, repeat.

- **Shoulder Circles.** Stand and raise your arms and shoulders straight up and move them in a clockwise circle several times. Lower your shoulder and repeat in a counter-clockwise direction.

Shoulders. If you are scheduled for shoulder surgery, you could expect

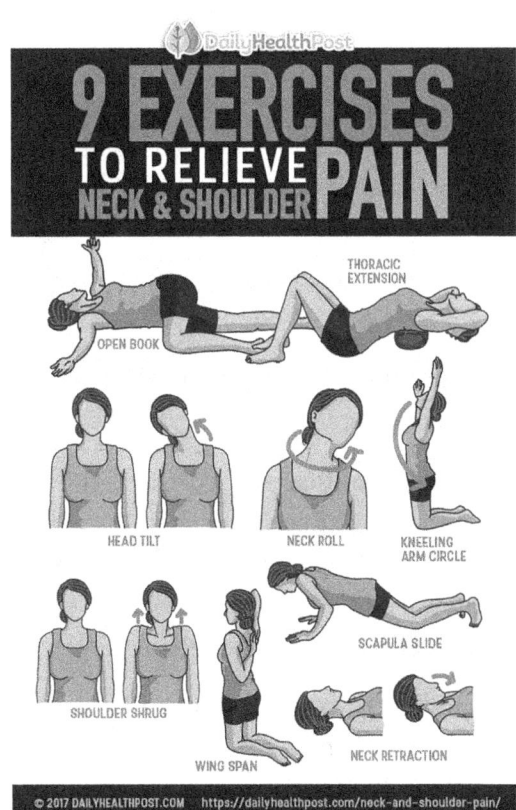

Do you have both neck and shoulder pain? If so, here are a few exercises to consider. Depending on your procedure, the scapula slide and wingspan may not be recommended by your therapist. Check that out before you do them.

Neck Strain Rehabilitation Exercises

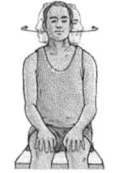
Active neck rotation

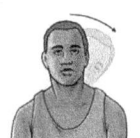
Active neck sidebend

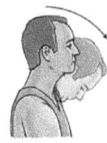
Neck flexion

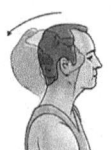
Neck extension

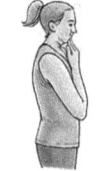
Chin tuck

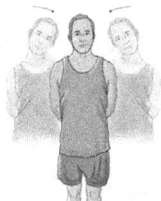
Scalene stretch

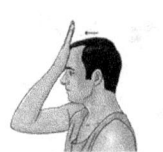
Isometric neck flexion

Again, note that some exercises could apply to different types of neck-pain issues.

your rehab to continue for six months or longer. You could return to some ADLs, such as typing and writing, in the first week after surgery so long as you do not raise your arm. Driving could begin in about a month after surgery. Returning to your ADLs such as golf or tennis and other activities that include the movement of your shoulder will only be allowed after a thorough examination by your surgeon. Don't rush it. The recovery period varies from person to person. Think in months, not weeks.

As always, check with your care-team about whether you can and should do the following exercises. Ask them to demonstrate how to do the exercises properly. Ask if they have an illustrated set of examples that you can refer to at home or work. Check out the reference provided by the Joint Replacement Center NYC, (Athwal and Elliot, *Orthoinfo.aaos.org*, 2017).

- **Pendulum, Circular.** Bend forward from your waist and place your hand on a table or the seat of a chair for support. Lower the arm of your affected shoulder so your hand is pointing straight down towards the floor. Rotate your arm in a clockwise circular pattern. This movement should occur through your shoulder joint, clockwise for about ten-times, then counterclockwise for ten-times. Repeat as directed.

- **Shoulder Forward Elevation.** Sit or lie down on the floor or an elevated table or bed. Clasp your hands together and lift your arms above your head, keeping your elbows as straight as possible. Hold for ten- to twenty-seconds, lower your arms, repeat. If you experience pain, raise your arms as high as you can without experiencing pain, keeping elbows straight, and progress to full elevation. Use your pain level to guide you as to how high you can go. Be careful, please.

- **Shoulder Rotation.** Keep your affected arm and elbow against your body. Move

EXERCISING FOR YOUR PRE- POST-CONDITIONING

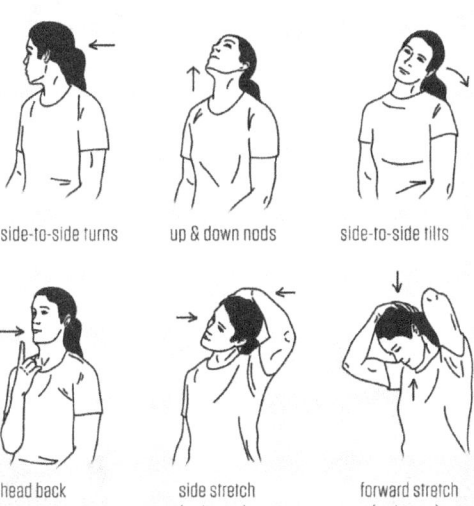

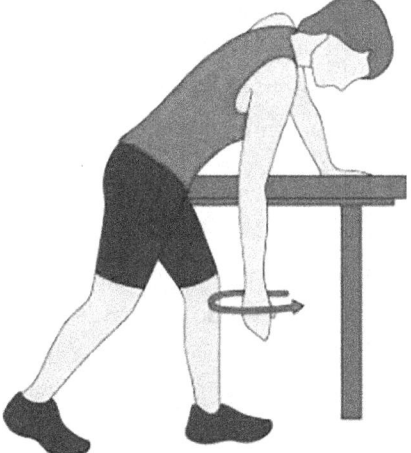

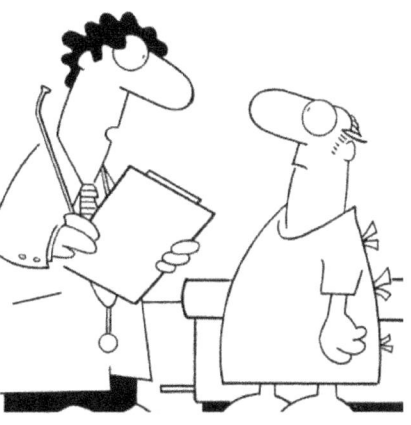

only your forearm back and forth, away from your body, keeping your elbow against your body. You could include a rolled-up towel tucked under your armpit to perform this movement, if you are cleared to do so by your care-team. Your surgeon may want to restrict the degree of outward movement (external rotation), depending on your situation. If you have not had your surgery yet, you should be able to do this exercise as a way to condition your shoulders.

- **Shoulder Abduction.** Stand and slowly extend your arm out to the side of your body, with elbow straight and palm facing the floor. Your arm should be parallel with the floor. Do not shrug your shoulder or tilt your body. Lower your arm, repeat. You may not be cleared to do this exercise after surgery, so check with your surgeon first.

You should be able to do any of the following exercises prior to surgery and include them as part of your warm-up to your ADLs- Walk-Up Exercise, and Isometric exercises, such as Shoulder Extension, Shoulder External and Internal Rotation, Shoulder Adduction and Abduction. For strengthening your shoulder, you could hold light weights, ten-pounds or less. You should only do these after surgery when cleared to do so by your surgeon and care-team.

- **Shoulder Internal Rotation (strengthening).** You could do this exercise standing or lying on your back or univolved (good) side. See the illustration on the next page. Keep your elbow bent at ninety-degrees and holding a light weight with your arm resting on a solid surface (your bed, raised table), raise your hand towards your belly. Slowly return, repeat.

- **Shoulder External Rotation (strengthening).** Lie on your *uninvolved side* keep your elbow bent at ninety-degrees and raise your arm with a light weight *away* from your belly. Slowly return, repeat.

- **Doorway Stretch.** Refer to the illustrations for neck pain in this module. Stand in an open doorway and spread your arms out to the side, touching or gripping the sides of the doorway with each hand at or below shoulder height. Lean forward through the doorway until you feel a stretch in front of your shoulders-chest. Keep your back straight as you lean into the doorway. Do not overstretch. An alternative is to sit on your bed, bench or the floor. Extend both arms behind you to support your body as you lean back and push out your chest.

- **Lawn Mower Pull.** Stand with your feet shoulder-width apart and place one end of a Thera-Band (resistance band) under the foot opposite your injured/sore/affected arm. Hold the other end with the injured/sore/affected arm so the band goes across your body, diagonally. Keep your other hand on a table or your hip or knee without

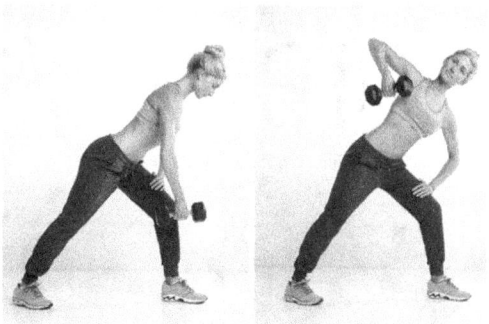

The lawn-mower pull could be recommended to you. Here you see weights included. You could also be given elastic ropes.

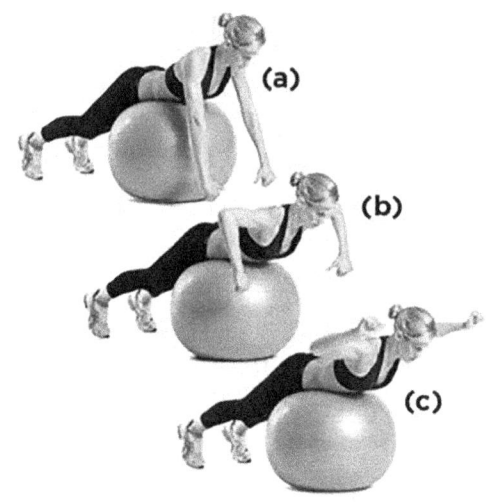

Lower Trapezium Arm raises. Modifications include resting on the ball (figure a) and extended your arms in a downward (b) or upward (c) goal-post position. Use a 55 or 65mm ball for this exercise. You exercise your trapezius, deltoid, external rotator and rhomboid muscles. Pretty good.

locking your knees, bend slightly at the waist so the hand holding the band is parallel to the opposite knee. Pretend you are starting a lawn mower and straighten upright while you pull your elbow across your favorite body to your outside ribs. Squeeze your shoulders as you stand. Repeat, slowly (Morrison, William, *Healthline*, May 13, 2016).

- **Lower Trap Arm Raise**

Isometrics. These exercises could be a bit easier for you. Isometric exercises are contractions of a specific muscle or group of muscles. During isometric exercises, the muscle doesn't noticeably change length and the affected joint doesn't move. Isometric exercises help maintain strength. They use your body to provide any resistance.

Shoulder Subluxation Rehabilitation Exercises

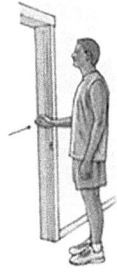
Isometric shoulder external rotation

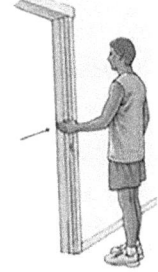
Isometric shoulder internal rotation

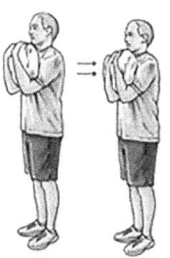
Isometric shoulder adduction

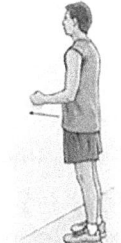
Isometric shoulder flexion

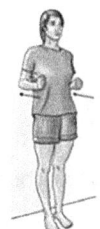
Isometric shoulder extension

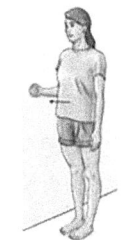
Isometric shoulder abduction

- **Isometric shoulder adduction:** Place a pillow between your chest and your arms. Squeeze the pillow with your arms and hold for several seconds.

- **Isometric shoulder flexion:** Stand facing a wall with the elbow on your injured (or painful) side bent 90 degrees and held close to your body. Press your fist forward against the wall. Hold this position for several seconds.

- **Isometric shoulder extension:** Stand facing away from the wall with the elbow on your injured side touching the wall. Press the back of your elbow into the wall, hold, rest, repeat.

- **Isometric shoulder abduction:** Stand with your injured side next to the wall and your elbow bent 90 degrees. Press the side of your arm into the wall as if you were trying to lift it. Hold, rest, repeat.

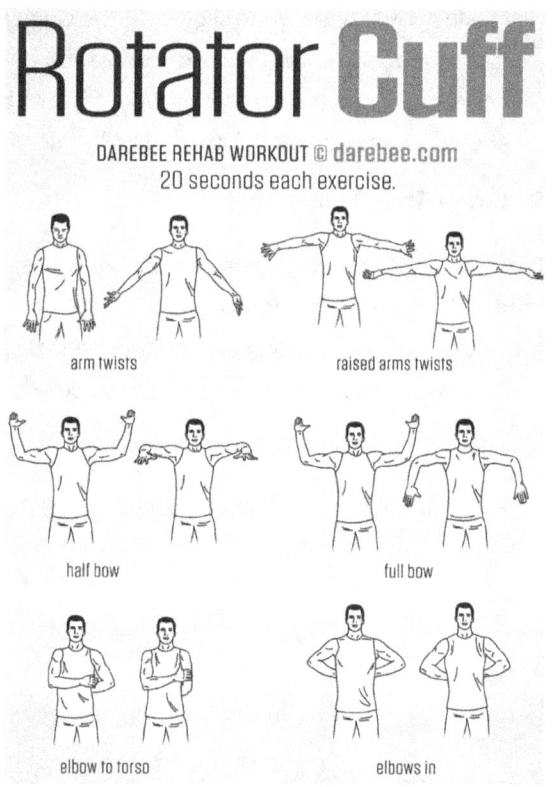

These exercises are often recommended for rotator cuff rehabilitation.

> **TIP:** Do you have a physical therapist now? If not, ask your favorite surgeon to give you a prescription for several sessions with a therapist. Your physician will identify what type of procedure you will be having. Your therapist will create a personalized exercise protocol for you. Check with your insurance company about coverage and whether you would have to pay a co-pay fee or any other fee. Check to be sure.

- **Rowing exercise:** Wrap an elastic band or tube around an immovable object, such as the leg of a sofa or a door-knob. Hold one end in each hand. Sit in a chair, bend your arms 90 degrees. Keep your back straight. Keep your forearms vertical and your elbows at shoulder level and bent 90 degrees. Pull backward on the band and squeeze your shoulder blades together. You may have access to a rowing machine. If so, check with one of the personal trainers about how to use it effectively. Make certain that you let that person know *why* you want-need to use this machine.

Push-ups. You will not be advised doing push-ups for the first weeks-months after surgery. At some point, depending on your progress, your surgeon may clear you to do them. One version that you could be cleared to do sooner is the wall push-up. Confirm this with your surgeon.

- **Push-up with a plus:** Lie on the floor or a wide and sturdy bench. Keep your hands a shoulder width apart and lift your

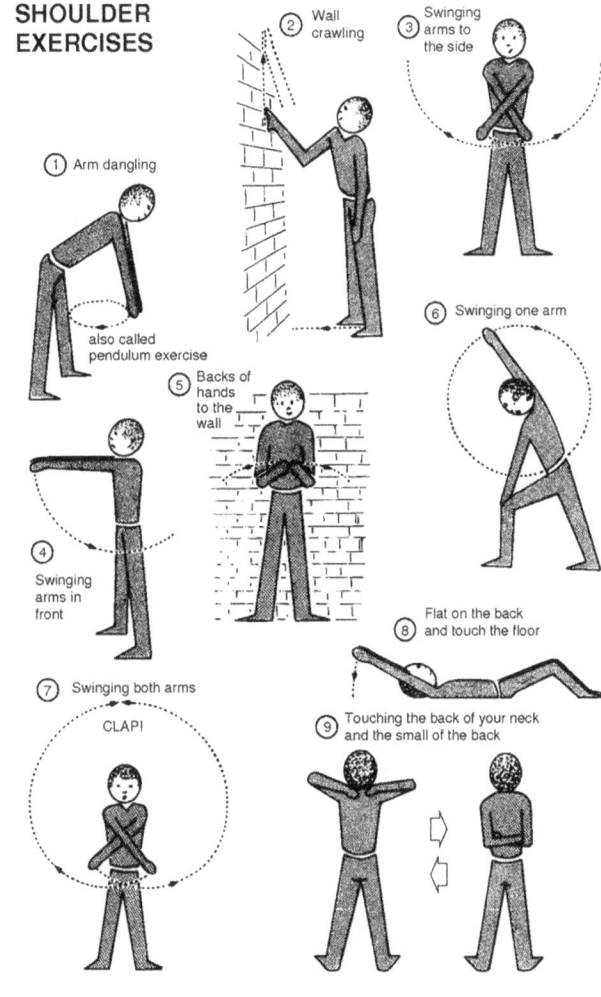

SHOULDER EXERCISES

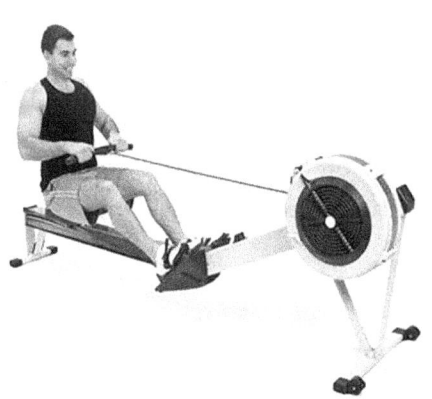

You can vary the tension on most rowing machines.

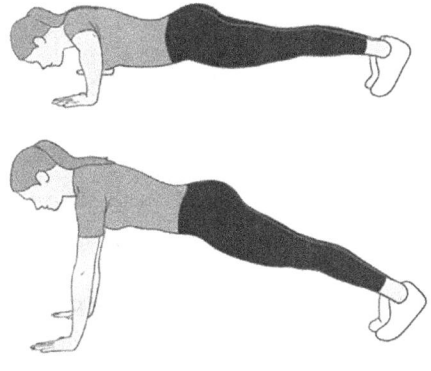

You are probably already familiar with push-ups. Your personal trainer could modify this exercise by having you keep your knees on the floor. One such modification could be doing wall push-ups.

feet off the floor. Arch your back as high as possible and round your shoulders (this is the *plus* part or the exercise). Bend your elbows and lower your body to the floor. Return to the starting position and arch your back again.

Tennis and Golfer's Elbow Exercises. If you have tennis or golf elbow you already know that it has limited your play. And it can be painful. But you do not have to play tennis or golf to experience pain doing very ordinary daily activities, such as opening doors or lifting a coffee cup. Tennis elbow is a painful inflammation of the tissue surrounding the outer side of your elbow. You can have this inflammation when you engage in other ADLs, sports and non-sports, if those activities require that you do repetitive hand, wrist, elbow and arm movements, especially while gripping something tightly, such as with a golf club, baseball, bowling ball, landscaping and gardening tools, or if you are an assembly line worker, mechanic or carpenter.

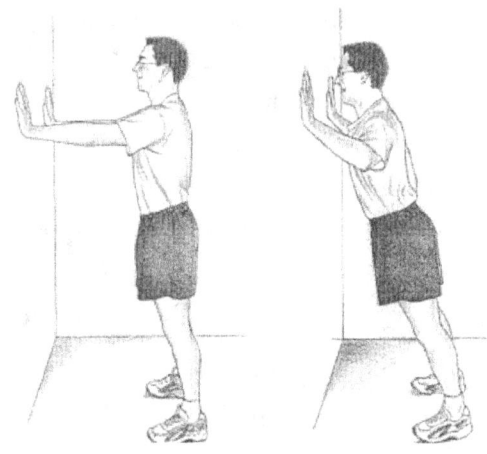

Wall Push-Ups. Are you not excited about putting your hands on the floor? Not sure you will be able to get back up, gracefully? Consider a wall. Wall push-ups may be easier for you to do, especially if you have trouble doing them in the typical floor-prone position.

Tennis elbow affects the *outer side* of your elbow and golfer's elbow affects the *inner part* of your elbow. Both describe a condition that is caused by "overusing the hand, forearm and arm muscles that result in a person having pain the elbow" (Johnson, *PTA Guide*, 2015).

If you have had (or will have) elbow surgery, your care-team prescribed a very specific protocol for you to follow. If you have not had that surgery yet, the following exercises could help you prevent and/or help your affected elbow pain from becoming worse and, perhaps, allow you to hold off surgery for a while. Check with your physician to see whether this applies to your situation.

- **Wrist Flexor Stretch (bottom of your forearm).** *Eccentric stretching* is one of the best ways to exercise for prevention. Sit or stand and extend your injured, sore or affected arm out in front of you with your palm facing the floor or resting on a table. Bend your wrist so that your fingers point up towards the ceiling. Then, with your other hand, place your palm on the tips of your injured arm's fingers and pull them back towards your body, stretching your muscles and tendons. You should feel the stretch on the underside of your forearm. This and the next three exercises are up and down movements.

- **Wrist Extensor Stretch (top of your forearm).** This is a reverse of the wrist flexor exercise. You may want to start with the wrist flexor stretch and, keeping the same position, restrict your fingers from being pulled back by your other hand. Bend your wrist in the opposite direction so now your fingers are pointing towards the floor. With your non-injured hand, place your palm over the back of your injured arm's hand and pull towards your body stretching the muscles and tendons in your forearm. You should feel the stretch in the top of your forearm.

- **Wrist Curls.** Use only small hand weights, between one- and five-pounds. No heavy lifting here. Sit and rest your affected forearm on your thigh so that the weight is hanging over the front of your knee. With your palm facing the ceiling, start curling the weight towards the ceiling. Reverse this motion and let the weight go back down towards the floor rolling to the end of your finger-tips, while still holding on to the weight. Do not use your biceps muscles. No biceps curls. You are working your wrist.

- **Reverse Wrist Curls.** Here you reverse the direction of your palm so that it faces the floor. Rest your forearm on your thigh and curl the weight up towards the ceiling. With both exercises use a slow and controlled motion with light weights. Start with ten-repetitions and increase the reps as you progress.

- **Tennis Ball Squeezes.** Hold a dead or used tennis ball in your affected arm and squeeze. Start with ten-reps, then increase up to about twenty-five reps over time. Rest after ten-reps, then repeat for a total of three-sets. You could use this exercise for prevention and during your recovery-rehab period. Check with your physician.

Golfer's Elbow (Medial Epicondylitis) Rehabilitation Exercises

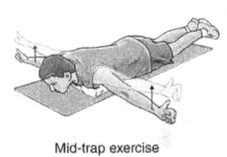
Mid-trap exercise

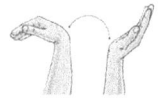
Wrist active range of motion: Flexion and extension

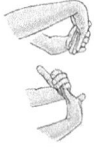
Wrist stretch

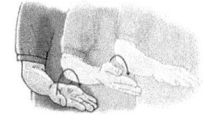
Forearm pronation and supination

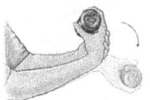
Eccentric wrist flexion

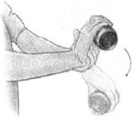
Eccentric wrist extension

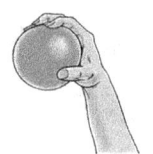
Grip strengthening

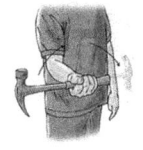
Forearm pronation and supination strengthening

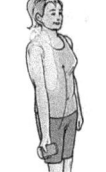
Resisted elbow flexion and extension

■ **Hammer Exercise (or forearm pronation).** Sit and rest your elbow on a flat surface or your thigh. Hold a hammer straight out and rotate your hand in a motion called *supination*. This is where your palm is facing upward or outward as though you were hammering something or turning a doorknob. You could use a light-weight dumbbell. Grip the dumbbell so your hand is at one end of the dumbbell. Turn your hand in a left and right motion. This provides torque and can help to strengthen your forearm. This is a side to side movement.

Other exercises include using a Thera-Band Flexbar, a Rubber Bar or a Broomstick with an exercise called the *Tyler Twist* (*www.bpp2*, Tyler-twist).

- Place your sore elbow by your side and bent at 90°
- Hold the Flexbar® in the hand of the sore elbow
- Extend or bend the wrist backwards
- Now grab the top end of the rubber bar with the other hand
- Flex or twist the bar forward with the top hand
- Don't let the bottom hand move while twisting the top
- Hold the twist and level the rubber bar in front of you
- Control the hand of the sore elbow side while letting it flex bend forward
- You should feel pain or discomfort at the outside of the elbow
- Complete fifteen repetitions of three-sets

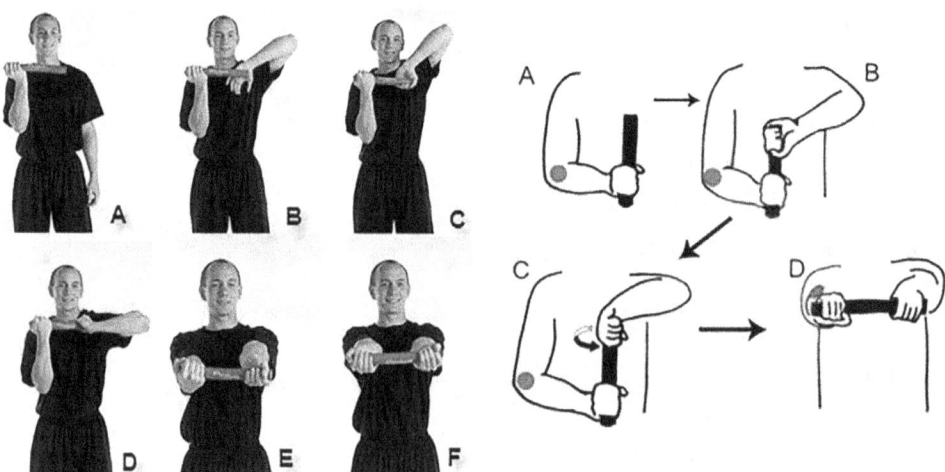

Illustrations of the Tyler Twist exercises.

Wrists and Hands. Exercises for rehabbing your wrists and hands often go together (and in some cases, your shoulders). Wrist exercises can increase flexibility and help to lower the risk of injury. Complete the exercises that are (were) recommended to you. If you have inflammation or serious joint damage you should check with your physician first. Misuse of these and other exercises could cause more harm to your hands and wrists (Minnis, *Healthline*, 2017).

- **Praying Position Stretches.** Stand and place your palms in a praying position. Your elbows and arms should be touching each other, and your hands should be in front of your face. Slowly spread your elbows apart while lowering your hands to your waist until they are in front of your belly button. You should feel a stretch. Hold for ten- to thirty-seconds, repeat. Then, extend one arm in front of you at shoulder height, with your *palm down* facing the floor. With your other hand grab your fingers and pull them back towards your body and hold for ten- to thirty-seconds. Repeat.

- **Extended Arm.** You can stretch in the opposite direction by extending your arm with your *palm facing up* towards the ceiling and with your free hand gently pull your fingers back towards your body. Hold for the same amount of time as above. Repeat both stretches with the other arm and repeat two- or three-times with each arm.

- **Clenched Fist.** Sit and place your open hands on your thighs with your palms facing towards the ceiling. Close your hands slowly into fists, but not too tightly. Raise your fists off your thighs and back towards your body, bending at the wrist. Think of this as doing a biceps or barbell curl, without the weights. Hold for ten-seconds, lower your fists and open your fingers wide. Repeat. The motion for this exercise is the same as wrist curls as described above without the weights.

- **Desk Press.** Sit and place your palms face up under a desk

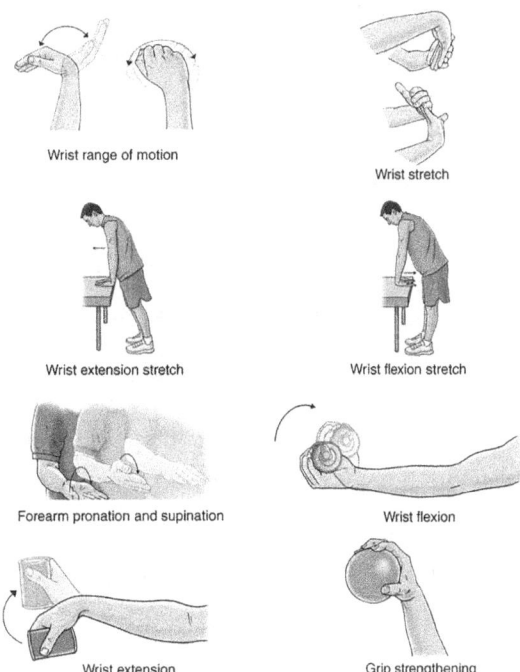

Wrist Tendon Injury Rehabilitation Exercises

or table, then press upwards against the bottom of the desk or table. Hold for five- to ten-seconds. This can build strength in the muscles that run from your wrists to your inner elbows.

- **Grip Strengthening.** Start with soft ball (maybe with one of those *stress-relief* balls) and work up to a firmer ball, such as a tennis ball. Squeeze, hold, rest, repeat.

For strengthening exercises, you can hold a can (pictured) or a hammer handle and increase the weight as you make progress (wrist extension). Hold a can or hammer handle and bend your elbow 90-degrees slowly bending your hand so that your palm is up, then down (forearm *pronation* and *supination*). Another option using the *wrist radial deviation* exercise involves placing your wrist in a sideways position with your thumb up. Hold a soup can or hammer handle and gently bend your wrist up, with your thumb moving towards the ceiling, keeping your forearm against your body.

Carpal Tunnel Rehabilitation Exercises

Wrist range of motion
Tension glide
Mid-trap exercise
Pectoralis stretch
Scalene stretch
Thoracic extension
Wrist stretch
Scapular squeeze
Wrist extension
Shoulder abduction

Note, again, you have seen these exercises for other upper body issues.

> **TIP:** Just for fun, do you want to check your blood circulation? Clench your fists, tightly, for a few seconds, then release and open your hand. Initially, your hand will be pale or lighter in color in most areas, then rapidly turn to your normal skin color within two- to three-seconds. If so, according to the folks at the Mayo Clinic, this is a good sign. If it takes longer, chat with your physician to see what (s)he thinks is happening and what, if any, next steps should take place.

Core Body Parts. Your core includes your abdomen, back and butt. When your core is strong and you are holding your head in a neutral position, that is upright and square to your shoulders, your neck should not have to work as hard.

Strengthening your core is important for your tennis, golf and other sports to alleviate or prevent back pain. Core muscles are important in the centralized area of your body because they provide you with the power to rotate your body and create greater club head speed and impact on the golf ball, for example. Baseball players, tennis players, gardeners and anyone else who need and want to have a more conditioned back with less pain while rotating their back, would benefit from core exercises. There are at least three exercises to consider: the plank, medicine ball and the Russian twist (Neighbors, *Golf Fitness Plan*, 2006).

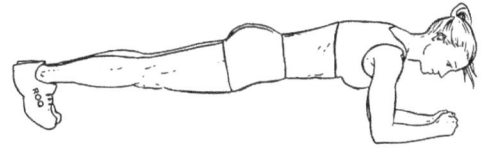

This is the typical position for a plank exercise. Your therapist can vary the positions for you and could include the use of weights. Keep your body parallel to the floor. No sticking your butt in the air. No bending your head-chin to the floor.

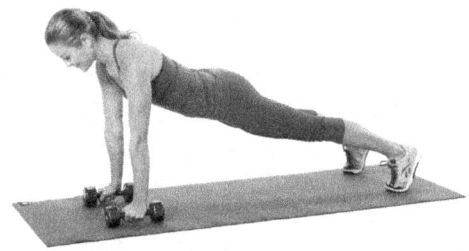

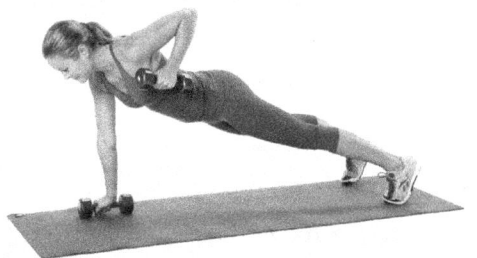

Variations of the plank and push-ups.

- **Plank.** One excellent core exercise to consider is the plank. Start with a goal of ten-seconds, then do the plank for up to sixty-seconds as you progress. Balance yourself on your hands and toes as though you were doing push-ups. Keep your back parallel to the floor mat or an elevated table for up to thirty- to sixty-seconds as a longer-term goal.

- **Medicine Ball (half-golf swing).** Stand with your feet at hip-width apart and hold the ball as though you were about to swing your club, bat or racquet. Swing the ball to the right and left side halfway up, then bring it back down and repeat. Start with a smaller, lighter ball and gradually progress to at least an eight- to ten-pound ball. You could progress to a heavier ball or increase the number of exercises. You can also swing the ball to the far left, then to the far right side of your body.

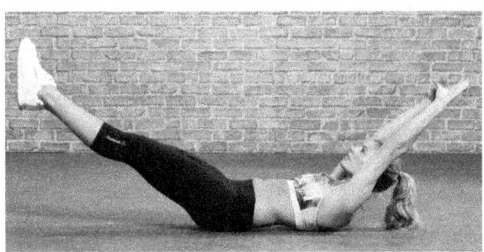

The Hollow-Man, Hollow-Men or Hollow-Body exercise is another great exercise for strengthening your core muscles.

- **Russian Twist.** Lie on your back, balancing yourself with your head, neck and shoulders. Your feet should be flat on the floor. Extend your arms to the ceiling and slowly twist to each side while keeping your balance on the ball. Note the alternative body position in this illustration.

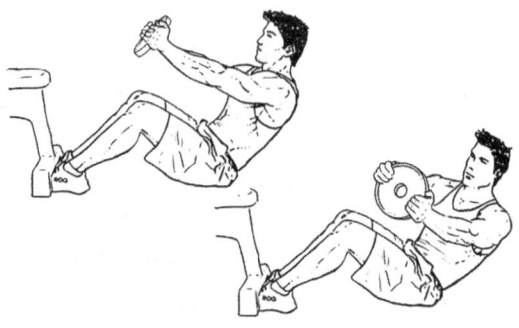

Russian Twist (WorkoutLabs.com).

- **Curl Ups (or crunches).** Lie on your back and raise or *curl* your shoulders about two-inches off the floor or bed. Keep your chin slightly tucked in towards your

- **Bird Dog, Side Bridge, Front Bridge, Push-Up Plus, and Planks** are also possibilities and are illustrated later in this module.

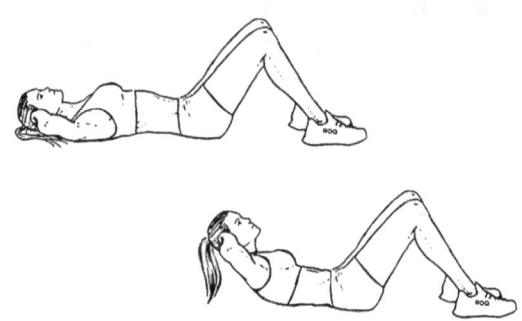

Compare the position of your body with curl ups, crunches and the Russian Twist.

There is a difference between an exercise that is for *prevention* versus one that is for *recovery*. Prevention exercises can involve weights to help build strength. Recovery exercises often focus on repetition without using weights. And when you use weights, you should *not* be thinking about weightlifting that cross-trainers, body builders, gym-junkies or others perform. Light weights are the rule. The muscles that you use to build up your post-surgery protocol need time to regain their full range of motion and strength. Start slowly, lightly with no herky-jerky motions. Be patient. If you believe the weights are too light for you, increase the number of repetitions.

Upper and Lower Thoracic Body Parts. As we travel down your thoracic highway you will learn about exercises for the mid-part of your back. Consider incorporating these exercises not just because you are having surgery, but also as an on-going part of your daily activities after surgery and well beyond after your rehab protocol has been completed.

Two core exercises to consider for multiple body-parts are the **Cat and Cow** and the **Bird Dog**. Both exercises target the deep stabilization muscles of your core building strength in the abdominal muscles, spine, back (upper, mid, and lower back), hip flexors, hip extensors and your glutes.

Upper Back Pain Rehabilitation Exercises

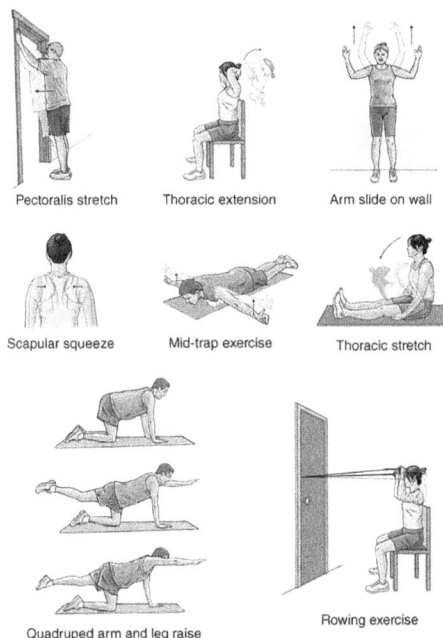

Note that many of the exercises apply to different body parts and can be incorporated to help ease your pain. For example, you could use these exercises to strengthen your shoulders and help you push, drag, to reach overhead, and pull stuff. As always, check with your physician and physical therapist.

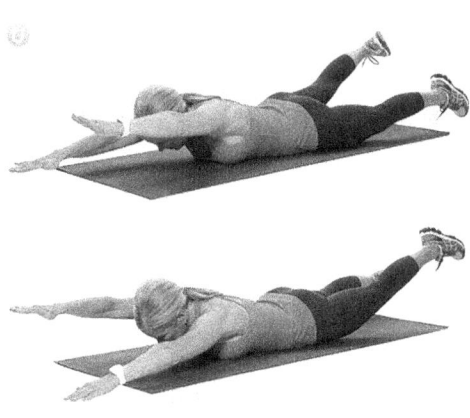

Pilates swimming exercise (**Gethealthyu, pilates**).

Low Back Pain Exercises

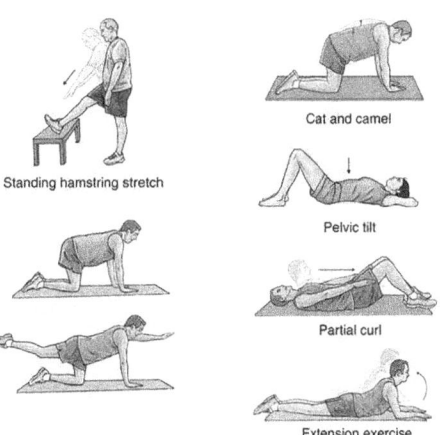

Low back pain can be another real pain that you may have lived with for a long time. You can do these and almost all the low-impact exercises in this module without the need for special equipment or fancy workout attire and maybe the best part is that you can do them at home.

Lower Back Stretches

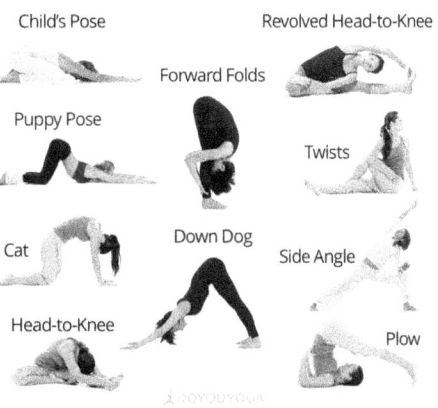

Yoga stretches. So *y*ou think you are flexible? You do not have to belong to a yoga class to do these exercises. Be careful with these exercises and check with your therapist if they apply to you.

GETTING YOUR ADL GROOVE IN GEAR WITH PAPS

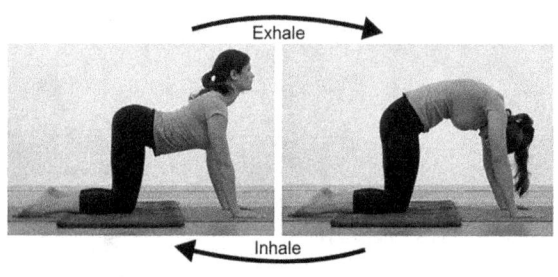

Use the Cat/Cow exercise to strengthen and stretch your abdominals and spinal muscles. Arching your back towards the ceiling (for the Cat portion of the exercise), strengthens your abdominals and stretches your spinal muscles.

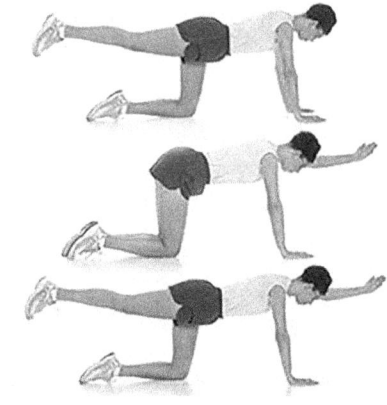

Bird Dog exercise can be called the quadruped arm/leg raise or the arm and leg extension exercise. Bird Dog is easier to remember.

Lower Spinal Body Parts: Want pain? Fracture your sacrum or coccyx and you will have your wish. The *sacrum* is located at the bottom of your spinal column. It is composed of five bones fused together. The sacrum helps anchor your lower back to your hip bone. Fracture the sacrum and you will experience some nasty pain and probably weeks or months of bed rest with some degree of immobility.

Your tailbone is called the *coccyx* and is the last three to five vertebrates at the bottom of your spine. You can injury the sacrum or coccyx by falling backwards on to the floor or stairs. A broken tailbone is very painful that may last for months

Spondylolysis and Spondylolisthesis Rehabilitation Exercises

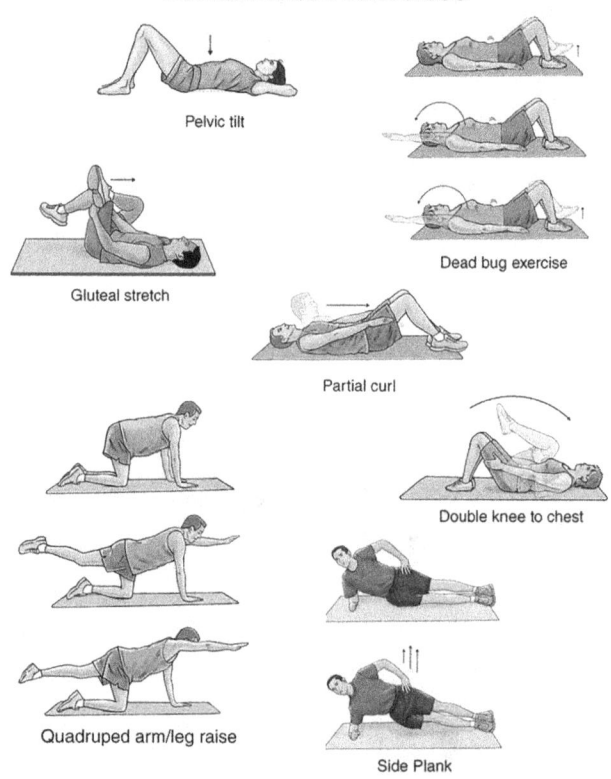

You may have more serious back-pain problems and, if so, perhaps these exercises would be approved for you by your therapist. Compare these exercises with those recommended for low-back pain.

or years. Some relief could be achieved through exercises described earlier and a relief pillow.

Doubtless, you have already seen a physician if either of these problems affected you. Your physician should recommend a very specific protocol for you based on the condition of your fracture or break and overall physical condition. Perhaps these can help you.

Sacrum and Coccyx (Tailbone)

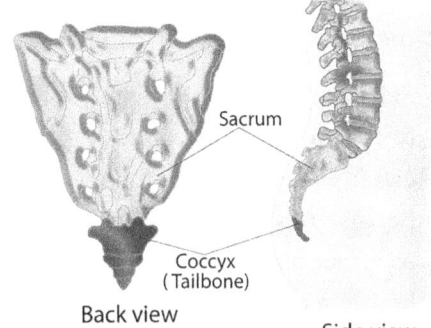

Bed rest and these exercises could be part of your rehabilitation process.

- **Squats.** Stand with your feet hip-width apart with toes slightly turned out. Extend your arms straight out in front of you and slowly sit back as if you were about to sit on a chair. Keep your heels on the floor and bend down until your knees are over your toes (check with your physician if you can-should go down to this position).

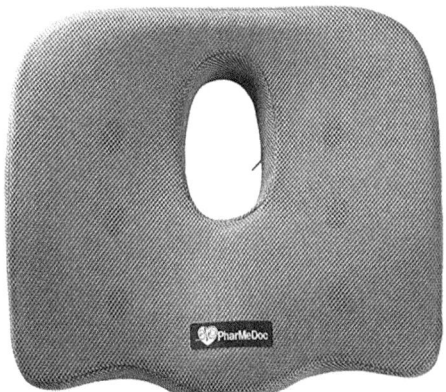

A relief pillow for fractured sacrum or coccyx.

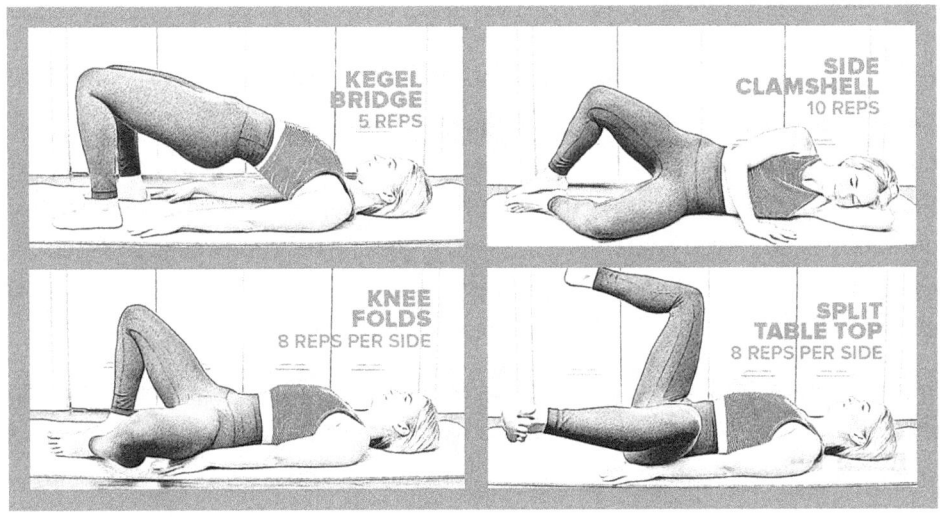

Compare the Kegel Bridge with the Pelvic Lift later in this module. Also, review the information about piriformis syndrome later in this module. Those exercises could be included in your tailbone protocol.

- **Cat/Cow Stretch.** Described above, this exercise stretches the spinal muscles.

- **Pelvic Lock** or **Mula Bandha** or **root lock.** Usually associated with yoga poses, one pose is to contract your core as though you wanted to hold in a bowel movement. Tighten those muscles as hard as you can and hold for ten-seconds. Release. Repeat.

These illustrations demonstrate other poses you may be cleared to do.

Exercises for Sciatica
A Way to Preserve Back Health

Sacroiliac Pain Rehabilitation Exercises

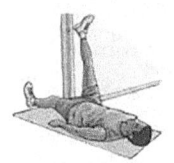
Hamstring stretch on wall

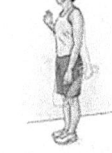
Quadriceps stretch

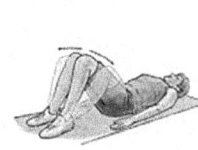
Hip adductor stretch

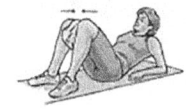
Isometric hip adduction

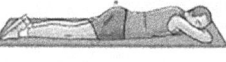
Gluteal sets

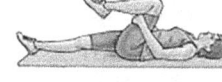
Single knee to chest stretch

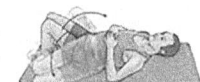
Lower trunk rotation

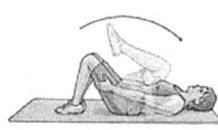
Double knee to chest

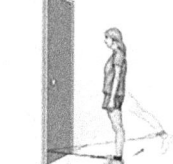
Resisted hip extension

Is it your lower back? Or, could it be your sciatica nerve that is causing your leg or foot to go numb or causing pain to shoot down from your hip area? Check with your physician about what is causing the problem and what types of exercises could help alleviate your pain and discomfort. These exercises could help relieve the pain caused by the sciatica nerve.

Lower Body Exercises: Hips to Feet

Hip and knee surgeries are relatively common. Any upper body issue can be a real problem, especially if reaching and pulling and pushing are part of your ADLs. Yet you should still be able to walk and have mobility. Maybe not so much with lower-body issues, especially those that affect your footsies and ankle areas. We'll start off easy with hips and knees and include a variety of exercises that can help strengthen joint and soft-tissue and provide you with more flexibility and movement and lower your pain level.

Hips and Knees. You should find these exercises very helpful if you are scheduled for either hip or knee surgery. Include them with your ADL routine. These exercises generally would be recommended to you both prior to and after a knee or hip operation. They can strengthen the muscles that support your joints, reduce fatigue and muscle soreness, improve circulation and speed up your overall recovery and healing process. All of these are low-impact and can be performed under the supervision of your physical trainer or personal trainer or by yourself in the comfy-ness of your home. Do them on your bed or elevated table or on the floor if you are able to get up and down easily. Do at least ten-repetitions at a time. Slowly. Safely.

- **Ankle Pumps.** This exercise helps with circulation and blood flow. Lie on your back and flex your foot up and down, with toes pointing down and away from your body. You can do one foot at a time or do both ankles at the same time, ten times.

- **Quad Sets.** This helps with circulation and blood flow and strengthens the front of your leg, your thigh muscles. Lie on your back with your legs straight out. Push your knee down into the bed or whatever it is you are lying on, tightening your muscles as you push down.

- **Gluteal Sets.** This is a bit racy, but simple. Lie on your back and clench or squeeze your butt-bum as hard as you can. Squeezing and releasing helps with circulation and blood flow while strengthening your hips.

- **Quadriceps (Wall squats).** Quad muscles are those big babies that live on top of your upper legs. Doing this exercise strengthens those muscles which provide stability to your legs. You can stand against a wall with or without a large exercise ball and with feet slightly apart slide down the wall, keeping your butt slightly higher than your knees.

- **Seated Quad Lifts.** Raise yourself from a sturdy chair *without* using your arms or any device, such as a cane or walker. Your natural tendency may be to use your arms to lift yourself up and off a chair, but don't do that if you are working on these leg muscles. Practice using your legs only, without any assistive device. Compare this exercise with the squats exercise described above. If you use your arms, you will be working your upper body rather than your lower body. There is no crime doing both and working upper and lower muscles is a wise move. Both are effective. Do both.

- **Short Arc Quads (Lying Kicks).** You can build strength and endurance of your quadricep muscle with this exercise. Lie on your back with a towel rolled under your knee. Slowly straighten your knee by lifting your foot up while keeping your thigh on the towel. Repeat for each leg.

- **Standing Hip Abduction.** This exercise targets the hips and knees. It builds strength, improves hip mobility and helps to increase your balance and core stability. Stand next to a chair or piece of furniture, a railing or your walker for support and safety. While standing (you can hold on to something if necessary), spread your leg out to the side. Keep your leg straight with your toes pointed forward. Return your leg to an upright position and repeat.

- **Heel Slides.** Another easy-peasy exercise. This is a ROM exercise that strengthens the muscles on the top of the thigh and builds knee flexion. Lie on your back with your legs straight out. Bend your affected knee by sliding your heel toward your butt. Repeat with the other knee.

- **Straight Leg Raises.** Lie on your back. Keep your legs straight and raise them a few inches off the surface of your bed or floor and hold for a few seconds.

- **Standing Knee Bends.** Steady yourself by holding on to the back of a chair or table and draw your leg up and behind you. Bend your knee so it is parallel to the floor.

- **Bridging (single and double leg).** Lie on your back. Keep your arms at your sides. Raise your hips-pelvis up towards the ceiling. Keep your knees and thighs parallel during the double leg procedure. For the single leg exercise, extend one leg straight out and perform the same hip-pelvic lift as you did for the double leg exercise. Note the similarities between the bridging and the straight leg raises. One difference is the height that you raise your leg.

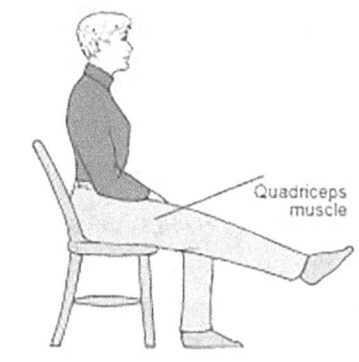

Straight-leg raise: sitting

- Other hip and knee exercises to consider include but are not limited to Sitting Knee Flexion (Knee Bending), Long Arc Quads (Seated Knee Extension), Standing Hip Extension, and the Single Leg Stance (McClure, *"Prehab Exercises", Peerwell,* 2016).

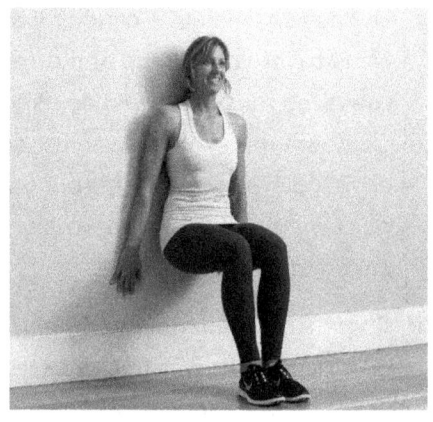

You will see illustrations or read about some of these exercises again in this module and in **Appendix Six.** Exercise both sides of your body—both hips, knees and feet—not just the side that is scheduled for surgery.

Quad Wall Squats. *You can simply use a wall to slide up and down on or use a large ball placed at the small of your back. You can also remain in the position you see in the photograph for thirty-seconds (or so), without sliding up or down.*

EXERCISING FOR YOUR PRE- POST-CONDITIONING

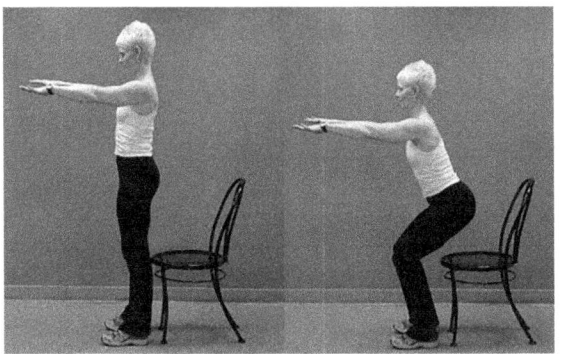

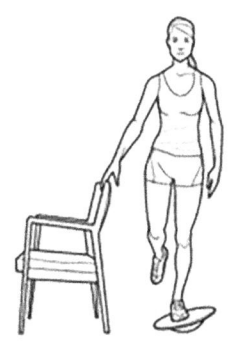

Seated quad lifts. Raise yourself from a chair with leg-power only. Do not push off with your arms or hands. Do not use a cane or walker or a piece of furniture to lift yourself. No grabbing unless you feel unsteady or unsure of yourself. Another great low-impact exercise.

Wobble-board. Use a stable chair to balance-support yourself as you rotate your feet on a wobble-board.

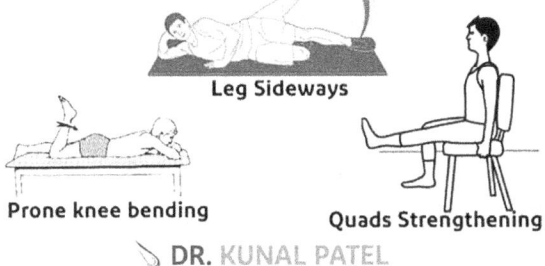

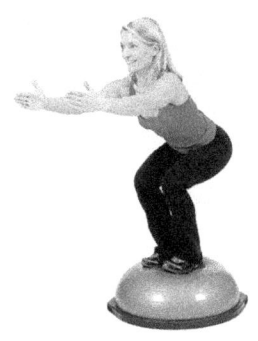

Bosu balance ball can help your balance. You may want to do this near something you can hold on to when you first decide to use it.

Use these low-impact exercises to reduce knee pain while strengthening your lower-leg muscles.

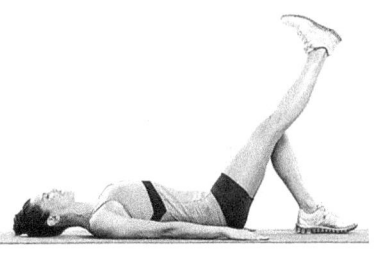

Straight leg, bridging and Pelvic Lift raises. There are variations to these leg raises. You can keep your back and butt flat on the floor or the bed. You can raise one leg a few inches and hold it for a few seconds. Repeat with the other leg. You can raise your butt while keeping your feet flat on the floor. You could raise one leg and your butt. Double-leg Bridging, Pelvic Lift and Single-leg bridging can strengthen your back and your core, hips, and thighs. For the Pelvic Lift you raise your butt as high as you can as noted in the illustration below. Use an elevated surface, such as a bed or exercise table, if you find it a bit difficult to get down and up from the floor.

Meniscal Tear Rehabilitation Exercises

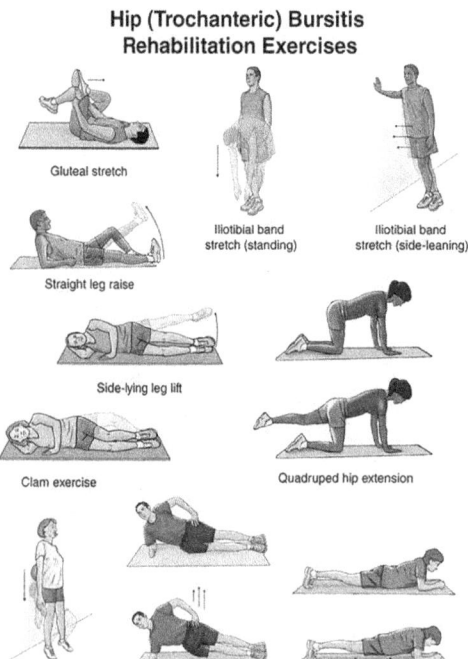

You can use any of these exercises if you are recovering from a Meniscus tear.

Hip (Trochanteric) Bursitis Rehabilitation Exercises

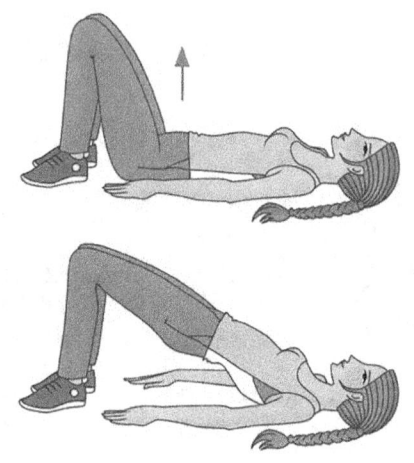

The Pelvic Lift.

Have you ever had a stiff or sore spot along the outside of your leg that ran from your hip to your knee? The culprit could be your IT band. The *iliotibial band* (IT band), also known as the iliotibial tract or Maissiat's band, is a long section of connective tissue, or fascia, that runs along the outside of your leg from the hip to the knee and shinbone. The function is to help abduct and rotate your hip. There are different stretching exercises you can do to alleviate the pain and stiffness. You can do the exercises with an elastic band, towel or rope.

IT band. Your therapist may indicate that IT band exercises could help reduce the pain you may be having. Often after hip (or knee) surgery any issues you were having with your IT band go away. Clarify that with your surgeon.

Notice that the plank and other exercises apply to other body parts and, therefore, provide you with multiple benefits.

EXERCISING FOR YOUR PRE- POST-CONDITIONING

Iliotibial Band Syndrome Rehabilitation Exercises

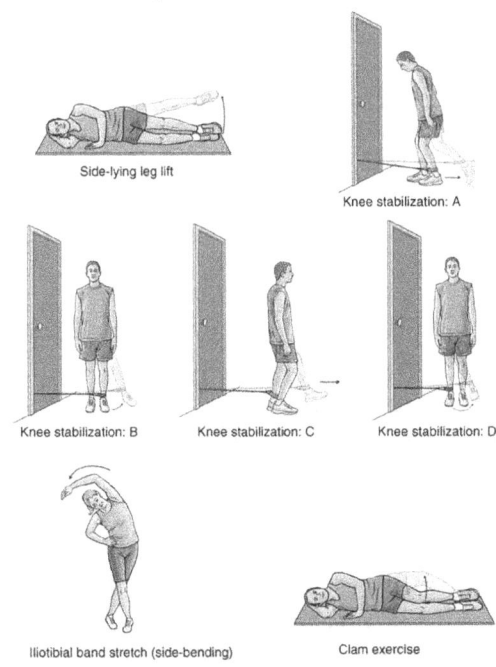

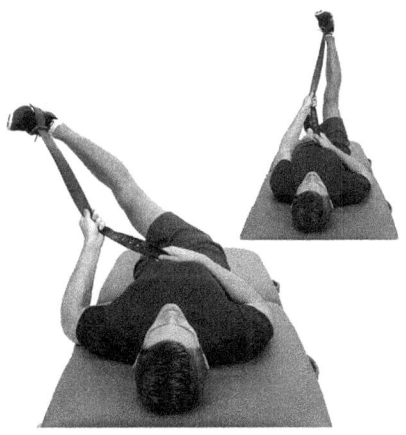

An easy IT-band exercise for stretching. Use an elastic band, towel, belt or other handy device and stretch your right leg over your left leg and vice versa as illustrated. While in this position you could work your hammies. If you want to work your hamstring muscles, bring your leg straight up to 90-degrees, or as much as you can. You can pull on your leg to get a good stretch using a band, towel or belt.

IT band. *Iliotibial stretch exercises with and without an elastic band. Again, note how one exercise can be used for multiple ailments. As you may have noticed, most of these low-impact exercises can be done in the comfyness of your own home, when you want.*

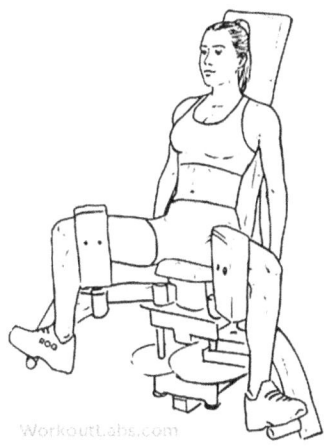

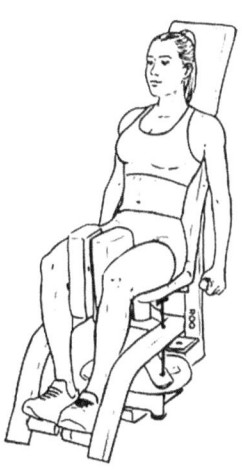

Exercising your thighs and butt with an adductor machine. You can adjust the weight resistance as you want. The adductor machine strengthens and develops your inner thighs, which is a difficult area to train because it is not overly used. The machine can provide exercise to the area by focusing (isolating) on these inner thigh muscles. Will this exercise help you condition your hip area? Ask your therapist.

Runner's Knee (Patellofemoral Pain Syndrome) Rehabilitation Exercises

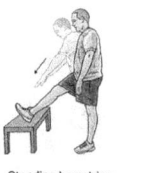
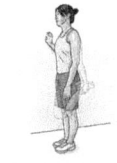
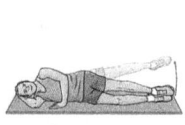

Standing hamstring stretch | Quadriceps stretch | Side-lying leg lift

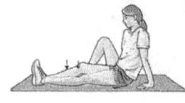
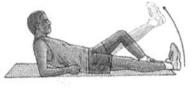

Quad sets | Straight leg raise

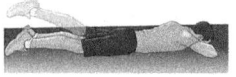
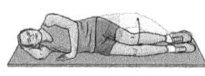

Prone hip extension | Clam exercise

Whether you are a runner or not, these are great exercises for your knees and lower body joints and muscles. Your pain could lessen as you gain flexibility with these exercises.

Hamstring Strain Rehabilitation Exercises

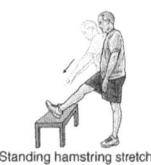
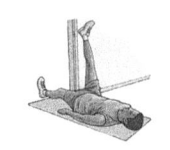

Standing hamstring stretch | Hamstring stretch on wall

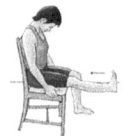
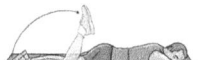

Slump stretch | Prone knee bend

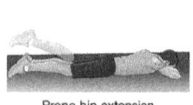
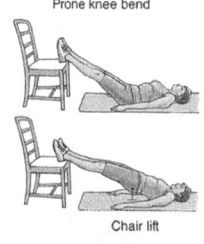

Prone hip extension | Chair lift

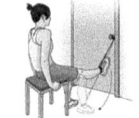
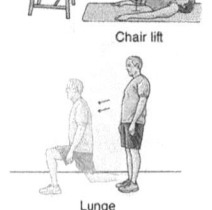

Resisted hamstring curl | Lunge

Butt Pain. Maybe some folks said that you are a pain in the butt or bum or words that approach that label. If so, the following exercises will not eliminate that moniker, but they can relieve butt pain that is the result of arthritis or some other infirmity.

Sometimes what you think is lower back pain is really *piriformis syndrome*. The piriformis muscle travels down your lower back to the top of your thigh. The sciatic nerve travels from your lower spine through your butt to the back of your thigh. If you have had an injury or inflammation in the muscle, you would have felt pain (called *sciatica*) especially if you have been driving for a while or standing

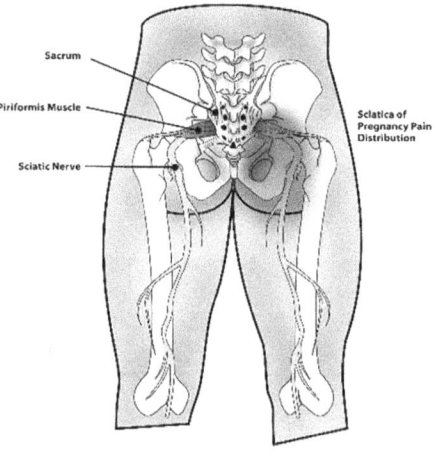

Sciatic nerve and Piriformis muscle. A pinched sciatic nerve could create numbness or tingling from your butt to your foot. Stretching exercises can help and you may want to consider the exercises shown here. Consult with your physician and exercise before you consider surgery. What does your physician say is the cause of your pain? What exercises do they recommend?

EXERCISING FOR YOUR PRE- POST-CONDITIONING

up or walking or running. You may also have experienced numbness or a tingling sensation. There are a series of piriformis stretches that could relieve some of the pain. These non-surgical exercises can help you stand, walk or drive your car with less pain and discomfort.

An article written by Stephanie Watson and reviewed by Suzanne Falck, MD identifies seven specific piriformis exercises you can do to help alleviate your sciatica and resulting pain (*Healthline*, 2017). In addition to those exercises, the exercises in the illustration are from *pbs.twimg.com/media*.

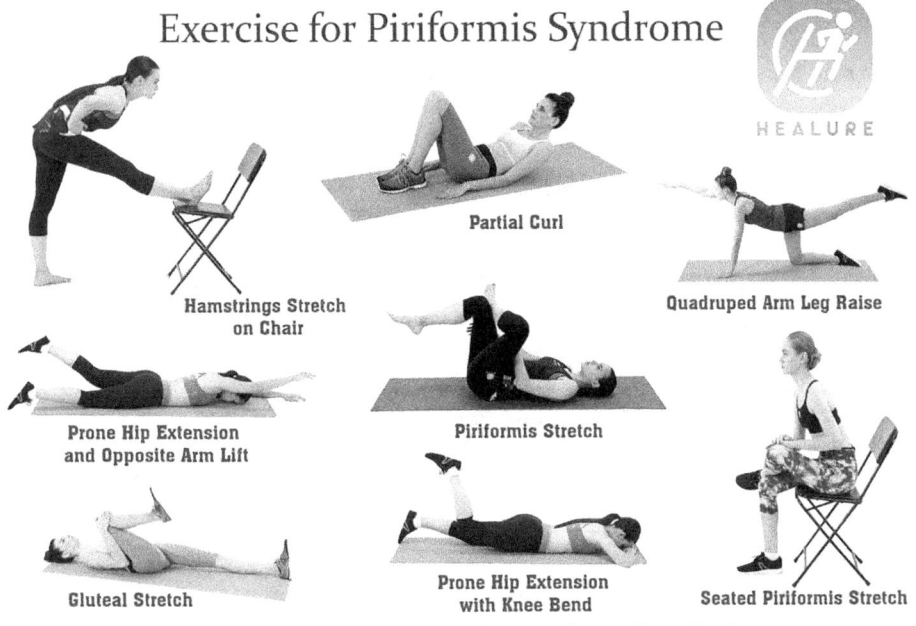

Again, note how you can use the same exercise for multiple body parts.

Knee to Chest. This exercise works your lower back, the front of your hip and inner thigh.

- Lie on your back on the floor with your legs extended straight out.
- Bend one knee and grasp your shinbone with your hands.
- Gently pull your knee toward your chest so long as you are comfy.
- Hold the stretch for 20 to 30 seconds and then relax for 20 to 30 seconds.
- Repeat on the other side; then repeat the entire sequence four times.

Piriformis Stretch. This will help open your hips and relieve your butt pain.

- Lie on your back with knees bent and feet flat on the floor.
- Cross one leg on top of the other, so one ankle is resting on the opposite knee.
- Grab through the legs and pull the bent-knee leg up toward your chest until you feel a stretch in your buttock and hip.
- Hold the stretch for 20 to 30 seconds, then relax for 20 to 30 seconds.
- Repeat on the other side; then repeat the entire sequence four times.
- Use a towel or elastic band to pull your leg up.

Hamstring Stretch. Exercise the back of your thigh and behind your knee.

- Lie on the floor with both knees bent.
- Lift one leg off the floor and bring the knee toward your chest. Clasp your hands behind your thigh below your knee.
- Straighten your leg and then pull it gently toward your head until you feel a stretch. (If you cannot clasp your hands behind your leg, loop a towel around your thigh. Grasp the ends of the towel and pull your leg toward you.)
- Hold for 20 to 30 seconds and then relax for 20 to 30 seconds.
- Repeat on the other side; then repeat the entire sequence four times. Do not pull at your knee joint.

Hip Abduction. Strengthen your outer thigh and buttocks.

- Lie on your side with your right leg on top and the bottom left leg bent to provide support.
- Straighten your top leg and slowly raise it to 45°. Keep your knee straight, but not locked. Hold for five seconds.
- Slowly lower your leg and relax it for two seconds.
- Repeat up to 8 to 12 times, then switch and repeat on the other side.
- Do not turn your leg in order to raise it higher. The outside of your thigh should be lifted toward the ceiling.

Bird Dog Stretch (Arm-Leg Raise). You read about this earlier. Here it is again.

- Start on all fours on the floor, with your shoulders directly over your hands and your hips directly over your knees.

- Raise your right arm out at shoulder height and level with the rest of your body.
- With your right arm still up, raise your left leg straight back so it's level with the rest of your body, tightening the muscles in your buttock and thigh. Hold for 15 seconds.
- Repeat on the opposite side, raising your left arm and then your right leg.
- Keep your stomach muscles tight and your back flat for balance.

Sitting Rotation Stretch. Exercise your bum and the oblique muscles in your core.

- Sit on the floor with both legs out in front of you.
- Cross your right leg over your left leg so your right foot is outside your left thigh.
- Twist your torso toward your bent leg, putting your right hand behind you for support.
- Hook your left arm around your right knee and use it to help you twist further.
- Look over your right shoulder and hold the stretch for 30 seconds.
- Repeat on the other side, then repeat the entire sequence four times.
- Sit up and keep your bum bones (sit bones) pressed into the floor during the stretch.

Feet and Ankles. We are almost at the end of our neck-to-toe journey. Any surgery is serious, especially if the surgery involves your body. Upper body procedures carry their own issues and risks, but normally you would still be able to motor around the house and engage in almost any ADLs that involve walking. With lower body procedures, your ability to walk requires crutches or a wheel- chair or knee walker and, in some procedures, you will be required to stay off your affected foot, with no weight-bearing for at least two-weeks or so. And your recovery protocol would probably be measured in months versus weeks. How are you fixed for patience?

Your care-team will create a nice protocol just for you and your situation. That protocol could include at least three goals: strength building, flexibility and targeting specific muscles. Strengthening muscles that support your lower leg, foot and ankle will keep your ankle joint stable, relieve your pain and prevent (hopefully) further injury. Stretching your muscles can restore your ROM and prevent injury, reduce soreness and keep your muscles long and flexible. Targeting specific muscles of the lower leg are part of your conditioning process and involve the tendons and ligaments that control movement in your feet.

The following exercises do not require any special equipment and once you learn how to do them you can easily do them at home and at work and whenever you choose to take time to do them.

- **Heel Cord Stretch (or Achilles Stretch).** You should feel a stretch in your calf and heel with this exercise. Stand facing a wall with your unaffected leg forward with a slight bend at the knee. Your affected leg is straight behind you, with the heel flat on the floor and the toes pointed in slightly. Keep both heels flat and press your hips forward toward the wall. Hold for about thirty-seconds, relax, repeat. You may want to do this exercise for both legs, affected or not, both in a preventive maintenance routine and after surgery as directed by your physician.

  One alternative is to stand on your toes and front part of your foot on the lowest step of your stairs with the heel below that step. Hang your body with your toes for at least one minute initially, then extend the time as you progress. Your Achilles Tendon and lower calf area should benefit from hanging for two- to four minutes. Do not do a bouncy-bouncy while you do this exercise. Hang on to the hand-rail to keep your balance. Ask your therapist for confirmation and advice and alternatives.

- **Tennis Ball Roll.** This exercise can work your *Plantar fascia* ligament. You should feel this along the bottom of your foot. Sit or stand and roll a tennis ball under the arch of your foot for about two-minutes. If you sit, sit up tall and straight; if you stand, do not lean forward. Place as much weight as you can tolerate. Use a dresser or railing or the back of a chair for support.

- **Calf Raises.** The two main muscles that comprise the calf muscle are the *Gastrocnemius-soleus complex.* The calf muscles live in the back portion of your lower legs attached to the heel courtesy of the Achilles tendon. You should feel the stretch in your calf with this exercise. Hold on to a chair or railing, furniture or a walker for support. Stand with your weight evenly distributed over both feet. Lift one foot off the floor so that all your weight is placed on the other foot. Raise your heel as high as you can, then lower it. Repeat, but do not bend the knee of the other leg.

- **Marble or Towel Pickup.** This is a dandy. You will exercise your *Plantar flexors* and should feel this exercise at the top of your foot and toes. You will need some marbles or other small round balls or one towel. Sit or stand and place the marbles (or towel) on the floor in front of you, within reach. Use your toes to pick up one marble at a time and place them in a bowl. Repeat until you can pick up all the marbles. If you use a towel or a sock, practice picking up and releasing the towel or sock multiple times without using any marbles.

EXERCISING FOR YOUR PRE- POST-CONDITIONING

- **Towel Curls.** Grab the center of the towel with your toes and curl the towel towards you. Do not pick up the towel, just drag it towards you. Relax. Repeat. You can make this a tad more challenging by placing a weight on the edge of the towel when you are in the process of grabbing and curling it.

- **Toe Splay (spreading your toes).** This exercise can help improve control over your toe muscles. Sit and spread your toes as far apart as possible. Hold for a few seconds, repeat. Once

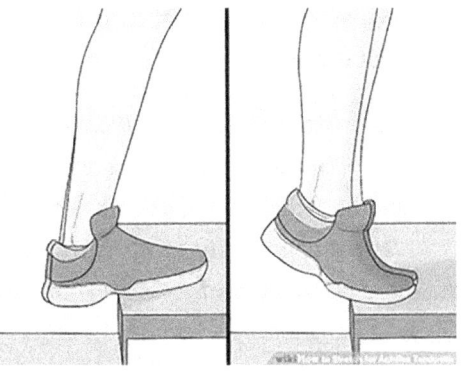

Achilles Stretch using a toe raise exercise on a step. Do not bounce. Hang your heel for a few minutes at a time. For toe raises, lift up as high as you can, hold, release, repeat. Hang on to a railing for support.

5 Simple Exercises to Help Keep Your Feet Healthy

1. Point Your Toes

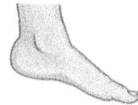

Sit in a chair with your feet flat on the floor. Lift one foot and point your toes toward the ground. Hold for 5 seconds. Repeat 3 times with each foot.

2. Raise Your Heels

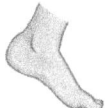

Stand up and lift your heels so that you are standing on the balls of your feet. Hold for 10 seconds. Repeat 3 times.

3. Curl Your Toes

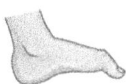

Sit in a chair with your feet flat on the floor. Lift one foot and curl your toes in. Hold for 3 seconds. Repeat 3 times with each foot.

4. Raise Your Toes

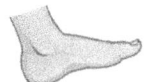

Sit in a chair with your feet flat on the floor. Keep your heels flat on the ground and raise your toes. Hold for 5 seconds. Repeat 3 times with each foot.

5. Spread Your Toes

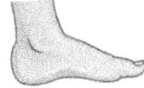

Sit in a chair with your feet flat on the floor. Spread your toes apart. Hold for 5 seconds. Repeat 3 times with each foot.

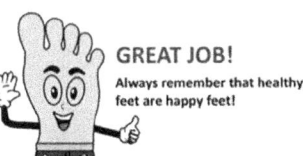

GREAT JOB! Always remember that healthy feet are happy feet!

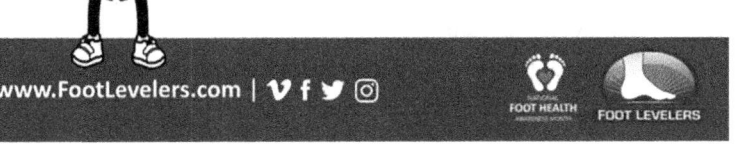

you feel comfy and want to go for something more challenging, add some strength resistance using a Thera-Band wrapped around your tootsies.

I have had PTTD surgery (Posterior Tibial Tendon Dysfunction) on my left foot and will have that same surgery on my right foot. Initially, I went to several doctors and foot-care folks who recommended that I use off-the-shelf orthotics. Use the soft variety so my foot would conform to the shape of the arch; no, use hard plastic so my foot would not conform but would remain in a set and stable position; no, use a Thomas Heel in my shoe to lift the foot up a bit. Yes, nothing worked for very long. Then I had surgery. That worked. On my back for about two weeks. Crutches. Wheel-chair. And one of the very few years that I could not get out into my yard and gardens. On to my right foot. Initially, I was given an orthotic with a felt-arch. That did not work. My current surgeon recommended a custom-made orthotic composed of a hard resin plastic with a softer liner to stabilize both my heel and tendon. I did some exercises for my calf and foot. That worked. Whew! Finally. Some of those exercises you will see below.

TIP: As a gentle reminder, whether you have had surgery or not, my suggestion is to involve both of your legs or arms to keep your body toned and in balance. Working on just one arm or shoulder or knee or hip because that is where your problem is, may not be in your best interests. Your therapist may focus on the problem area but best to confirm whether (s)he believes you should involve both legs, both arms, both shoulders and so on.

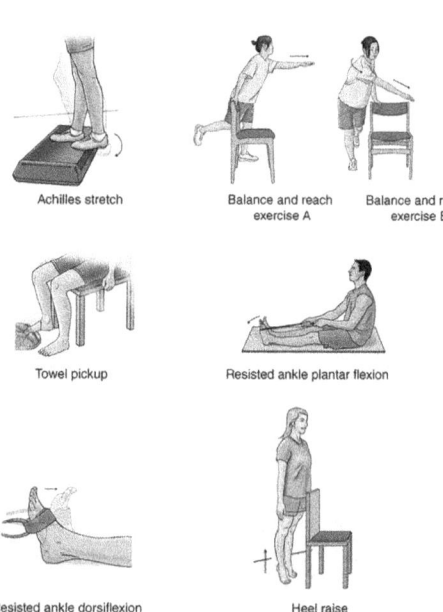

Arch Pain Rehabilitation Exercises

Achilles stretch

Balance and reach exercise A

Balance and reach exercise B

Towel pickup

Resisted ankle plantar flexion

Resisted ankle dorsiflexion

Heel raise

If you have a Plantar Fasciitis problem, perhaps your therapist will recommend one or more of these exercises.

Cross-Training

You have a problem there and you want it to go away now, so you select a specific machine or exercise to make you feel all better. And that can work. You have your routine down. You do it a couple of times a week. If you tend to get bored doing the same exercises in the same sequence, consider cross training, whether you are a runner or walker or jogger or golfer or pickle-baller. Cross-training could improve your cardiovascular fitness. It can help balance different muscle groups. It can help balance weaker muscles with the stronger ones. You can incorporate cross-training exercises with any sport, with any ADL, including gardening and your favorite exercise class. You can cross-train with a wide-range of exercises, with or without machines.

You will see high-intensity interval training exercises (HIIT) on television or on Y-tube. They are fantastic if you are younger, in fantastic shape to begin with, are willing to endure the different strenuous exercises, from running to doing push-ups to doing pull-ups to jumping up on to an elevated bench or platform to lifting heavier weights and other heart-pounding sweat-inducing activities in a relatively short period of exercise-time. Great. If you are not keen for all of that, consider these low-impact and effective exercises.

- **Cycling or Spinning.** Both can improve your cardio-fitness and increase your hamstring strength. Also consider it for leg cramps and for quad or knee pain. You can join a spinning class where the instructor directs the speed and intensity. Granted, spinning and cycling can get your heart-beating going and could be a tad strenuous for you. Cycling could be better. You can ramp up your speed on your own, on a good-old-fashion stationary bike. Your local YMCA or club usually has both.

- **Swimming.** Increase your upper body flexibility by helping to reduce your neck and upper shoulder pain and even if you are having (or recovering from) hip or knee or ankle surgery or pain in those areas.

- **Yoga, Pilates, Tai Chi.** Each could help with flexibility and balance issues with their stretching and ROM exercises.

- **Strength Training.** *Resistance training* involves using your own weight, such as when you do push-ups or plank exercises or sit-ups. *Weight training* involves using weights, such as free-weights (e.g., barbells, dumbbells) or machines (e.g., leg presses, lat-pull downs). Strength training is a great way to tighten your core and help with over all muscle toning. Weight training

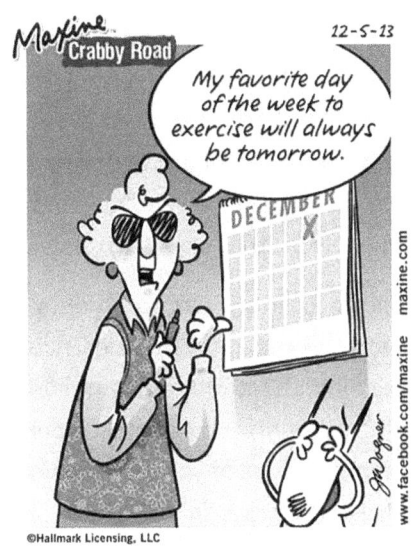

should be included in your daily-weekly exercise routine. Start (and continue) with lighter weights. Increase the number of reps you do as you feel more comfy. Weight training has at least one added benefit: you continue to burn calories even after you have stopped lifting for that session. And as you get older, include weights in your exercise class or do them on your own, several times a week.

Module Summary

Pre-surgery exercises can help condition your body. Post-surgery exercises can help you recover quickly and help you live and enjoy your life after surgery. You will be given exercises to do with a therapist or on your own. How comfy and cooperative will you be when you work through your PROM, AROM, ARM and LRE exercises? Will you be compliant or combative?

Depending on your procedure and the recommended post-surgical protocol, you will begin with a therapist who does the work for you, PROMs. Progress to an assisted set of exercises, AROMs, then on to a fully active, you-control-it process, ARMs. It will not be in your best interests to lift as much as you can for as long as you can. And stop if you experience pain. Build some endurance. Re-build your strength and flexibility. Rehabilitation is not a race. If you over-extend yourself at the beginning you could end up extending your recovery process longer than you want and, in a worst case, subject your surgical area to further injury. Not good. Forget the no pain, no gain thing. Conversely, if you baby yourself and do not exercise as prescribed, you could prolong your recovery period.

You will find additional low-impact exercises in **Appendix Six**. Most can be performed in the comfy-ness of your home or at your local YMCA or club. They can help you maintain the levels of strength and flexibility you need to live with less pain and discomfort. Always check with your personal trainer and medical care-team to identify which exercises you could incorporate, the level of intensity and duration and any other issues that would be relevant to your situation.

Weight Training. Lifting weights, even light-weights, is a form of strength training that helps keep your muscles strong. Strong muscles support your joints. This book started with arthritis and its relationship to joint problems. We have come full-circle. Lifting weights will not make your arthritis worse. Muscle-building exercises are an important part of your arthritis management plan. Muscle tissue will not turn into fat tissue, nor will fat tissue turn into muscle tissue.

EXERCISING FOR YOUR PRE- POST-CONDITIONING

Worrying about something is a lot like sitting in a rocking-chair.
You feel good about the movement,
but there is no forward progress.
You aren't going anywhere
You sit and stare.
You worry.
You procrastinate.
You sit and stare some more.
What is more important to you:
Where you are now?
What your life-style is now?
Where you would like to be?
Are you rocking in a rocking chair?
Or are you rocking ahead?

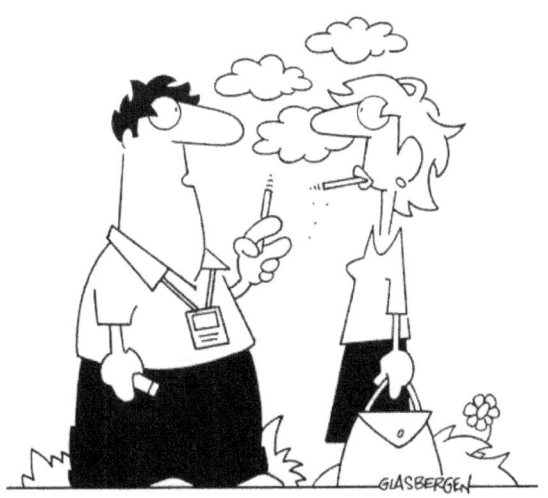

"My doctor told me to stop smoking cold turkey. That was easy, because I never smoked cold turkey in the first place!"

Your Notes

APPENDICES

MODULE A1

PREPARING MIND AND BODY

Arthritis: Natural Remedies

There are many treatments for easing arthritic pain. Some work. Most do not, regardless of the marketing and advertising. You may be familiar with many of these *remedies*.

- **Acupuncture.** You may find relief as others have. Or not. If it works for you, continue using it. If not, save your money. Asians, especially the Chinese, have used this for centuries. It is becoming popular in the USA. You may want to consider a person who has experience and a positive treatment record. While many people can provide this service, the Asians have been doing it longer and seem to be the most successful with it.

- **Assistive devices.** Shoe inserts, custom-made orthotics, canes, splints, braces can help redistribute your weight and take some pressure off your arthritic joint. You will need to wear them daily.

- **Capsaicin cream.** This can relive osteoarthritis pain and is available without a prescription. It is made from the substance that gives hot peppers their heat. It could benefit you. Wash your hands after applying it. Do not even think about rubbing your eyes or touch your lips-tongue.

- **Chiropractic therapy.** This will not help relieve your arthritis. However, it can help treat muscle spasms that can accompany arthritis. Check with your insurance company about your coverage. If it works for you, continue doing it. Otherwise, save your money.

- **Chondroitin.** Initially, this seemed promising, especially when combined with glucosamine. Recent studies indicate that it is not effective. If you have bone-on-bone, it may not work for you. You decide.

- **Exercise.** Walking is an excellent exercise as is swimming and biking. If you are a runner and are experiencing pain, cut down on the mileage; cross-train; run on softer more even surfaces, such as a tread-mill or track. Golfers, tennis players and any other sport-folk can benefit from doing some simple stretch exercises. Check with your physician or personal trainer. Most clubs will encourage you to chat with a trainer, no obligations, about what exercises to do for what ails you. Ask them to demonstrate the exercise for you so you can do them on your own at home or at work. Exercise is a great non-medication remedy. Just do it.

- **Glucosamine.** This can help, depending on the type of glucosamine you use. Glucosamine sulfate is beneficial, but glucosamine hydrochloride is not, which is what is mostly sold in the United States. There are no scientific-medical definitive trials that indicate the benefits of this to people with osteoarthritis.

- **Physical therapy.** You probably do not need this, but it can help.

- **Supplements.** Avocado soybean *unsaponifiables* (ASU) are not reliable. Rose hips and concentrated ginger could be helpful. Fish oil has anti-inflammatory properties, but more research is needed. Eating the fish provides greater benefits than swallowing the pill and usually tastes better.

- **Topical remedies.** Mentholated rubs make your skin tingle but have limited value to arthritis.

- **Weight Loss.** Easy to say but dropping poundage may not be the easiest for you. Yet, for every pound you lose, there is four pounds less pressure on your knee joints. No knee problems? No hip problems? Well, then maybe just for your overall health lose the weight anyway.

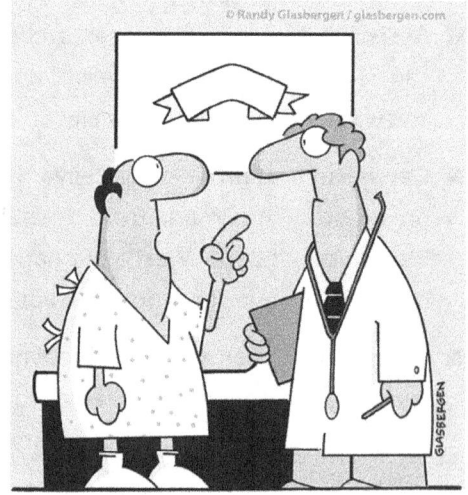

"I would be a lot healthier if you'd stop finding things wrong with me!"

Additional resources and more information about arthritis can be found on the Internet and from the Arthritis Foundation and Centers for Disease Control and Prevention. If any of these remedies work for you, great. If not, then maybe surgery could be on your wish list.

C and A Words

I have mentioned some issues related to the potential need for elective orthopedic surgeries—pain when you are bending, kneeling, lifting, even walking, twisting and generally problems with arthritis that can affect your ADLs. *Medica Magazine* had a recent article (Summer, 2019) about how exercise relates to cancer. You can get cancer in any part of your body, including bones and soft tissue. Is there a 100% preventable solution? Probably not. But you can do exercises which can keep you healthy and, ideally, reduce your chances for contracting this dreadful disease. Exercise as a cure for cancer? No. Exercise is good for your heart, muscles, bones, lungs, brain and pretty much every part of your body. According to the article, research shows that exercise leads to:

- Twenty-four percent lower risk of colon cancer
- Twenty percent lower risk of endometrial (uterine) cancer
- Twelve percent lower risk of breast cancer

Does this look like a 100% fix? No. 100% lower risk of contracting cancer? No. Not too keen about exercising? And what is sitting in a chair doing for you? Specifically, the authors recommend that you do at least 150 minutes of moderate-intensity activity per week. That is twenty to thirty minutes per day over a five or seven-day period. Walking is one activity. Riding a stationary bike is another. Engaging in an aerobic or exercise class is a third option. There are others. Do not let the 150-minute figure discourage you. Break up that time into five, ten or fifteen- minute sessions, multiple times per day. Getting up out of your chair to walk to the refrigerator does not count. Walk around your home or the hallways of your condo. Walk around with some light weights in your hands and do biceps curls at the same time. Multi-task. Climb up and down your stairs a few times. Sitting is not an exercise, even if you are watching television and snacking on a snack and clicking the remote.

The article further recommends that should you get cancer, keep up your exercise routine to the extent that you are physically able. Many years ago, people "were discouraged from being physically active if you were undergoing cancer treatments." Exercise. Keep physically active. Check with your physician about the types of activities will benefit you. Resources to consider include the National Cancer Institute, National Institutes of Health and the American Cancer Society.

Exercise can also help you with Alzheimer's disease. According to an article in *Current Psychiatry* (January 2019), "physical exercise may have a positive impact on

Alzheimer's disease (AD) symptoms. Compared with being physically inactive, low levels of weekly physical activity were associated with a 29 to 41 percent lower risk of developing AD, while higher weekly physical activity was associated with a 37 to 50 percent lower risk."

Great. But is gardening considered exercise? For the most part, yes. According to the University of Virginia, gardening rates up there with other moderate to strenuous forms of exercise, like walking and bicycling. According to the author, like any other form of exercise, you have to be active for at least 30 minutes for there to be a benefit (Spruce, 2019). But you can still get many benefits from an aerobic exercise such as gardening if you pursue it regularly. Even the less strenuous forms of yard and garden upkeep – weeding, trimming, raking – can burn off about 300 calories an hour. Spading, lifting, tilling, and raking can improve muscle tone and strength.

Can you benefit from hitting a bucket of balls at a golf hitting range? What about pickle-ball? The short answer is yes. You do not have to run a marathon or play 16 rounds of golf or play at your favorite sport as though you were competing for the World Cup. Can exercising until you sweat (or glow) help? Sure. But maybe you cannot do all that high-intensity stuff. Simply, get up and off your butt and do an activity that gets your body moving. Overweight? Smoker? Couch potato? Chat with your physician. What can you do to move and help yourself?

Superfoods versus Cancer. There are many foods that you can eat that can help reduce your risk of cancer. Look for foods with *phytochemicals*. Beans and cruciferous, such as broccoli, cauliflower, cabbage, brussels sprouts, and kale have it. Dark green leafy vegetables, such as spinach, romaine lettuce and collard greens are packed with fiber, *lutein*, and *carotenoids*, all cancer-fighting substances. Other foods that have levels of vitamins C, E, and A, can protect you from cancer by preventing the growth of free radicals in your body. And, by the way, if you choose to smoke, eating these superfoods may not provide you with much protection. You decide which habit you prefer-smoking or eating.

Here are just a few foods that you may want to include on your menu:

- Avocados
- Beans (kidney)
- Berries (especially strawberries, blueberries)
- Broccoli (raw or cooked)
- Cabbage (coleslaw)

- Carrots (cooked)
- Dried Apricots
- Garlic
- Olive Oil
- Onions (the smaller yellow and red varieties)
- Pasta (whole wheat)
- Peppers
- Spinach
- Sunflower seeds
- Tomatoes (sauce, paste and juice)
- Watermelon

Dining Out. The Mayo Clinic has some excellent advice for healthier eating, especially if you plan to dine out. First, review the menu on the restaurant's website. Do they provide any nutritional information? Second, avoid these less than healthy words: Au Gratin, Battered, Buttered, Crunchy, Fried, Glazed, Scalloped and Smothered.

Instead, look for these healthier food-words that describe how your food will be prepared: Baked, Broiled, Charbroiled, Grilled, Poached, Roasted, Seared, Steamed.

Third, hold off gorging on the bread on your table while you think about what you want to order. Drink water. Avoid the booze. If you want a drink, drink at home. It's cheaper. Fourth, are the portions a bit large for you? Ask them to pack what you don't eat and take it home. Eat it the next day.

MODULE A2
PREPARING YOUR INSIDE WORLD

Mobility Devices and Aids

Make sure you have the assistive device(s) you need to give you the mobility and stability you require during your recovery process. Walker, crutches, a kneel-walker or a cane would be good to have ahead of time. Your physician will identify what you need.

Plan ahead. Locate a human mobility device, aka your spouse or partner or big-strong person. Who can help you around the house? Who can help you move stuff and drive you to where you want to go? Do you have a coach who can give you support and feedback about your exercise and rehab program? Are there mobility vehicles that can take you shopping or to the doctor's office? Keep phone numbers handy. Contact the local VA or VFW. They may loan you the device(s) you need, sometimes for free, sometimes for a small fee or donation. Or, check out the yellow pages for assistive devices to buy or rent.

Re-Organizing Where You Live

Earlier you learned about moving small tables and chairs and things that could cause you to go bump-in-the-night. Clear a path so you can use your walker or crutches without having to worry about banging and bumping into things. Keep loose stuff away from the edges of your counters so you can do your furniture-walk without worrying about dropping stuff on the floor, which you will then have to stoop and bend down to pick it up. If you live in an apartment or condo, get your daily exercise walking in the halls with your walker or crutches or kneel-walker. Go outside and get some Vitamin D and those rosy cheeks while you walk around the parking lot (careful of wayward moving vehicles).

The first two weeks of most operations are the most trying. Your head and body need this time to heal and get used to your new prosthesis or whatever the surgeon stuck and jammed into or pulled and yanked out of your body. Put at least two weeks of food in your refrigerator and freezer. If you live alone or your spouse-partner has trouble locating the stove, stock up on meals that you can use in a microwave or that require very little preparation and are easy to open, especially if you have difficulty using your thumb and forefinger to pry open the box or plastic wrap. Some of the packaging on certain foods require a crow-bar or machete to get open. Keep a good pair of scissors handy in case you need to break into that type of packaging. Of course, sometimes saying some bad words helps.

If you think you will have a problem or think that climbing a set of stairs will be a challenge, consider making a temporary bed out of a couch or a recliner on your main floor. Bring down some blankets and a pillow to make yourself comfy. Or, rent an adjustable bed and use your family room or living room as a temporary bedroom.

Regardless where you bed down at night or rest for a nap, keep your phone, charger, a nightlight and a flashlight handy. Your phone may have a light within the unit. A nightlight is handy to have in the bathroom. If you have a tub that has an opaque curtain, consider turning on the light in the tub and close the curtain. This will give you plenty of light during the dead of night when you need to get up in the dead of night, but not so much that it will hurt your eyes.

Preventing Falls

You can break or bruise something when you fall and are young. You generally heal quickly. As you get older that break can be close to serious. You could break a hip or have head trauma. Falling is not an inevitable aspect of aging and there are some things you can do as a preventative measure. Falls can occur whenever and wherever and to whomever. They do tend to rise during the winter months especially if you live where there is snow and ice. *Medica Magazine* (Fall, 2019) has some great tips for you.

- Avoid walking on ice and if you do walk slowly and take smaller steps. Walk like a penguin using slow, short, shuffling flatfooted steps. You can buy slip-on cleats for your shoes that can help as well.
- Remove (or have removed) snow from your steps, walks and driveways.
- If possible, wait for better weather before you venture out to do your errands.

- This may sound far-fetched but carry a zip-top bag filled with sand and spread it ahead of you if you see ice or the area seems a bit slick-slippery.
- Wear shoes and boots with good traction.
- Engage in exercises that improve your balance, such as yoga or Tai Chi, so long as your physician clears you to do so.
- Prevent falls at home by reviewing the tips and suggestions mentioned in **Module Two**.
- Keep stuff off your stairs.
- Keep stuff, such as papers, shoes, books and other objects off the floor.
- Place a lamp close to your bed so you can reach it easily before you get out of bed and walk around.
- Do not, as in never, use a chair, especially a folding chair, as a step stool to climb up to grab something. Use a grabber-thingy or grab a helper-person to do it for you.
- Keep your hands free and out of your pockets to help you balance.
- Do not carry anything heavy or big that could affect your balance or block your vision.
- Be careful getting out of cars. Put both feet firmly on the ground and steady yourself on the door frame before you get up and go vertical.
- Stay awake and aware regardless of the weather and look ahead about six feet and watch for any cracks or bumps or other hazards.

MODULE A3
PREPARING YOUR OUTSIDE WORLD

If God made it, consider it good to eat
And without a doubt a yummy treat.
If Man made it best beware
There is beasty stuff out there
That can give you a nasty scare
And at your health especially tear,
Maybe more than you can bear.

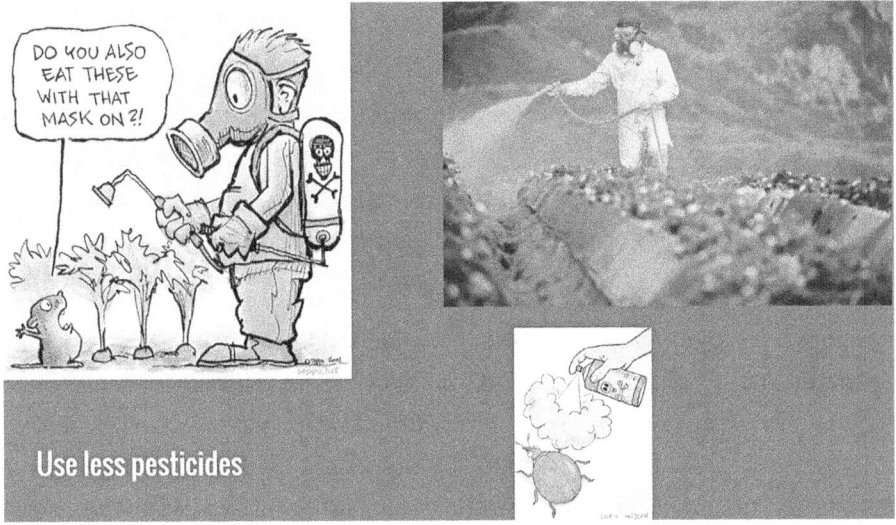

There are situations when spraying the bad-bugs is essential for our health and for keeping critters off our food crops. However, all too often we grab the spray bottle, nuke the yard as far as the eye can see, giving little thought to what we are killing, except to kill it. That spray that you use to kill the critter-bug is non-discriminatory. It kills the good-bugs as well. Yes, there are many good bugs. In addition, it can also be taken up by the plant, which you were planning to eat at some point. Read the directions. Enjoy your lunch. (Seppo.net)

Yard and Gardening Benefits

Your ADLs could include many different activities, such as exercising, cooking, playing cards, using the computer and gardening. For many folks, competitive sports are not a relaxing form of entertainment. Who knows maybe it is relaxing for you when you are doing whatever it is that you are doing better than the other person is doing it and especially so if you are beating the heck out of that person.

Working in your yard may be one of your ADLs. You may be an avid gardener or not. If you enjoy gardening, you know there are benefits. You do not need to join a club or gym or buy fancy clothes or drive anywhere unless you belong to a community garden. Go outside in your yard and reap the benefits and have fun picking off those creepy crawlers who relish attacking your plants.

Are you aware gardening can help lower your blood pressure and cholesterol? It can prevent diabetes, heart diseases, even depression. When you are working in your yard weeding or planting or harvesting, you are working different muscle groups by lifting, pulling, bending, kneeling and reaching. Gardening is good for your mental health and general well-being. There is no clock to punch. You can garden for as long as you want. Then rest. You are the weed-killer of your weeds. You are the care-giver to your plants. You can very easily tune out the world and not have to tax your brain very much, especially if you are pulling weeds.

What could be more fun than ripping out a weed down to its roots so your favorite veggie, herb, or flower plant can grow? It is a great way to zone-out and to relieve tension and stress. There is not a lot of thinking you need to do. You can day-dream, sing to yourself and your plants, and if you can, crawl along the ground on your hands and knees weeding and loosening up the soil and getting all nice and dirty as much as you want. And because you are older, you do not have to worry that someone will yell at you because you got all nice and filthy dirty.

Gardening can help you get in touch with your five senses. As you relax in your garden be aware of all the sights, sounds, and fragrances. Grab a leaf of lettuce and eat it (you don't really need salad dressing). Smell it. Taste it. Connect with nature and your part of the world. Did you hear that bird? Can you identify that sound with the name of that bird? Elizabeth Hurley, mother and model, is fit and in great shape, mentally and physically. She does not have a personal trainer or engages in an active exercise program. She attributes her well-being to gardening. Image that.

Gardening can be a solitary hobby or one that involves your whole family. Involve others, but do not use it as a punishment or as a disciplinary act. Sending the kiddies out to weed because they did something naughty will not give them a real joy and love for gardening. Condemning them to sit in a naughty corner because they pulled a few carrot plants, which can be easily mistaken for a weed (that would be the wild carrot which looks and smells like a carrot and which so happens to be an immature Queen Anne's Lace plant, aka bird's nest and bishop's lace), will not instill a love of gardening. Mend your ways. Set aside a small portion of your yard or a container or two and let the kiddies plant, weed, water, harvest, prepare and eat what they grow. Make the connection between a growing plant and your dinner table. Let them get all nice and dirty.

Another benefit comes with your harvest. What is more exciting than planting seeds and some plants, watching those little guys grow, feeding them, nurturing them, talking, singing and taking care of them by keeping the bug and bunny critters away and sympathizing with them when nasty weather approaches until the day of their reckoning when your expected reward finally comes as you grab and snatch and rip them up out of their comfy growing-zone so you can enjoy them for your next meal and be in your comfy zone? Are we are talking about joy and ecstasy or what! And you get to do that all over again during the next growing cycle.

The best place to find God is in a garden.
You can dig for him there.

—GEORGE BERNARD SHAW

Beware: Botanicals and Allergies

Do you have allergies? Are you allergic to some foods? Does your skin itch when you use certain shampoos? Do you have a rash? No? Yes? You may be allergic to something. But what?

Allergies are the body's reaction to certain substances. When you contact something that you are allergic to your body's immune system identifies it as harmful and releases chemicals, such as *histamine*, which is what most people are familiar with. Typically, folks take an anti-histamine over-the-counter pill. Perhaps the most common allergies are to foods, dust, pollen, mold, insect stings and even some medications. Check with your dermatologist and physician about any botanicals you are taking. Some folks can develop an allergic reaction to certain plants-botanicals and fragrance-infused products.

> *I am a master gardener and have been gardening for many years. In addition to vegetables, I grow several herbs that I use for cooking. I have never had an allergy*

from food. I eat almost everything, except lima beans and Brussels Sprouts which are not high on my wish-list.

The only plants I was allergic to were poison ivy and poison sumac. As far as I can remember, I contacted poison ivy almost every year when I was young by playing along the edge of our woods and burning brush where PI grew. When I was older and knew what to look for, I avoided it and have not have an outbreak for over forty-years.

About six years ago (circa 2014) I developed a serious rash around my waist. The incredible and painful itch and my scratching caused (?) the rash to spread to my back and arms and in areas here and there. Doctor #1 said I was allergic to sulfur and had me switch from the one medication I was taking to another one. That, along with using a topical cream, hydrocorisone, seemed to help a bit. I went to Doctor #2 who took a biopsy, which indicated that I had a dermal hypersensitivity reaction. Swell. But there was nothing more specific. I could have a food allergy, but they did not know from what. Topical cream was the remedy. I had a second biopsy, with the same inconclusive result and that I should go to another specialist to test for food allergies. Doctor #3 thought it could be a food or fabric issue and recommended that I see a specialist and thought that having a test for latex was a good thing. The rash was very pronounced around my waist and my undies had an elastic band, which probably had latex or latex-type material. That seemed logical. Topical cream was the remedy and that I should see another specialist, Doctor #4. The latex test came back negative: no allergic reaction. On my way to another doctor.

Doctor #5 said that Doctors #1 and 2 were not correct that I was not allergic to sulfur, which is used in many foods, especially a type of red grape-juice that I am fond of, and that I was not allergic to food or latex. That I did not need a patch test to determine which foods could be the source of my problem and within a ten-minute interview-examination concluded that I was not allergic to latex or food or sulfur, but rather it was the products I was using—shampoo and laundry detergent and synthetic materials in my clothing—were the cause. Stop it! I was given a list of what to stop using and a topical cream. My condition cleared almost 100% within three weeks. One of the key ingredients that was causing my problem (maybe not yours) was lavender. Lavender, that fragrant plant; that flower that attracted pollinators; that nice plant was causing my rash and itch and scratching? Yes. I changed my soap and shampoo and laundry detergent and tossed and donated all my polyester-synthetic undies and shirts and clothing not made from 100% cotton or wool. And there is now no lavender in my yard.

Do you have an allergy? Maybe not. Are you allergic to lavender and chamomile and perhaps other botanicals? Maybe not. But ...

Allergens and You. "Chamomile and lavender, common ingredients in cosmetics and many other household items, sometimes cause people to develop allergies after repeated exposure. The European Union is considering a warning label for just that reason." An article by Rebecca Guenard (January 21, 2015), caught me by surprise. She is not the only person who has raised a note of caution (alarm?) about these two botanicals. I always grew these plants, but not anymore.

Dr. Cindy Jones, a biochemist and natural-beauty formulator, says that "a lot of people think if you buy a natural product then you are not going to have any allergies to it. No, that's not what natural means." Chamomile and lavender are known allergens and if you are allergic to this family of plants (daises and ragweed) you could be affected. Chamomile is thought to soothe and relax people. If it causes an allergic reaction, you could end up with hives.

Like chamomile, lavender can relax you. It can also cause enough skin irritation that "in May 2014 the Swedish Chemicals Agency (SCA) proposed a health warning on lavender products." A compound within lavender extract, *linalool*, produces lavender's "fragrance and reacts with air to form the skin irritant." Some varieties of lavender growing in your garden contain about twenty- to forty-percent linalool. Chemists who formulate your natural beauty products can synthesize linalool "at a purity of 97 percent." Wonderful.

An allergic reaction may suddenly appear on your skin one day, but it has been long in development. "The more people use natural products, the more likely they are to develop an allergy to them, since reactions often occur with regular contact. These types of allergens are called *sensitizers*." According to Dr. Michael Stierstoffer, a dermatologist, an allergic reaction is not something new. [And] "But often it's something that they have been repetitively exposed to and then at some point in time the immune system just decides to become allergic to it." Lovely.

Some types of allergies induce hay fever and asthma as your body's immune system dumps histamine and other inflammatory response chemicals into your blood stream to counteract the allergen. Stierstoffer says that many people believe that natural is the better, but the more "you get exposed to an allergen, the higher the chance that your body's immune system will see it as something it doesn't [eventually] like and react to it." He says that an allergy does not go away.

Read the labels on the products you buy. Whether you have a lavender allergy or not you may want to buy products listed as *fragrance-free*. Products listed as *unscented* may still contain linalool to hide other odors within that product. Be careful out there as you troll the aisles.

Scientist-folks are not sure why some people become sensitive to linalool and others are not. The popularity of lavender has grown dramatically over the years and is touted as natural and therefore presumed safe by the consumer thanks to the marketing of those products. *"Lavender is present in 90 percent of cosmetics products sold in the U.S. It's found in places you would expect, like detergents and air fresheners, but it is also a common ingredient in less intuitive products, such as adhesives, plasters, and inks. Any scented product, be it cosmetic or stationary, most likely contains lavender. And, because of its proven sleep-inducing effect, products marketed to children—bubble bath, shampoo, lotion—contain lavender 70 percent of the time. It is this omnipresence that provoked the SCA to warn consumers of lavender's potential harm."* [Emphasis is mine.]

Lavender's Bad Side. There's more. According to an article in *Livestrong.com* (Picincu, 2019), "Lavender oil has emerged as a natural remedy for pain, anxiety, inflammation, acne and other common health complaints. Thanks to its therapeutic properties, it's widely used in aromatherapy and skincare. Like everything else, though, this natural cure has its risks. The dangers of lavender oil include nausea, vomiting and allergic skin reactions, among other side effects. A lavender overdose may cause poisoning and severe adverse reactions." Well, that is a nasty surprise.

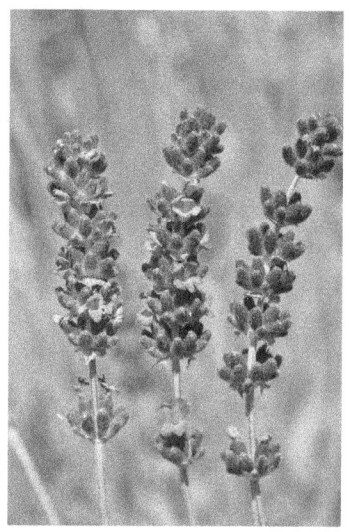

Lavender: lovely to look at and lovely to smell, but it can create an allergic reaction in some folks. Be careful out there.

Lavender oil is distilled from the flowers or spikes of *Lavandula vera, L. spica, L. officinalis* and other varieties. Folks have used it for thousands of years to treat digestive disorders, relieve stress and anxiety and ward off fatigue and fight depression.

While safe for most people, lavender can cause hives and breathing problems and other allergic reactions when ingested. When used as a topical cream, it can irritate the skin. "According to *Examine.com*, lavender oil *may worsen contact dermatitis* [emphasis is mine] when used topically." And it can interact (not in a good way) with certain medications, such as sedatives, *benzodiazepines, antihypertensives* drugs, cholesterol-lowering drugs and blood-thinning drugs. Before taking lavender pills or using lavender oil, check with your dermatologist. Don't have one? Get one. Those products can interact (not in a good way) with over-the-counter drugs, prescription drugs and even herbal supplements.

Used in large doses, lavender oil can be toxic. Use the lowest effective dose. "Watch out for any signs of lavender oil poisoning, such as burning pain in the throat, rashes, diarrhea, confusion and blurred vision. According to *MedlinePlus*, these symptoms are typically due to *linalool* and *linalyl acetate*, two naturally occurring chemicals in lavender oil." People can suddenly develop an adverse reaction to something, even if it is a so-called *natural something*, though they may have used that something for many years.

Allergens: Safe and Avoids. Here is a very short list of products dermatologists consider to be safe, that are botanically-free, and some products that you may want to consider avoiding. Some of the companies and products listed may surprise (shock) you. Again, you may not develop an allergic reaction from some of the listed products. Dermatologists treat patients with skin rashes. Their Go-To-Safe and Avoid recommendations are for your information. You decide. You choose. Be consumer-wise. Just for the heck of it, read the label. If you develop something *funny*, bring the product when you see your dermatologist.

- **Safe** hair care products include Free and Clear, Suave (non-botanical), Pantene (non-botanical), Neutrogena Anti-Residue and Head and Shoulders Classic Clean.
- **Safe** soaps and cleaners include Neutrogena products, Dove (non-botanical), Cetaphil Cleansers, Vanicream and CeraVe.
- **Safe** moisturizers, creams and lotions include CeraVe, Cetaphil, Vaseline and Vanicream.
- **Safe** cosmetics and makeup include Almay products.
- **Safe** laundry detergents include Tide Free detergent, Cheer Free detergent and ALL laundry detergent.
- **Safe** toothpastes include Colgate cavity prevention, Crest original (cavity protection) and Cavity Protection toothpaste.
- **Avoid** hair care products from Aveda, Herbal Essence, Herbal 'Natural', AXE and Moroccan Oil.
- **Avoid** soaps and cleansers from Bath & Body Works, Natural Homemade Soaps, AXE and LUSH soap and 'bath-bombs'.

- **Avoid** moisturizers, creams and lotions from Aveda and many salon-marketed products, Bed Bath & Beyond, Burt's Bee products, and LUSH lotions.
- **Avoid** cosmetics and makeup from Aveda and AXE body spray.
- **Avoid** laundry detergents that are fabric softeners, 7th Generation Detergents and Method Laundry Detergent.
- **Avoid** toothpastes such as Whitener toothpaste, Tartar Control Toothpaste and Thom's of Maine toothpaste.

Critter Control and You

A friend and fellow master gardener (Theresa Rooney) wrote a book, *The Guide to Humane Critter Control (Amazon.com)*. She talks about attracting animals to her backyard. She talks about what plants will attract pollinators and beneficial insects. She talks about the joy of seeing critters of all sizes and shapes coming to her yard scampering about hither and thither. Then she talks about getting upset when those same critters and their pals take a chomp out of the veggies she was planning to have for dinner that day. Then, after some thought, she remembers why she planted what she did.

If you want to reap the benefits of seeing critters, remind yourself that they are there because of what you did (planted). Critters have a nasty habit: they like to eat. They have this thing about wanting to survive and thrive, just like we like to eat and want to survive and thrive. Who knew?

Bunny critters are just darling when they are small and are hopping hither and thither all over your back yard. Cute. Cuddly. And tasty when all grown up. They are not especially selective about what you think is yours and what you know is not theirs. Your yard and the plants you are growing with tender loving care are part of their world. And, no doubt, their ancestors were there first, long before you moved in.

I like to see a bounding, care-free bunny
But in my garden yard 'tis not so funny.
Bounding about is when I savor
Their mild, fat-free flavor.
I like them baked or broiled,
But never in water boiled.
I like them nice and roasted,

But not so burnt or toasted.
Done up in a hearty stew,
Covered in a favorite brew,
Such as with a fine red wine
Adding flavors mighty fine.
I like them skinned and whole
Or cut and chopped into a bowl.
Bounding-bunny you are no more.
Day in and day out I told you way before,
You should have stayed away and gone next door.

Identify the critter. Who is stealing your veggies? You should know who is eating your crop before you call in an air-strike. Are they rabbits? Deer? Woodchucks-groundhogs? Look for the signs: deer leave tracks and usually make clean snips on herbaceous plants. Rabbits make sharp cuts as well and leave pellet droppings. Groundhogs create large mounds of soil at the entrance of their burrows (there are usually two entrances by the way). They eat greens versus woody shrubs. Birds peck holes in fruit and like raccoons and chipmunks and squirrels, they will eat all or some of your veggies and fruit before you even knew they were ripe. Knowing what you have will determine how to control it or at least protect what you are growing as much as possible.

Fence it. A fence, ugly or not, is usually the most effective and ecologically-safe way to keep critters out. Put the fence up from day one so it prevents them from finding the food source in the first place. A fence that is only about twenty-four inches high should keep out most bunnies. Groundhogs will attempt to climb over that fence or burrow underneath it. A fence of forty-eight inches, buried a bit in the ground, should prevent bunnies and groundhogs. If burying the fence is a problem for you, buy a roll of chicken wire that is twelve or twenty-four inches wide and lay it on the ground, outside your garden, along the fence line, to prevent critters from digging. You can cover the wire with mulch—wood mulch, composted material or rock. The critters may dig, but soon get discouraged when they realize there is something preventing them from digging deeper (the wire). Got deer? Eight feet is a good starting point. A mature stag can easily clear that height standing just a few feet away. They do not need a running start.

Motion Activated Devices. You can squirt water at critters when they cross into your territory. One product, Scarecrow Sprinkler Motion Activated Animal Deterrent, hooks up to your garden hose. (I met the inventor and his wife in 2019 and had dinner with them. They currently live on Vancouver Island, Canada.) You keep the water on, but nothing squirts out until an unsuspecting critter (or person-critter) crosses the sensor and they get a couple of shots of water. Surprise. That usually is enough to scare them away. Sometimes not.

Animals have evolved on this planet far longer than we have. Most animals we label as dumb. Most are not. Devices such as these will scare the first time, almost always. After a few times, they will move or run away from the spray and then determine that the spray has its limits. And once they notice the device, they will walk around it or find another way into your yard. If you are lucky, they will take up residence in your neighbor's yard. Regardless, if you are looking for some entertainment consider a device such as this. Of course, some critters may even look back at you and smile because they out-foxed you.

Most veggies are yum-yum food-beacons. Herbs, not so much of a problem. If your garden is mostly flowers, plant deer and bunny resistant varieties. Not all Hosta are deer yum-yum food. Plant critter resistant plants.

Protect your plants. You can use floating row covers and bird netting to protect your plants. Some of these can be left on all growing season. Otherwise, remove them when the plants are half-grown and not as tender to the critters.

There are sprays that will keep critters away from your ornamental plants-Deer Off and Liquid Fence are two options. Spray those plants as soon as they break through the soil in early spring. Do not wait until they are half grown. If critters have eaten that plant, spraying may not prevent them from returning. It has become a food source. Spraying very early will create a behavior change in them, just like with humans. The shoots are very tender when they emerge and by spraying early you associate those tender shoots with a bad smell or taste or both. And, under no circumstances should you spray anything you intend to eat, unless of course you have a perverse liking and attraction, to food that smells and tastes awful.

Beware of Jumping Earthworms. Another new something to worry about. Earthworms in your garden and raised beds and containers are a good thing. None are native to Minnesota (and other states). Our forests developed in the absence of earthworms. All earthworms probably arrived from Europe in soils and plants that settlers brought with them. Earthworms are good because they decompose leaves and other organic materials. They are great decomposers in your garden (and lawn). That is the good news.

Earthworms in the forest are not so good because they eat what is called *duff*, a spongy layer of leaves and other matter. While more mature trees survive, the

MODULE A3: PREPARING YOUR OUTSIDE WORLD

younger trees, ferns and wildflowers die without that layer of duff. Soil erosion can increase. Fisher-folks have helped to spread this problem by dumping their excess fishing bait, e.g., earthworms, in the woods. All these bait worms are non-native species, including worms that are sold as *night crawlers, Canadian crawlers, leaf worms* and *angle worms*. That is the bad news.

Now gardeners have something else to worry about—jumping worms (*Amynthas agrestis*). If regular old earthworms are considered as invasive in the forest, the jumping worms are invasive wherever they are found-in your garden, in your lawn and in the woods. They will eat your mulch and more. They will take over and make it difficult (impossible?) for earthworms to survive.They earned the name of jumping worm because when disturbed they become very active, move like a snake and appear to be jumping. Nice.

According to Laura Van Riper, a Terrestrial Invasive Species Coordinator at the Minnesota DNR, you should never buy worms advertised as *jumping worms, snake worms, Alabama Jumpers or crazy worms* for any reason or purpose. And how do you tell a jumping worm from a non-jumping worm? Note the illustration below. The position of the *clitellum* is a key identifier.

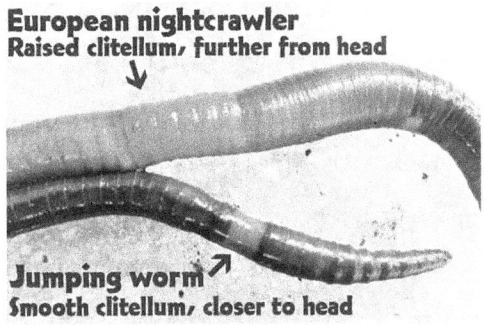

What's in your soil? And how do you know?

> **NOTE:** If you find these worms, collect them (they do not bite or sting) and put them in a plastic trash bag for your favorite trash-person to cart away. If you have a university extension office or a master gardener office close by, bring those rascals there for positive identification. Folks there are in the process of tracking their location.

Ticks and Bites. There are some critters you can see bounding about your yard and garden. Some come in at night. Others arrive whenever they get the urge. Most of them do not do damage to your favorite body. Yes, they attack your plants, but generally not you. Not so with deer ticks (blacklegged ticks). If you garden hydroponically you should not experience ticks. Likewise with your soil-based garden, though if you have plants along the edge of your garden or have a wooded lot you could experience them. Lyme disease is a bacterial infection that should be taken very seriously.

The easy recommendation is to avoid them. Thank you. Stay out of their habitat, such as long grass or brush or leaf litter. If your property (or any area) has a walking path, keep to the center. Ticks do not bite through clothing. You would do well to wear long pants and shirts. You may want to keep a wood pile or your bird feeders (guilty as charged) away from your house. These are nice feeding grounds and safe places for tick-carrying mice. Light colored clothing should make it easier for you to spot them. They are very, very tiny. You can also use insecticides and repellents. My suggestion is that you use an insecticide on your clothing (Repel) and a repellent on your skin (Deet), so long as your skin that does not have an open cut. Some products may cause a reaction in you and you should stop using them if that happens to you.

Permethrin. Spray this on your clothing (Repel), but not on exposed skin. Usually, it remains effective for two- to four-weeks, even through multiple washings.

Picaridin. It is as effective as DEET and will not harm fabrics and materials in general. It is also safe for children of all ages.

DEET. You can purchase it in concentrations of 30 -100% on unbroken skin. You may not want to use this on young children.

Oil of Lemon Eucalyptus. This is a natural repellent and you can use it on unbroken skin. Of all the herbal repellents, this is probably the best.

Not all ticks carry the Lyme disease (named for a town in Connecticut where it was first discovered). Yet a safe tick is a dead tick. Remove them as quickly as you can and if in doubt or nervous about removing them, contact your doctor within 48 hours. You could remove the critter by:

- Remaining calm. Right, sure.
- Grasp the tick as close to your skin as possible.
- Pull the critter straight up with steady pressure until it is out of your skin.
- Wash the area with soap and water.
- If you can, save the critter so your doctor can examine it. (S)he may be knowledgeable about the type of tick and what is your next best step.

And to add to your tension, an article written in the *Wisconsin Medical Journal* (April 2011) says that "a single dose 200mg dose of doxycycline is not highly effective and can cause subsequent blood tests to be unreliable." The article is "The Management of Ixodes *scapularis* Bites in the Upper Midwest," *PubMed ID: 21560562*.

Tetanus and You. Not that you need something else to worry about but check your health records. As if worrying about bug bites and stinging plants and botanicals and creepy-crawlers are not enough, make sure your tetanus shot is up to date. According to the U.S. Department of Health and Human Services, gardeners can be prone to tetanus infections. Tetanus, or lockjaw, can be serious.

"Tetanus lives in the soil and enters the body through breaks in the skin, especially when using sharp tools, digging in the dirt, or handling plants with sharp points." Before you start gardening after surgery, please make sure your tetanus, diphtheria, and pertussis (Tdap) vaccinations are up-to-date. Use a good set of gardening gloves to help lower the risk of skin irritations and cuts.

MODULE A4
PREPARING YOUR WATER WORLD

Foodies for Food

Sugar in Veggies. Yes, that sugar. All things being equal, it seems that more and more folks are getting hooked on foods that are sweet (sugar). I am not talking about processed foods, candies, muffins, pastries, junk foods or the usual suspects. I am talking about the higher levels of sugar (sweetness) in our veggies. Our preference for sweeter veggies has prompted plant breeders to develop varieties with higher percentages of sugar content. Pick up a seed catalog and you will find that many tomato and carrot varieties talk about the sweetness, the *Brix* level, in those varieties.

That description of sweetness now applies to onions. Onions? An article published in the seed catalog, *Seeds 'n Such* (*Gardener's Greenroom*), stated that "in many cases this [trend of plant breeders] has led to varieties that are lower in the precious *phytonutrients* that transfer protection from the plant's pest-and-disease-immune system to our body's immune system. This is especially true in the case of onions, according to nutritional research reported by organic gardener and author Jo Robinson..."

Way back when almost all the varieties of onions grown and sold in the United States were stronger tasting (pungent) and potent (real tear jerkers), with respect to their level of phytonutrients and antioxidant properties. Now, not so much. The trend towards larger, sweeter, milder, and less nutritious onions started around the middle of the 20th century. Perhaps the most famous or infamous variety available on the market is 'Walla Walla Sweets', developed over multiple seasons by Peter Pieri, a French soldier who discovered an "unusually large, mild and sweet variety of onions growing on the Mediterranean island of Corsica in 1900," (Robinson, 2013).

In a marketing effort to meet consumer demand, other varieties invaded our grocery stores, such as 'Vidalia Texas', 'Bermuda', 'Jumbo Sweet', 'Sweetie Sweet' and 'Candy

Cane'. Some of these and other sweet-onions can have as much as 16% sugar, the "same percentage found in our sweetest apples," which is another variety bred for higher Brix (sugar) levels. Interestingly, the larger the onion, the less concentration of phytonutrients. If you are concerned about the health benefits from, say onions, buy and grow the smaller varieties, which contain less water and "therefore the greater its concentration of phytonutrients."

Robinson recommends choosing varieties that are red and pungent, yellow and pungent and all varieties of scallions. "All varieties of red or yellow pungent onions are rich in antioxidant values, and their flavor mellows dramatically when cooked. All varieties of scallions are one of the most nutritious of all the different species of onions."

One yellow variety to consider for your own garden and health is 'Copra', a yellow, slightly pungent variety that grows to about three to four-inches and is an excellent storage choice. Some red varieties that are slightly pungent and grow to about three to four-inches include 'Red Zeppelin', 'Red Marble Cipollini' (four inches), and 'Red Wing'. 'Red Creole' is a dark red variety that is more pungent and grows to about three to four inches. Other pungent varieties include 'Western Yellow', 'New York Yellow', 'New York Bold', and 'Northern Red'. These varieties and shallots, which are a botanical variety of the species Allium *cepa*, had the greatest antioxidant content. These pungent onion varieties (and shallots) are the most potent inhibitors of human cancer cells (*WebMD* 2004).

Garlic and Your Health. I know what you are thinking: garlic? Stop it. You may not want to chomp on a clove on your first date. But if you do, give one to your spouse, partner or date to equalize things. Garlic and onions can be big-time healthy additions to your grocery cart. If you are interested in establishing (or maintaining) a healthier lifestyle, consider garlic, especially the *red* or *purple* varieties. While varieties in the Allium family have multiple health benefits (white, yellow, or red), those that are reddish in color have the highest antioxidant levels.

The antioxidant *resveratrol* gives purple garlic is color and according to traditional Chinese medicine practitioners, purple garlic is one of the best nutritional supplements. When eaten on a regular basis, one benefit is that it increases insulin secretions, which can reduce the risk of Type II diabetes. It is also known to reduce your cancer risk. Its high levels of *germanium* and *selenium* block the synthesis of *nitrosamine*, a carcinogenic agent, and the *allicin* in purple garlic inhibits the growth of cancer cells. Sounds good to me. There is more.

Purple garlic reduces the nasty lipids in your blood and can help prevent *atherosclerosis* or coronary heart disease. It is said to temper wrinkles in your skin. And, perhaps best of all as it applies to orthopedic and joint issues, it can help prevent rheumatoid arthritis.

Purple garlic may be hard to find in your grocery store. Check out your organic food stores and your local farmer's market. You can certainly buy it online, though that is usually more expensive. Eat the real stuff. I am not sure that garlic pills or supplements have the same positive health benefits. The folks in the *pill-bottle shops* will say yes, of course. Best to check that out with a bona fide nutritionist first. In the upper Midwest you would plant the cloves in the fall, which would be convenient if you are having surgery during the first part of your growing season. They emerge very early in the spring, with harvest around the end of July. You can plant them in the spring, but the bulbs will probably not be as large as a fall planting. You cannot plant garlic hydroponically. They do much better in soil.

Some red-purpose varieties to consider include:

- Anka
- Bai Pi Suan
- Belarus
- Bogatyr
- Brown Vesper
- Chesnok Red
- Duganski
- Estonia Red
- Jovak
- Metechi
- Monshanskij
- North #3
- Pacer
- Persian Star
- Purple Glazer
- Romanian Red
- Russian Red
- Spanish Roja (Ajo Rojo)

When shopping for garlic you may notice that some bulbs have a stiff stalk attached to the bulb. Those are hard neck varieties. The primary difference between hard neck and soft neck garlic is their appearance. "Hard necks have a long flowering stem growing through the center of the bulb. Called a *scape*, this stalk produces an *umbel*, a terminal pod within which bulbils are produced. Bulbils can be removed from the scape when mature and planted in the same way as cloves, although they usually need two or more season's growth before they produce a differentiated bulb. The bulb surrounding the scape of a hard neck variety consists of a single layer of regularly-shaped cloves. The

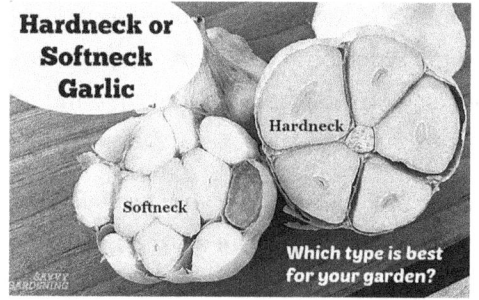

number of cloves vary between hard neck cultivars but tend to fall between four and twelve." If you see garlic braided in long strands, those are soft neck varieties. All (most) soft neck varieties have very good storage abilities.

Hard neck varieties tend to grow and thrive better in regions with more severe winters. They require a greater period of vernalization than soft neck cultivars, so a prolonged period of cooler weather is ideal. In turn, soft necks tend to perform better in regions where the winters are significantly milder.

"Hard neck cultivars tend to have a more complex flavor profile than soft necked ones, being richer, spicier, and generally more 'garlicky'. Hard neck cultivars also tend to have a larger average clove size, which, due to their plumpness, regular shape, and thicker skin, are easier to peel. Soft neck varieties on the other hand, tend to be milder and more vegetative in their taste. Although delicious when eaten fresh, a great proportion of soft neck garlics are used for processing into products, including garlic powder, and as the garlic seasoning in many processed foods. The cloves of soft neck cultivars are also more difficult to peel, given their irregular shape and tight, thin skins. There are few more mouth-watering sights than a big beautiful soft neck, drizzled with olive oil, roasting on the BBQ" (*Mother Earth* "Garlic").

Food and Ailments

Veggies and Pesticides. As a society, we tend to nuke our food more than could be necessary. You, me and other consumers tend to select fruits and veggies that are blemish-free. We don't want to buy all bumpy, bruised or banged-up food. Most vegetables (and fruits) are sprayed on a regular basis to keep what you and I eat insect and blemish free. You can avoid those pesticides and other chemicals when you grow your own. Granted, that may not be feasible for many folks.

Does it ever end? The Environmental Working Group, a non-profit advocacy agency recently released their list of the most contaminated fruits and veggies with pesticides (April 2018). These fun chemicals remain on fruits and vegetables "even when they are washed and peeled." I get the part that washing may not always rinse those pesticides down the drain and that peeling will not remove them either. Peeling! If peeling won't remove the pesticide, that tells me that those chemicals are strong

MODULE A4: PREPARING YOUR WATER WORLD

(and dangerous) enough to penetrate the skin of the product, the part you eat. That bit of news spoiled my day.

Eat your fruits and veggies. They are good for you. Okay. Be aware that some products have much higher amounts of pesticides than others. If you can buy organic, do it. If you can grow some yourself, in your own soil-based garden without pesticides, do it. Better yet, if possible, grow them hydroponically the year-round so you won't be tempted to buy them in the dead of winter from a source from who-knows-where. Buy locally if you can. Find out what that local grower has done to the produce before you buy it.

> *You said you grow organic,*
> *Now no need for me to panic.*
> *And though you said it was true*
> *And though you said you knew,*
> *A fib a day keeps the devil away.*
> *So, before you I pay,*
> *I'm asking anyway,*
> *About your organic best*
> *To keep my mind at rest.*

It may be difficult or even impossible for you to grow fruits in your own yard or in your condo. You may have limited space. And, your favorite spouse-partner-pal may not be happy about you growing veggies or fruit in the living room. Nevertheless, here are some *fruits* with the highest amount of pesticide residue. You may want to keep this in mind when you are thinking about buying them from your favorite grocery-person.

- Apples. An apple a day keeps the doctor away. Maybe not so much.
- Peaches. With or without the fuzz it doesn't matter.
- Nectarines. Say it isn't so!
- Strawberries. Test results identified thirteen different pesticides per sample. Whew!
- Grapes. Fifteen different pesticides identified on a single grape sample. Not good.

Here is the list of *veggies* with the highest amount of pesticide residue. Most of these you can grow yourself, hydroponically and in your soil-based garden, pesticide-free.

- Celery. Best grown in soil, your soil, in your backyard.
- Spinach. Easy to grow. Consider a Japanese variety called 'Komatsuna'.

- Sweet peppers. Fifteen pesticides identified per sample. Grow them yourself.
- Cucumbers. Grow the bush or vining varieties.
- Cherry tomatoes. Thirteen different pesticides per sample.
- Snap peas (imported). Thirteen different pesticides found per sample.
- Potatoes. "The average potato had more pesticides by weight than any other produce."

Leafy greens, collard greens, hot peppers and kale, are not on the dirty pesticide list, but are contaminated with insecticides that are particularly deadly to the human nervous system. "Research conducted by USDA scientists in 2007-2008 found 51 pesticides on kale and 41 pesticides on collard greens. Several of those pesticides … are extremely toxic." Some of those pesticides [insecticides and pesticides are the same thing] kill both beneficial and bad bugs and creepy crawlers and can damage children's intelligence, brain development and nervous systems even in low doses.

Well, on that happy note, please be careful about what you grab in the grocery store. Grow you own. Hydroponics is one option to consider for you and your family. Organically grown produce and fruit is another option. Before you spray and nuke the world, hand-pick the critters and give them a nice soapy bath in warm water. Most should be killed-dead within thirty-seconds.

All of that said, there are some fruits and veggies that are less contaminated than others. Really! According to Dr. Mercola and the Environmental Working Group (EWG), the Clean 15 include:

- Asparagus
- Avocados
- Cabbage
- Cantaloupe
- Cauliflower
- Eggplant
- Grapefruit
- Honeydew melon
- Kiwifruit
- Mangos
- Onions
- Papayas
- Pineapples
- Sweet Corn
- Sweet Peas (frozen)

Have a nice day and grow some of your own food. At least you can control what you spray on your food and know for sure what you are eating.

E. coli (Escherichia coli). There are more than 700 types of E. coli, most of them are harmless or cause brief bouts of diarrhea. A few strains, however, can cause more severe abdominal cramps, bloody diarrhea and vomiting. Nice. The other bad news is that rain can cause an increase in the content of this bacteria by washing lawn fertilizer and animal feces into the water—lakes, rivers, well-water, ponds, et al. And if that is not enough, boat owners who illegally dump human waste into the water also contribute to the problem.

Perhaps you are more familiar or have read about E. coli because of contaminated water or food, especially if you have eaten raw or undercooked ground beef (hamburger). The cause was probably a strain called E. coli 0157:H7. Healthy adults can usually recover from infection within a week, but much younger and older adults have "a greater risk of developing a life-threatening form of kidney failure called hemolytic uremic" (Mayo Clinic 20372058).

According to recent article in the *Minneapolis Star Tribune* (November 2018), hydroponically grown and greenhouse grown veggies "does not appear to be related to the current outbreak [of E. coli in romaine lettuce]." As of this writing, there have been at least three major problems with that lettuce and E. coli. E. coli is a bacterium that lives naturally in the intestines of cattle, poultry and other animals. It is not a problem for animals. It is a major problem for humans who consume products infected by E. coli.

The source of the contamination is (or has been) on farms located in California and Arizona, though it can occur anywhere. The E. coli is, probably, the result of using fresh manure on the land. Be very careful about using fresh manure as a compost or soil additive. You may be doing the right thing about recycling but only use manures that have been processed by reputable companies and/or that has been in a pile on a farmer's property or your own property for at least a year or more. And folks may want to wash their hands, thoroughly, after a trip to the bathroom.

Oxalic Acid and Stones. You could develop kidney stones when calcium and magnesium salts combine to create higher levels of *oxalates* than your body can handle. If you have had them, they are a tad painful. Sometimes they pass within a few days and all is well. Other times, not so much. For most folks, oxalic acid is not a problem. Not everyone will be affected by eating veggies and fruits with higher levels of oxalic acid.

The acid can also prevent some minerals from being absorbed especially when combined with fiber. Some veggies that are high in oxalic acid include spinach, swiss chard, beet tops, parsley and rhubarb. Some fruits include the berries, such as blackberries, blueberries, raspberries and strawberries. Great. All my favorite foods.

Some diseases can create serious health problems, even death, for people across all age groups. You may not be able or willing to grow your own vegetables and fruits. You can, however, minimize your risk to foods purchased outside your home when you garden hydroponically. You have control over what you grow and how you grow it. If you choose to use pesticides and other chemicals, that is your choice. But at least you know what you used and how much of that chemical you used on your food. You have control. You forfeit that control when you purchase food from others, whether that includes small vegetable and fruit stands, farmer's markets, organically grown or other sources. Become more aware of what you are buying and eating, regardless of the external source.

Hydroponics

At Home. Shopping at a grocery store is easy. All you need to do is grab up what you want and tuck it into your grocery bag, pay the nice cashier-person and drive home, doing your best to contribute to air pollution. Of course, you could grow some of your own veggies and herbs. How about gardening in water in your own backyard or in an under-used room?

If you garden hydroponically, you can set up your buckets or totes or PVC units where you want them. Set up your system, add your water, then if your surgery is within sixty-days, you can start your seeds (if you start your plants from seeds) at that time and a week or two prior to surgery you can transfer them to your hydroponic units, add the nutrient solution and walk away. You should not have to add any additional solution (fertilizer or water) for at least three weeks. And if you do garden hydroponically, you will not have to use any big-boy or big-girl tools. There is no weeding or cultivating the soil. No heavy lifting. No heavy hauling. Your main task will be to add the solution and harvest the produce. Easy-peasy.

- There is a hospital system in Minnesota that has a hydroponic system. They provide a range of veggies to folks to ensure they are eating a healthier diet while they are there and, ideally, to continue doing so when they return home.

- Residents in high-rise units have set-up low-cost hydroponic systems. The produce is shared with those who help to maintain the system.

- Schools use hydroponics. Rather than wait on the weather, teachers (with help from master gardeners) set up systems in September and grow small quantities of produce, up to forty-eight plants, on a standard four-foot by six-foot table or elevated surface. They realize a continuous harvest of salad greens before their holiday break, then start the cycle again when they return in January. Students choose what they want to grow based on what they want to eat. Lettuces and salad greens, collards, kale, peppers, chards and herbs and strawberries are some of their selections.

- Some schools integrate hydroponics with their science classes to reinforce the circle-of-life concept. Others have expanded their system to grow enough produce for the school cafeteria. Still others have expanded (or plan to expand) their systems and offer pesticide-free food to local restaurants and grocery stores and farmer's markets.

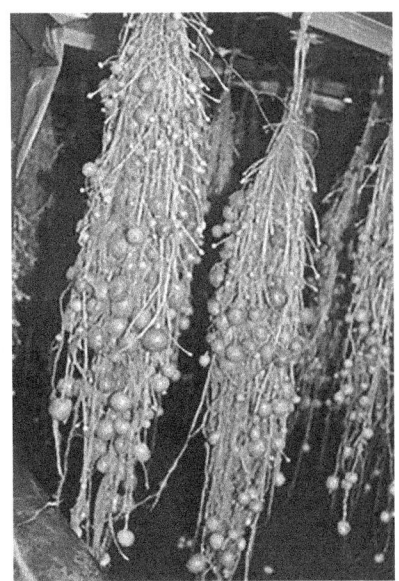

Hydroponics can be grown indoors throughout the year, without regard to the elements, which means they can be grown anywhere and at any time. Artificial lighting allows growers to produce market-ready produce in a short time period and because of its portability and flexibility, plants and hydroponic units can be grown locally, even on roof tops in cities and towns across the USA (and around the world).

*Organizations around the world, including NASA, are experimenting with potatoes and other vegetables as a potential food source for astronauts using aeroponics. Aeroponics is a viable alternative. This photograph illustrates how large volumes of potatoes can be grown from a single **eye**. No soil-based potato comes close to this kind of productivity.*

In Outer-Space. As of this writing, NASA is experimenting with a method known as aeroponics in outer space to produce a food source for future astronauts. They are growing potatoes. Water is too heavy to transport to the Space Station. Soil is too heavy. Aeroponics suspends the potato eye (tuber) and spritz it every few seconds

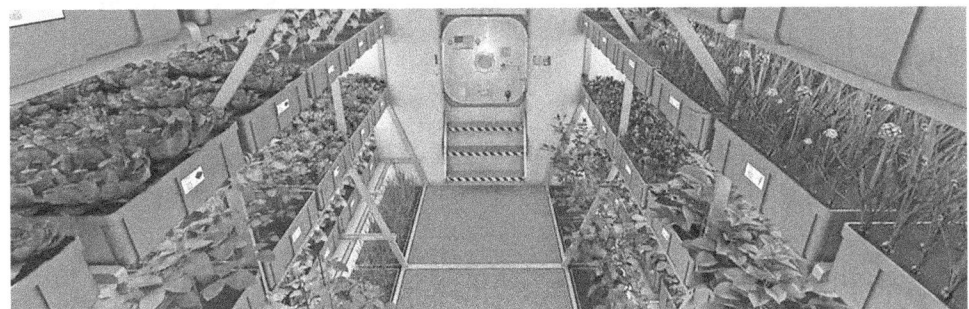

*'Outredgeous' is an organic non-GMO lettuce variety that is part of the **Open Source Seed Initiative**. This variety has been grown and eaten by astronauts while orbiting the earth. There are other plants growing in outer space as well.*

with a hydroponic solution. Results are close to amazing. A recent article (July 2019) mentions that NASA will experiment with growing peppers for use by astronauts. And scientists in Antarctica are growing vegetables.

Sustainability. Man has used hydroponics for thousands of years. The advantages of hydroponics are multiple.

- Plants grow in a self-contained environment that is easily controlled and is not at the vagaries of the weather—temperature, rainfall, wind, hail and flooding.

- Less nutrient material, fertilizer, is needed to feed the plants. Excessive use of fertilizer is not an issue and does not run off to pollute waterways—rivers, lakes, ponds, wells and drinking water.

- Less water is needed (only ten-percent) when compared to soil-based farming methods. There is no excessive evaporation and the water is recycled, reducing water costs to the farmer.

- The rate of plant growth rate is higher given the controlled environment. Plants are in constant exposure to more oxygen, water and the nutrient solution.

- Plants grow faster and larger because the plant does not need to expand their root system to search for nutrients. The nutrient solution is always within the controlled container-environment.

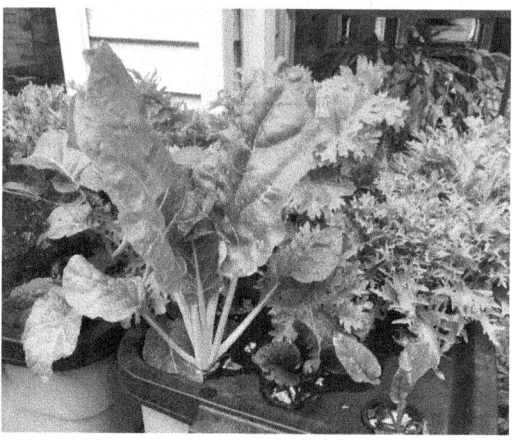

Complement your soil-based garden with hydroponically-grown veggies, herbs and flowers. Grow chards, mustards, and deep red lettuces in a ten-gallon tote.

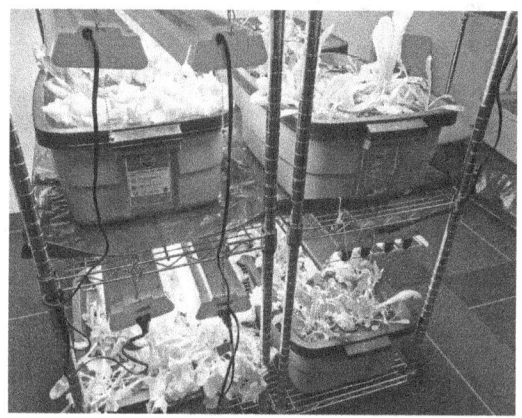

Got space limitations? Grow vertically, indoors. You can grow up to twelve lettuce plants or Asian greens in a standard ten-gallon tote. You can use resin or metal shelving units. Attach the LED (shop light) on the underside of the shelf with "S"-hooks or electrical ties. Artificial lighting with energy-saving, standard low-cost LED bulbs provide the necessary light. A multi-bulb lighting unit could include a 4100K bulb (for flower-fruit development) and a 6500K bulb (for vegetative growth). Plants should receive fourteen- to sixteen-hours of light each day.

- Plants can be grown vertically, from floor to ceiling, thus producing a much higher yield, more food per acre, than can be realized with soil-based methods.

- Less labor intensive because of the absence of weeds. Personnel can check the nutrient levels in minutes. Harvesting can be done quickly and manually, without expensive, heavy soil-compressing machinery. Planting, maintaining and harvesting is not hindered by heavy, wet (or flooded) acreage.

- Indoor hydroponic systems reduce the damage from insects and plant-eating animals, thus reducing (eliminating?) the need for pesticides and deterrent chemicals.

- Crops can be grown almost anywhere in cities allowing local growers to bring their products to market quicker and with less transportation and spoilage costs.

Regardless whether you are a soil-based gardener or someone who augments and complements your efforts with hydroponics, hydroponics is here to stay. It is not a fad. There will always be soil-based farms that stretch as far as the eye can see. Yet, given the excessive use of fertilizers to maintain acceptable yields and the excessive use of pesticides and herbicides to control damage done by insects and weeds, and constant depletion of forests and draining of wetlands, hydroponics is a much more viable and environmentally-favorable option.

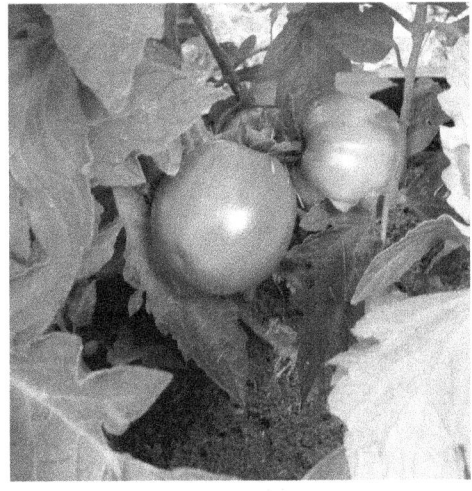

Do you like to eat tomatoes? Grow them indoors or outdoors hydroponically. A tomato variety, 'Cipolla's Pride', growing hydroponically (available through Johnny's Selected Seeds, Maine).

The ever-growing populations around the world and the need for food to sustain those populations will require options other than just soil to sustain the masses. Hydroponics will be that option.

Taste or Toss. There is no question that many years ago hydroponically-grown veggies were not high on peoples' taste buds. Grown somewhere and shipped to somewhere else required that produce such as tomatoes be shipped green or certainly not fully ripe. Soil-based produce suffered the same fate and so long as they were shipped across distances taste and texture suffered. Locally (and backyard) grown food, hydroponic or soil-based, has a significant taste advantage. And hydroponics has an advantage not always available to soil-based produced.

"Plenty, Bowery, Aerofarms and 80 Acres Farms are among young [commercial] companies that see a future in salad greens and other produce grown in what are called vertical farms that rely on robotics and artificial intelligence, along with LED lights. While the first versions of modern vertical farms sprouted about a decade ago, in recent years the introduction of automation and the tracking of data to regulate light and water has allowed them to get out of lab mode and into stores. Now they are trying to scale up."

"Plenty and others say their customized, controlled lighting – some more blue light here, some more red light there – makes for tastier plants compared to sun-grown leaves and that they use 95% less water than conventional farms, require very little land, and use no pesticides, making them competitive with organic farms. And because vertical farms exist in windowless buildings that can be located in the heart of urban areas, produce does not have to travel far by fossil-fuel-guzzling trucks to reach stores."

These newly formed companies are competitive with organically-grown (soil-based) produce. Investors, such as Amazon founder, CEO Jeff Bezos, Japan's Softbank and Alphabet Chairman Eric Schmidt have invested in hydroponics. 80 Acres Farms in Cincinnati says it already grows and sells tomatoes and cucumbers, and Plenty is testing cherry tomatoes and strawberries in the lab. "We use no pesticides," said Nate Storey, co-founder and chief scientist at Plenty. "We don't even have to use things like ladybugs, because we go so fast in our production that we out-race the pests themselves." (Reporting by Jane Lanhee Lee; editing by Peter Henderson and Leslie Adler, Vertical farms).

NPK: A mnemonic to remember. There are six macro nutrients and eight micro-nutrients. Most of these elements are found in hydroponic fertilizers. The macro nutrients include:

- Nitrogen (N)
- Phosphorous (P)
- Potassium (K)
- Magnesium (Mg)
- Calcium (Ca)
- Sulfur (S)

The micro-nutrients are:

- Iron (Fe)
- Boron (B)

- Copper (Cu)
- Zinc (Zn)
- Chlorine (Cl)
- Molybdenum (Mo)
- Nickel (N)
- Manganese (Mn)

Kauahi Perez has created a *Nutrient Mnemonics for Plants* that could help you remember fourteen of these elements, on the assumption that you want or need to remember all fourteen. It goes like this:

Never **P**unch a **K**itten, [N-P-K]
They'll **Ca**-ll Aunt **Mag**, and then you're **S**crewed. [Ca-Mg-S]

Cousin Clemb is coming in February for money
Cu-Zn Cl-e-Mb is coming in **Fe-B**ruary for **Mo-Ni**. [Cu-Zn-Cl-Mn-Fe-B-Mo-Ni]

Diet Pyramids

Okay, there are a plethora of diet programs that promise you will lose anywhere from a few pounds to a couple of tons if you buy into their program. Your call. There are *diets* that you can include just because they have proven to be healthy in other cultures. Below is the Mediterranean food pyramid followed by illustrations of other food pyramids—African, Asian, Latin America, Vegetarian/Vegan, New Diabetes Food Pyramid and a model from Dr. Willett. —that can help you sort out the types of foods to eat and how frequently to eat them. All illustrations are from *www.oldwayspt.org*. Mediterranean Food Pyramid *www.oldwayspt.org* (Oldways Preservation and Exchange Trust).

But keep in mind that regardless of what diet you follow the best and most effective long-term solution to losing weight and staying healthy is to eat less and exercise more.

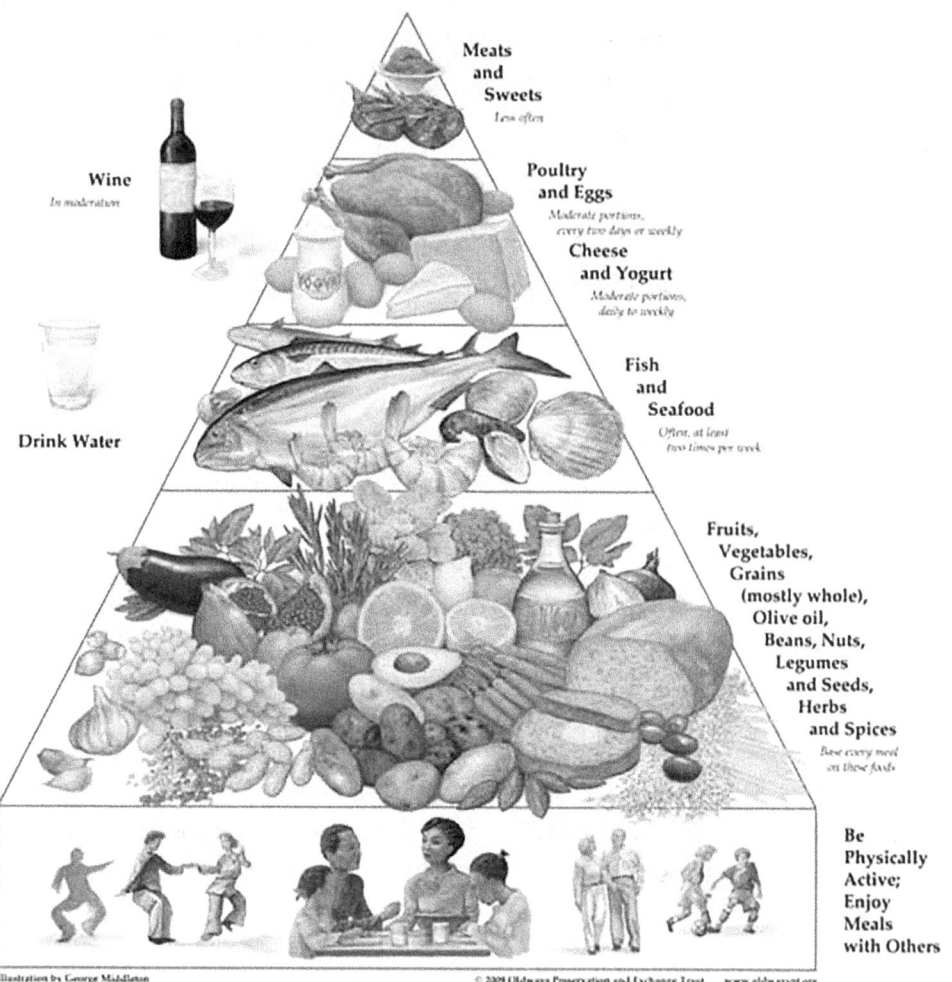

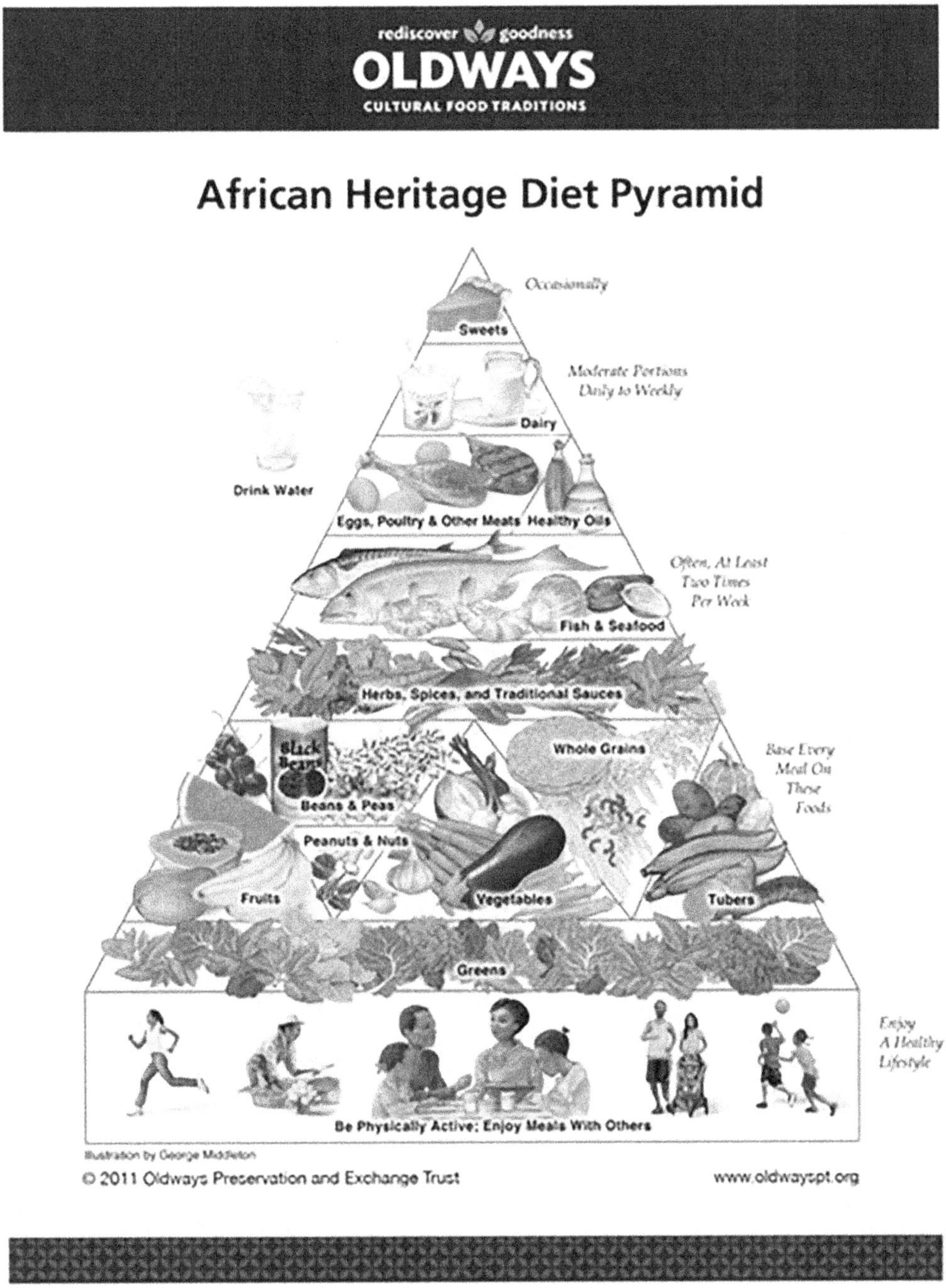
rediscover goodness
OLDWAYS
CULTURAL FOOD TRADITIONS
African Heritage Diet Pyramid
Occasionally
Sweets
Moderate Portions
Daily to Weekly
Dairy
Drink Water
Eggs, Poultry & Other Meats
Healthy Oils
Often, At Least
Two Times
Per Week
Fish & Seafood
Herbs, Spices, and Traditional Sauces
Whole Grains
Base Every
Meal On
These
Foods
Black Beans
Beans & Peas
Peanuts & Nuts
Fruits
Vegetables
Tubers
Greens
Enjoy
A Healthy
Lifestyle
Be Physically Active; Enjoy Meals With Others
Illustration by George Middleton
© 2011 Oldways Preservation and Exchange Trust
www.oldwayspt.org

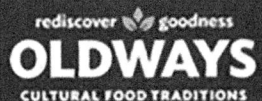

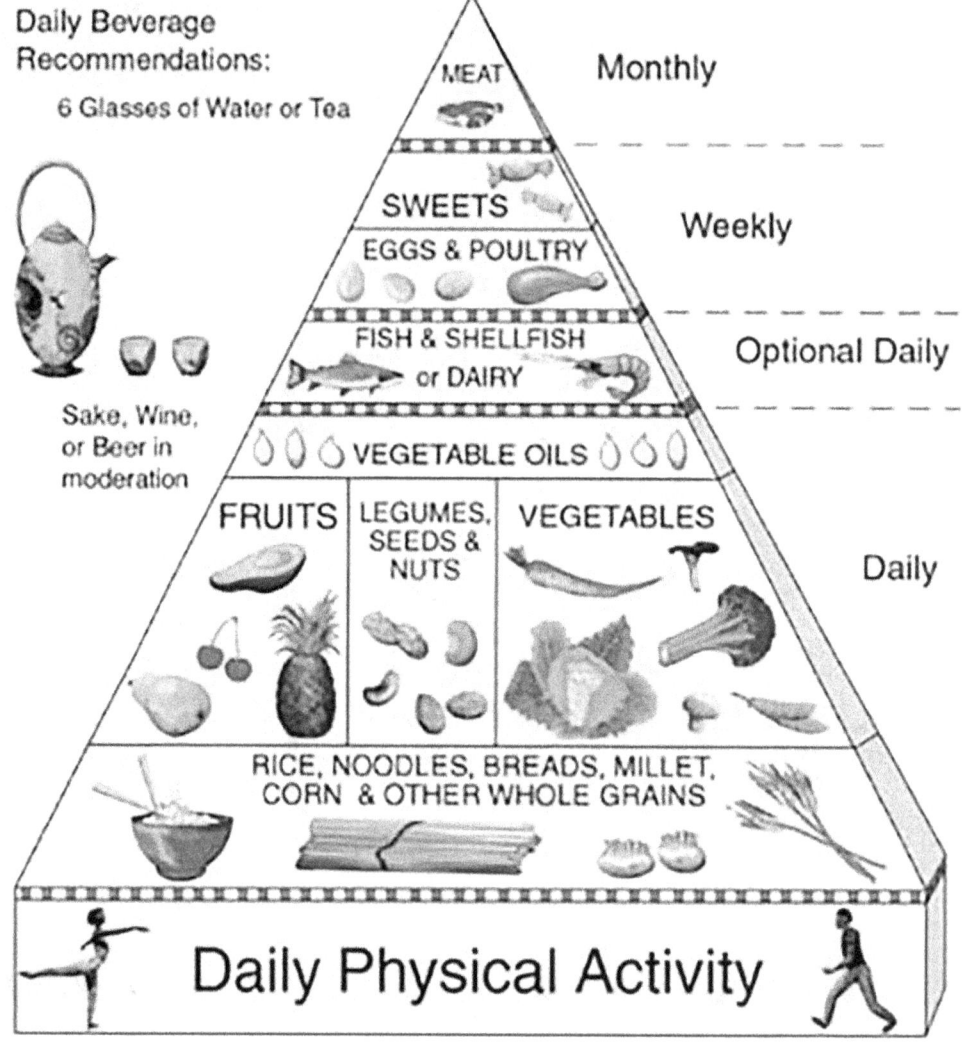

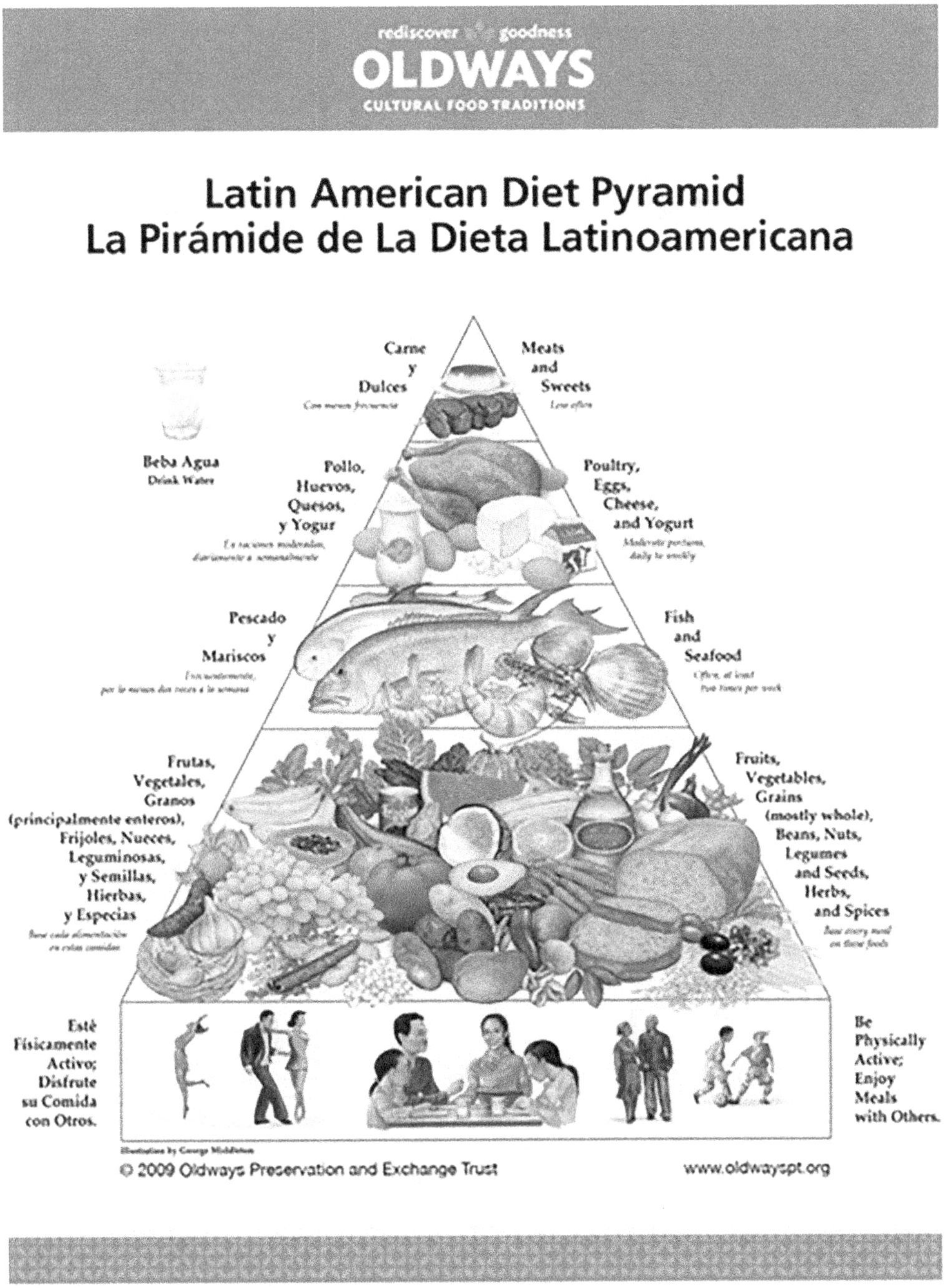

MODULE A4: PREPARING YOUR WATER WORLD

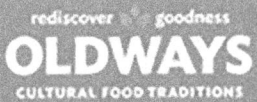

Latin American Diet Pyramid
La Pirámide de La Dieta Latinoamericana

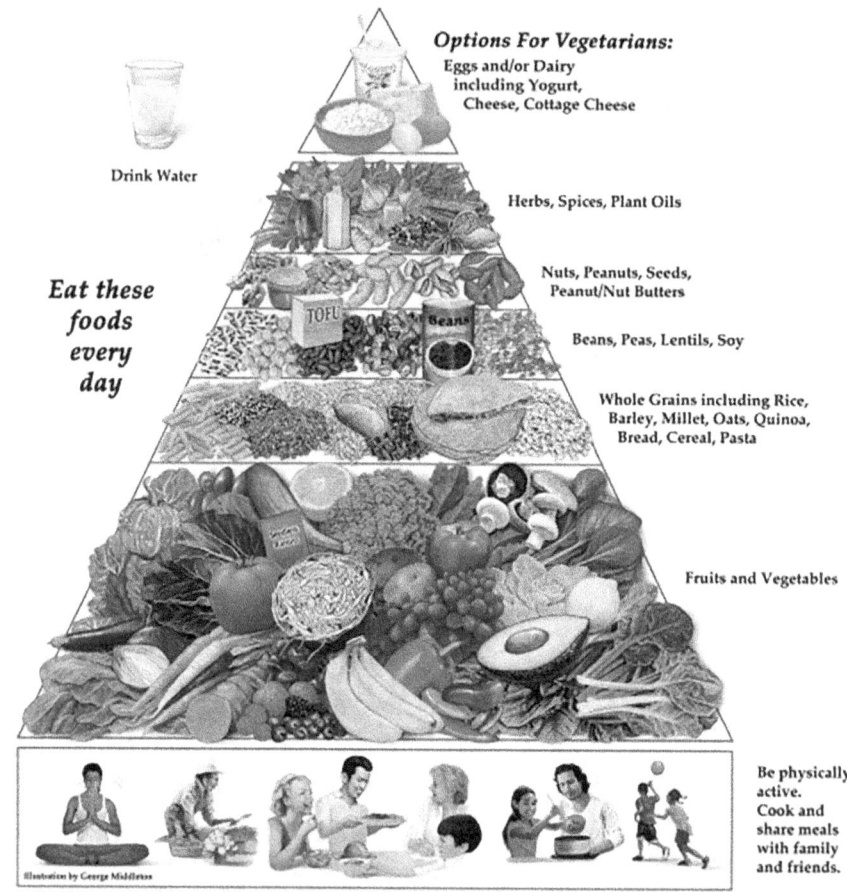

MODULE A4: PREPARING YOUR WATER WORLD

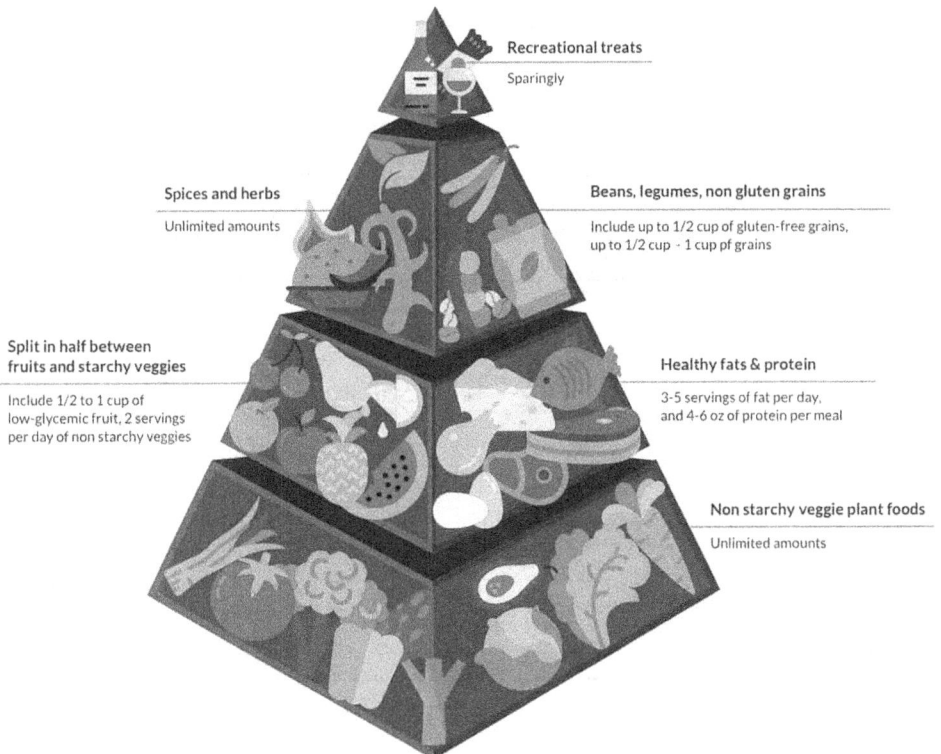

New Diabetes Food Pyramid

Recreational treats — Sparingly

Spices and herbs — Unlimited amounts

Beans, legumes, non gluten grains — Include up to 1/2 cup of gluten-free grains, up to 1/2 cup - 1 cup pf grains

Split in half between fruits and starchy veggies — Include 1/2 to 1 cup of low-glycemic fruit, 2 servings per day of non starchy veggies

Healthy fats & protein — 3-5 servings of fat per day, and 4-6 oz of protein per meal

Non starchy veggie plant foods — Unlimited amounts

Enjoy a variety of foods and be active every day!

*Inspired from Dr. Mark Hyman's Pegan Food Pyramid

GETTING YOUR ADL GROOVE IN GEAR WITH PAPS

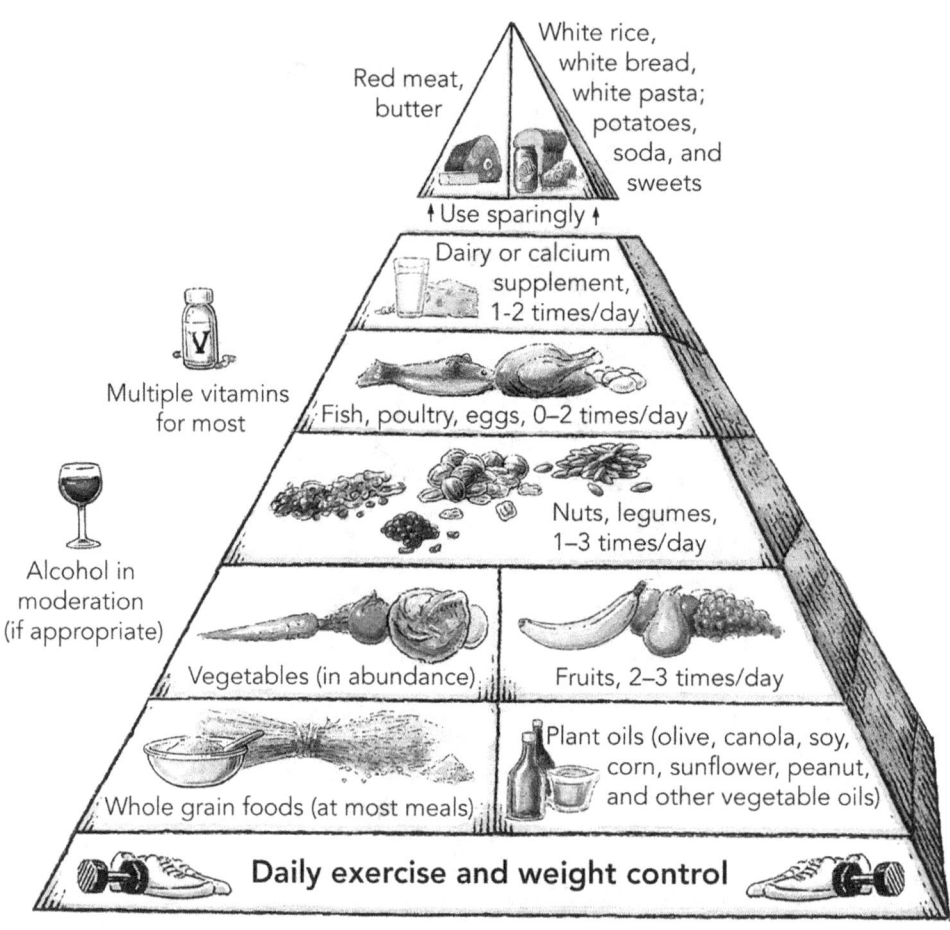

Dr. Willett, professor of epidemiology and nutrition at **Harvard School of Public Health**, a professor of medicine at the **Harvard Medical School**.

MODULE A5

COLLABORATING WITH YOUR CARE-TEAM

Your Guide to Elective Surgery

We often act differently when we need surgery because of a sudden accident or an unforeseen problem. Something broke or is severely sprained. There is pain. We want relief. And, if surgery is needed, we want it now. We want the pain to go away. We may not have much time to dwell on issues other than to resolve the problem now.

With elective surgery our attitudes may be different. We have endured pain and compensated for that pain by walking differently or by not being as active socially or athletic as we once did for a long period of time, maybe for years. We had time to think about our situation. We had time to conjure ways to cope with our situation. We ignored it. We had time to worry and get all stressed out. We made excuses for why we limped or could not lift our arms over our head or open the cover on a glass jar of our medicine bottle.

We listened to the experiences of others. We procrastinated having surgery based on the negative or less than optimal results of those we listened to. We took non-surgical remedies to minimize the pain and for a time that seemed to work. We tolerated our pain and situation. Then, at some point, for whatever reason, we knew the problem had to be fixed. Maybe we asked the surgeon to schedule surgery. Maybe the surgeon made that decision for us.

Once the decision was made to have surgery, we might feel a bit overwhelmed by the preparations we need to make; by the apprehensions we have about the surgery; perhaps some concerns about the extent to which the surgery will in fact resolve the pain and discomfort we have endured over these last months and years; and about the adjustments we may need to make in our daily lives after the surgery.

Any elective orthopedic surgery, and surgery in general, can have its risks. It is serious stuff. The surgery may be advertised as non-invasive (there is no such thing) or minimally invasive (that's better). Your body is about to be cut. It may be a big cut or a little cut. But a cut, nonetheless. Your body may not react kindly to being cut. It could respond by giving you the gift of swelling and soreness and stiffness and maybe pain, a different pain from what you had before surgery, but pain, nonetheless.

In a worse case of something akin to revenge, your body could present you with inflammation or an infection or rejection. And, given these gifts, you wonder why you ever decided to have surgery in the first place. Then at some point relatively soon, your original pain and discomfort disappears. Maybe two weeks go by and your new pain from the surgery disappears.

You wonder why you ever waited this long to have the surgery. The decision to have surgery can do scary things to your brain and emotional state. The rehabilitation process is tough. It is hard work. No one knows the pain *you* have experienced, regardless how many of your friends have had that same or similar procedures. You toughed it out alone. Well, almost. Your behind-the-scene team of doctors, nurses, assistants, physical therapists coached and convinced you to do the proven exercises and recovery protocol. You made it. And you wonder why you ever decided to wait as long as you did. You are living life after surgery.

Post-Surgery Protocol

Let's assume that you had your surgery. If you did, maybe you had to stay overnight for a day or two. Maybe you had out-patient surgery and went home a few hours after surgery. At some point you were discharged, after waiting for all the paper work to be completed and the nice medical-person came to your bedside to talk about your post-surgery protocol—what you need to do for the next few weeks. Then you got into a wheel-chair and were motored out to a car or van and were on your way back home or to a care-facility. You decided to go home. Home! At last. Now what?

Well, maybe your haven't had your surgery. Use this checklist and any recommendations from your medical-team about what you will need to do, what you need to be careful about doing or not doing the next few weeks (or longer) to ensure that you have a great recovery.

- ☐ Get some rest. Take naps. Sleep is a restorative mechanism for your body, especially a body needing healing. Keep your legs or arms raised if that is what you are supposed to do. Elevating your limbs will reduce swelling from blood circulation and, in the process, reduce your pain level. Ice your surgical area. Drink plenty of liquids.

- ☐ Remember R.I.C.E. – Rest, Ice, Compression, Elevation.
- ☐ If you find it difficult to sleep, take several deep breaths and hold each one for about five seconds, then exhale slowly. Keep any sound from the radio or television as low as possible so it relaxes you but doesn't interfere with your nap.
- ☐ Keep your dressing or plaster cast dry. It will probably be removed at your doctor's office within two weeks. Even after that time, take showers versus submerging yourself in a bath for at least the first month. Your physician will give you the all-clear signal.
- ☐ Monitor your incision for any infection. Contact your doctor if you notice any ...
  - Redness
  - Swelling
  - A foul odor (or stinky smell if you prefer)
  - Drainage from the incision
  - Chills
  - A temperature of 101 or more
- ☐ Take your medications as directed. Get off your opioids as soon as possible.
- ☐ Probably for most people, constipation is a given with pain medications and the effects of the anesthesia used during surgery. Drink plenty of water each day. Eat high-fiber foods, such as fruits, vegetables, bran, beans, lentils and prunes. Doing your exercises, walking and staying mobile throughout the day will help you. Stool softeners will help. If you think you have a problem, if your constipation lasts more than three days, ask your doctor or a pharmacist to recommend a laxative or something.
- ☐ Circulation problems should not be a problem, but here is what to look for during the first weeks of recovery. Contact your physician if you experience the following ...
  - Cold feet or ankles or hands (extremities)
  - A pale color in or around the surgical area
  - Tingling or numbness
  - A sharp increase in your level of pain

- ☐ Get up and walk around every hour for five to ten minutes.
- ☐ Do ankle exercises to prevent blood clots.
- ☐ Keep a positive attitude. Keep your distance from the stinkin' thinkin' folks.
- ☐ Keep yourself entertained. Read a book. Write a book. Keep a diary. Be thankful that you are alive and on the mend.
- ☐ Think about how and when you can get back into gardening or smacking your golf balls or tennis balls. Make a list of plants you intend to grow. Visualize yourself walking around your yard, gardening, enjoying the sights and smells of flowers, yours or your neighbors. Visualize making that hole-in-one. Visualize slamming your fuzzy yellow ball over the net, first to the right, then to the left, then tapping it just over the net as you watch your foe (or opponent) scramble to return that fuzzy yellow ball. Great fun.
- ☐ Think about how and when you can get back into sports or a favorite exercise class.
- ☐ Think about what other exercise classes you will sign-up for.
- ☐ Depending on your procedure, you may need physical therapy after surgery. You need to get that body part back functioning so you can get back doing what you want to be doing.
- ☐ You may not start therapy until after your first follow-up session with your surgeon. In the meantime, make sure you continue doing the exercises the medical discharge person gave you to do. You can do those. You do not need a therapist to show you how.
- ☐ What should you expect during your first therapy session? The first session will be nice and easy and comfy and low-key. You will share your level of pain, concerns, and apprehensions about your surgery or recovery period. Your therapist is a good listener and probably will take notes on a computer. Towards the middle to end of your first session, that nice-good-listener-person molts into a physical terrorist. Time for your real protocol to begin.
- ☐ (S)he will contort parts of your body in ways you never thought possible. (S)he will rub your scar (if you have one) until you are sure the incision will split wide open. Pain? Stop me before I scream. Okay, go ahead and scream.
- ☐ Then from the sessions that follow, depending on your progress, your terrorist sheds that hard-core demeaner and becomes that nice-good-listener-person again. Pain? What pain?

☐ Continue with your protocol and give yourself an atta-boy or atta-girl as you improve and gain more mobility and flexibility with less pain.

Force Field Analysis: Making Decisions

They told me to stop
Or else I'll drop.
No more smokes
And no more tokes.
No more chews
And no more brews.
No more sweets
And no more treats.
Guess it's time for me to quit,
More than just a little bit.
I'll quit and forever end,
All over once again.
Then once more to quit again,
And again, to my very end.

Did your medical-team recommend that you lose some weight? Stop smoking? Cut back on drinking, at least for a while after surgery (or a long while after surgery)? Did you make the decision to follow their recommendations or did you decide to do what you want to do because you know what's best for you and they do not? How did you decide to make that decision?

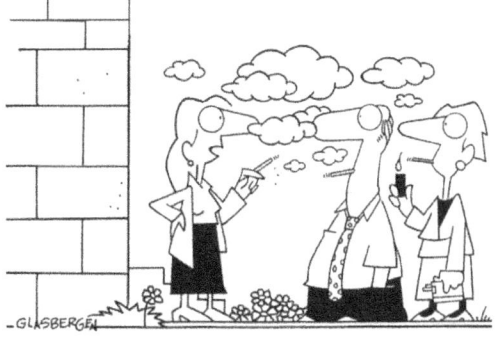

"That's what I like best about smoking—it gets me out in the fresh air a couple times a day."

You read about Force-Field Analysis in **Module Five**. You could apply this technique to almost anything. You could use it to make behavior and attitude changes. Buy a car? A house? Change jobs? Move to another state? Deciding about having another surgical procedure? Starting an exercise program? The Force-Field Analysis process is an excellent and relatively easy way to decide whether you have a GO or NO-GO decision.

Note the illustration below. Identify what you are thinking about now-present state, your goal or where you want to be or do-your future state. What decision are you faced with? Then, identify what driving forces will help you move towards your goal and what restraining forces could prevent you from achieving that goal. Your decision will be easier when you weigh whether your driving forces are greater than your restraining forces.

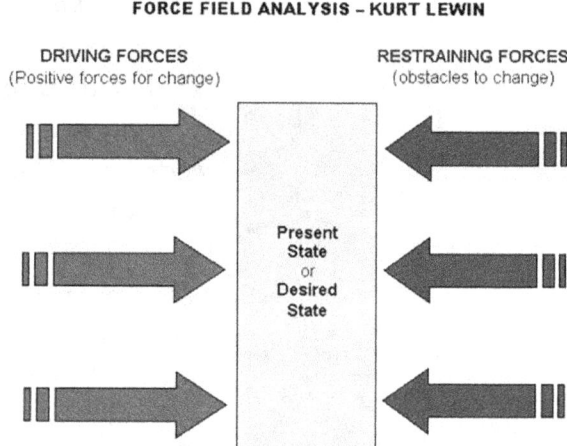

The greater the number of driving forces, the greater you would be inclined to move forward and realize success. Conversely, the more restraining forces you identify, the less likely will you succeed or move forward, but rather reject buying that car or house or change jobs and so on. Finally, identify what you could be doing differently to reduce forces restraining you. Your decision to GO or NO-GO will be there in front of you. Of course, then in spite of all the *facts* you have to *decide* if you are willing to go forward or not.

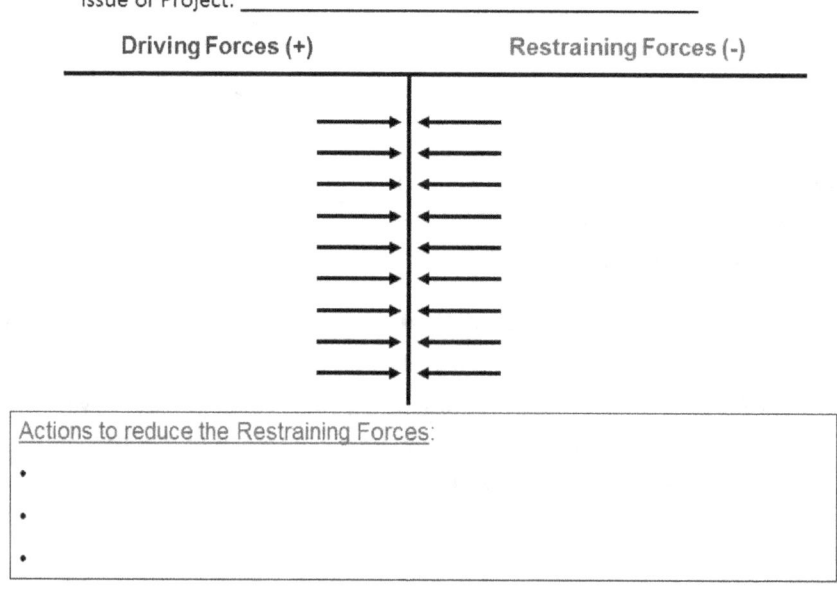

MODULE A6

PROTOCOL EXERCISES

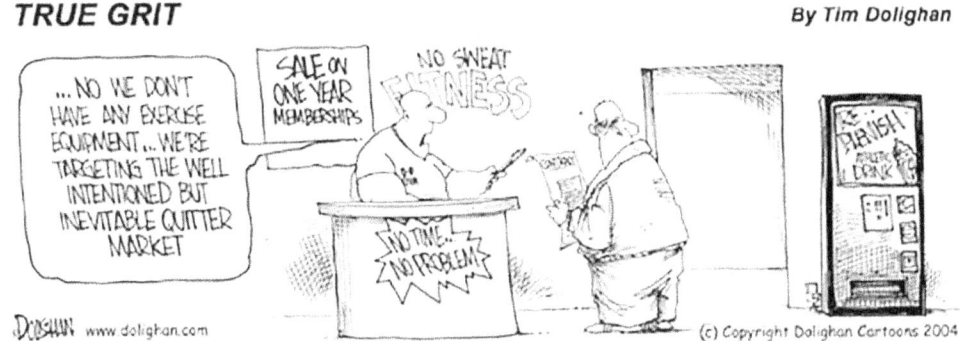

Do Not Make Resolutions

Have you decided to quit smoking? Lose some weight? Lose a lot of weight? Cut back on sugar? Eat less chubby-food? Become a Vegan? Get in shape? Improve your golf game? Improve your tennis or pickle-ball game?

Those all sound great. Making a Res or two is the thing to do. Lots of folks decide to pick New Year's Day to turn the page and go on the straight and narrow. Don't do it. Don't make resolutions. Absolutely not. And especially not after New Year's. Your success rate will be close to none or zero. How many resolutions have you made that quietly died on you? Well, you did follow-through for those first few days or weeks, but by the end of January, zip.

Making a resolution to, say get in better shape or lose weight, is having the cart before the horse.

Why not just join the YMCA or your club or the senior center where you can exercise. Just exercise. Yes, but for what purpose? Why are you going there? Just to exercise.

And that's it. No resolution. Nothing noble or socially-worthy. Just get up and out there and exercise. Forget about making a resolution for now.

The key to success is to change your behavior and attitude. The only activity you need to add to your ADLs is to just get up and out and do it (behavior change) and maybe why you want to do it (attitude change). Get in the habit of exercising every day or at least a couple of days each week. Your commitment will turn into a habit, a positive habit. At some point, you will feel more comfy and find yourself increasing what you do—the time, the number of repetitions, including more routines and machines. Your attitude changes as your behavior changes. Your behavior changes as your attitude changes. You may have found folks to socialize with. Exercising is now one of your ADLs. It becomes an integral part of your active daily living activities. Now you can make that resolution. Your body is ready. Now you can get your brain ready to put your new behavior and attitude to work. Now you can tell the world about your resolution to lose weight or stop smoking or whatever it is that you believe will be something you are able and willing to do.

What you say on New Year's Day
May not last or long stay.
Your heart may pave the way
And lead your brain astray.
But then your brain will say
Enough and keep you away.
Saying so will not make you go today.
So just get up and out this day so,
You get into a comfy flow.
Until the day you know
You can make that resolution
For your daily solution
And create a healthy constitution.

Low-No Sweat Exercises

All the exercises in this section are easy and low-impact. You can up your game by doing more repetitions and more sets and extending the time for each exercise and by using light weight dumbbells or elastic bands. No special equipment or clothing is needed. You can do these exercises at home, at work or in a group session with your friends and neighbors.

MODULE A6: PROTOCOL EXERCISES

Include these exercises in your rehabilitation protocol. Check with your medical-team about them and ask for their recommendations and what other exercises you can do to make your life after surgery as safe and enjoyable as possible.

Tai Chi. I have been to China and Taiwan and Singapore and other countries in Asia and South-East Asia and wondered how people could benefit from the slow, gentle, choregraphed movements of Tai Chi. No weight-lifting. No heavy breathing. No pounding-heart. No sweating or moist skin. How could that be beneficial? What is wrong with this picture? Nothing.

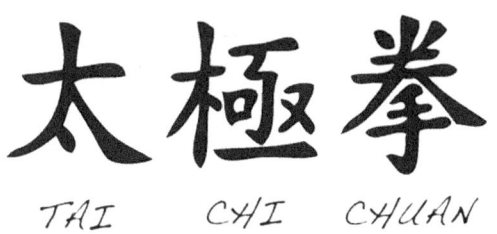

Tai Chi is an ancient martial art without the gravity-defying, strenuous moves associated with Kung Fu (thanks to movie-makers). You can easily learn all the Tai Chi moves and do them whether you are a senior or in a wheelchair or suffer from arthritis or other ailments. It is a gentle and relaxing activity that involves deep breathing without the sweat and without that breathless feeling. There is no undue stress on your joints and muscles, which is fantastic for an arthritic condition. As a result, Tai Chi is unlikely to cause you pain or injury and, best of all, requires no special equipment or fashion-forward outfits.

Many health clubs, senior centers and the Y's around the USA, have included Tai Chi as part of their exercise and flexibility programs. And once you learn the proper form from a qualified Y (or other) instructor you can practice it anywhere and anytime. Fantastic.

Tai Chi has several benefits. It can help your balance and prevent falls. If you do fall you could be less likely to get hurt or injured. The exercises strengthen your lower body, improve your posture, promote flexibility, and improve your ability to move around obstacles while walking. It can also significantly reduce bone loss and the risk of getting fractures.

Got painful joints? Think Tai Chi. One of the problems associated with first-time exercise folks is that exercise can hurt. The more it hurts, the less likely are you to look forward to more pain caused by exercising. Sitting in a chair may have more appeal to you. Tai Chi movements minimize stress and painful areas and by improving blood circulation can provide you with relief. Are you scheduled for hip or knee surgery? Tai Chi could be one excellent exercise to include in your pre-surgical conditioning.

Perhaps one of the better benefits of Tai Chi is psychological. As you get your body in shape with Tai Chi and other exercises, you should notice an improvement in your

GETTING YOUR ADL GROOVE IN GEAR WITH PAPS

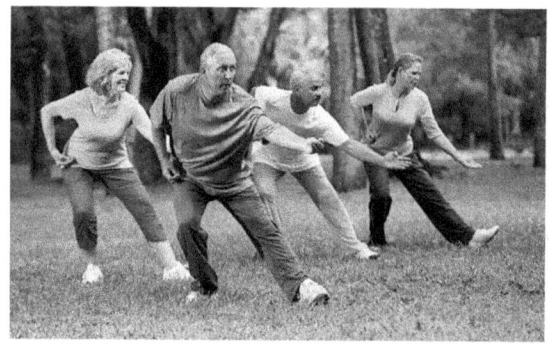

Tai Chi at any age is easy. It is commonly practiced outdoors, in an open space, such as in a park, usually with a group of people. Tai Chi can be a very beneficial exercise program that conditions the body without creating pain or stress. It is low-impact which helps to lubricate your joints, especially if you suffer from arthritis.

mental state. Your self-confidence improves when you realize you are performing various activities without pain and discomfort. You realize you can do this. You then feel more inclined to continue doing Tai Chi and perhaps other exercises even after your procedure. You make it an integral part of your daily activities. It can help you engage in the kinds of sports and activities you enjoy doing.

Tai Chi Chaun, or simply Tai Chi, meaning *supreme ultimate*, came from China in the year 1300. It is a gentle martial art, "designed to work the muscles and joints using a method of soft and low impact." It revolves around a person's *Qi* or *Chi* a life force that drives all living beings and forms. Your feet move your body, while your "arms are moving slowly and gracefully in the air. The posture is continuous. Your body is in constant movement. The movement must come from the inner part of

Tai Chi Chuan Simplified 24 Forms

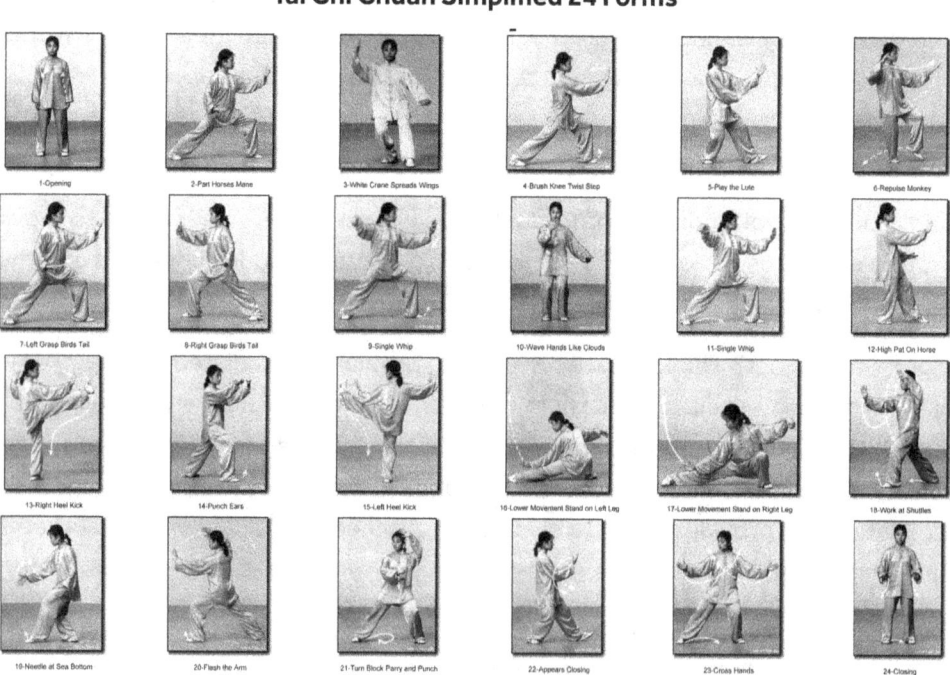

Simplified 24 Tai Chi Form

1	Starting Postures: Both arms float up then sink down with body 起势
2	Part the wild horse mane: Hold ball, step out then spread arms 左右野马分鬃
3	White crane spreads its wings: Cross wrists, lift up then open arms 白鹤亮翅
4	Brush Knee and Step Forward: Raise arms, brush knee then push 左右搂膝拗步

the body (abdomen and back), and not from the outside (arms and shoulders)." The constant flow of Chi in a person is what "keeps a person's body healthy and fit. If the flow of Chi is interrupted, then the body becomes sick."

Learn the movements. Just as with any exercise or activity, if you do not do them properly you will not receive the benefits of doing them correctly. Learn from your instructor. If you experience pain, move on to other poses. Tai Chi can provide you with relaxation and concentration. It "helps develop strength, balance and flexibility."

Yoga and Tai Chi. Yoga is bit more aggressive than Tai Chi. Yoga is native to India and Tai Chi comes from China. Tai Chi uses your legs to support the weight of your body, while in yoga your body weight usually falls on your arms. "Yoga is an exercise of body and mind, while Tai Chi is more mental. The postures of Tai Chi can be practiced by people of any age, while in Yoga there are postures and positions that can be quite complicated for the elderly."

Yoga is said to be more than 3000 years old. The most common yoga practiced in Western countries is the Hatha yoga. Modern yoga became popular during the mid-19th century when it was introduced by Swami Vivekananda. "Yoga is most commonly associated with meditation and the *'prana'* or *'life'*. Yoga can provide benefits in at least three aspects: the physical, mental and spiritual. The physical includes flexibility and good balance. The mental aspect includes relaxation and contributes to foster positive thinking and self-acceptance, while the spiritual aspect promotes one's own feelings of the body and environment. Yoga can help increase energy, improve breathing and circulatory health, relieve pain, increase vitality, help weight loss and provide a feeling of greater joviality."

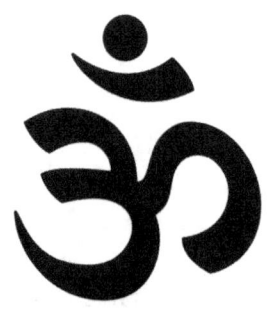

Yoga symbol for 'breathe'.

Yoga could cause stress on your neck, shoulders, spine, legs and knees if you over-exert yourself. Check with your instructor about alternative poses. Yoga is generally practiced in a group setting on a mat with an instructor.

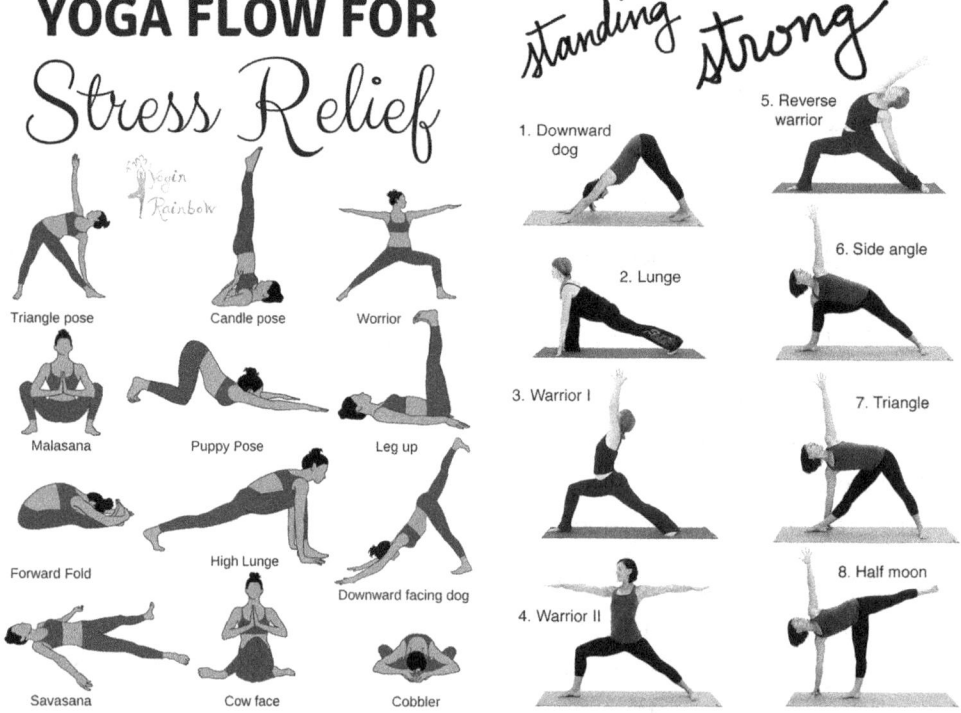

Some basic yoga poses to include in your ADLs.

Aerobic and Anaerobic Exercise. *Aerobic* means with oxygen and *anaerobic* means without oxygen. Aerobic exercise implies a moderate rhythm regarding the use of oxygen, to generate the necessary energy. Muscles use oxygen to burn glucose and fat to generate *adenosine triphosphate* (*ATP*). Exercises that are aerobic include walking, running, swimming, cycling, skiing and just following the rhythm of an exercise video.

Aerobic exercise helps tone your muscles, improves circulation, lower blood pressure, improves lung capacity, strengthens the heart and increases the number of red blood cells. Anaerobic exercises help your body increase its performance, strengthens bones, improve speed and strength, which can reduce the risk of muscle atrophy as you increase in age. Anaerobic exercises include tennis, weightlifting, speed races, jumping, among others. Include both aerobic and anaerobic exercises in your ADLs.

As always when you decide to engage in exercise activities that you may not have been involved with in a while, consult your physician about how and when you can engage in those activities in a safe and healthy way.

Heart Rate Zone Chart. Refer to this chart when checking on your heart rate as you work out on a treadmill or other machine that allows you to monitor your heart rate. I decided to shorten the chart and start at Age 50.

YOUR AGE	ZONE Warm-up Recovery	ZONE 2 Aerobic Base	ZONE 3 Aerobic-Anaerobic	ZONE 4 Anaerobic Threshold	ZONE 5 Peak Training
50	85-102	102-119	119-145	145-162	170
55	82-99	99-116	116-140	140-157	165
60	80-96	96-112	112-136	136-152	160
65	78-93	93-109	109-132	132-147	155
70	75-90	90-105	105-128	128-143	150

The lower the aerobic range, e.g., between 90-105, the more fat you should lose. The higher the anaerobic range, e.g., greater than 105, the more your heart should benefit. There are at least two ways to use this chart. (1) Locate the age closest to yours and use the corresponding heart rate zones. (2) Multiply your age by 0.67 and subtract that number from 206.9, which will give you the peak training Zone (5) to work towards.

Stretch Exercises: Sitting or Standing

Are you a desk-potato? You don't have to be in road construction or an aspiring athlete to experience pain. You may be experiencing pain because of repetitive motions, poor posture or having to remain in the same relative position on a production line or sitting at a desk or standing behind a customer service counter.

According to the Mayo Clinic, "more than four hours a day of screen time can increase your risk of death by any cause by 50 percent. There's also a 125 percent risk for cardiovascular disease." Now you tell me. Some of what you do at your desk-computer can contribute to a variety of health issues, including but not limited to:

- Neck and Shoulder pain
- Obesity
- Musculoskeletal disorders
- Stress
- Lower back pain
- Carpel Tunnel

If you have experienced any of these issues, you can resolve or reduce the severity of many, non-surgically, by simply getting up and walking around a bit or stretching. You can apply these exercises before starting your ADLs—gardening or non-gardening—to loosen up a bit. Make sure you continue to breath while you do these exercises. Turning blue is not part of the process. Sit on a sturdy chair (not a sofa or lounge chair). You read about some of these exercises earlier.

- **Triceps Stretches**. Raise your arm and bend it so that your hand reaches towards the opposite side. Use your other hand and pull the elbow toward your head. Repeat on the other side.
- **Latissimus (Lat) Stretch**. Keeping your arms straight, extend the arm up, over and behind your head and reach to the other side of your body. You can do one arm at a time or do both simultaneously.
- **Upper Body Arm Stretch**. Clasp hands together over your head with palms facing outward. Push your arms up and stretch upward. Hold. Repeat.
- **Upper Back Stretch**. Extend your arms straight out from you at shoulder height. Grab one hand with the other and push outwards while pulling your back and shoulders forward.
- **Shoulder or Pectoralis Stretch**. Clasp hands behind your back. Push your chest outward and raise your chin. Hold. Repeat.
- **Shoulder Circles**. Place fingertips on your shoulders and circle your shoulders for several seconds, then reverse the circle—maybe starting clockwise, then counterclockwise.
- **Forward Stretch**. Clasp your hands in front of you and lower your head in line with your arms. Press forward and hold. Repeat.

MODULE A6: PROTOCOL EXERCISES

- **Torso or Trunk Rotation.** Keep your feet firmly on the ground, facing forward. Place one arm on the back of a sturdy chair. Twist your upper body in the direction of the arm that is resting on the back of your chair. Try not to twist your hip area. Hold. Repeat.

- **Tummy Twists.** Hold a weighted ball, say three to ten pounds, close to your belly, with elbows slightly bent. Slowly rotate your torso to the right, be comfy while keeping the rest of your body stable. Return to center. Repeat to the other side (left). Hold. Repeat.

- **Hip and Knee Flexion Stretch.** Grab one knee and pull it up to your chest. Hold. Repeat with the other knee.

- **Knee Lifts.** Slowly draw both of your knees towards your chest at the same time. Touch your chest or until your legs touch your abs. Hold. Repeat.

- **Hamstring Stretch.** Extend one of your legs outward. Reach towards your toes as far as you can. Careful. Hold. Repeat. You could do this lying on your bed or floor or standing and bending down towards your toes.

- **Sit and Reach Stretch.** Sit at the edge of your chair and extend your legs forward, bending your knees slightly. Keep your heels on the floor and your toes pointed toward the ceiling. Extend both arms in front and touch your toes, slowly bending your body at your waist. No bouncing. Hold. Repeat.

- **Head and Shoulder Stretches (shrugs).** Raise both shoulders at the same time towards your ears. Hold. Drop them back to your side. Repeat.

- **Neck Stretches.** Lean your head forward and drop your chin down towards your chest. Slowly roll your head toward one side toward your shoulder. Hold. Repeat to the other side. Relax. Lift your chin back to your neutral or starting position. Repeat.

- **Front Arm Raises.** Hold a ball in both hands with your palms facing each other. Extend your arms forward so the ball rests on your legs, elbows slightly bent. Slowly raise your arms to lift the ball to shoulder level, lower back down. Hold. Repeat.

- **Side Bends.** Keep your feet flat on the floor. Place one hand behind your head and the other arm stretched out to one side, a little away from your body, leaning over on the side as though you were going to pick something off the floor. Lean straight to the side, keeping your chest from leaning-falling forward towards your knees and still keeping your feet flat on the floor.

Note that some of the exercises described on the previous pages are illustrated on the following pages. One of the interesting aspects of exercising, whether you do it with weights or not, is that while you are conditioning one part of your body you could be *automatically* conditioning another part. And, depending on the energy you are expending you could be realizing some cardio benefits as well.

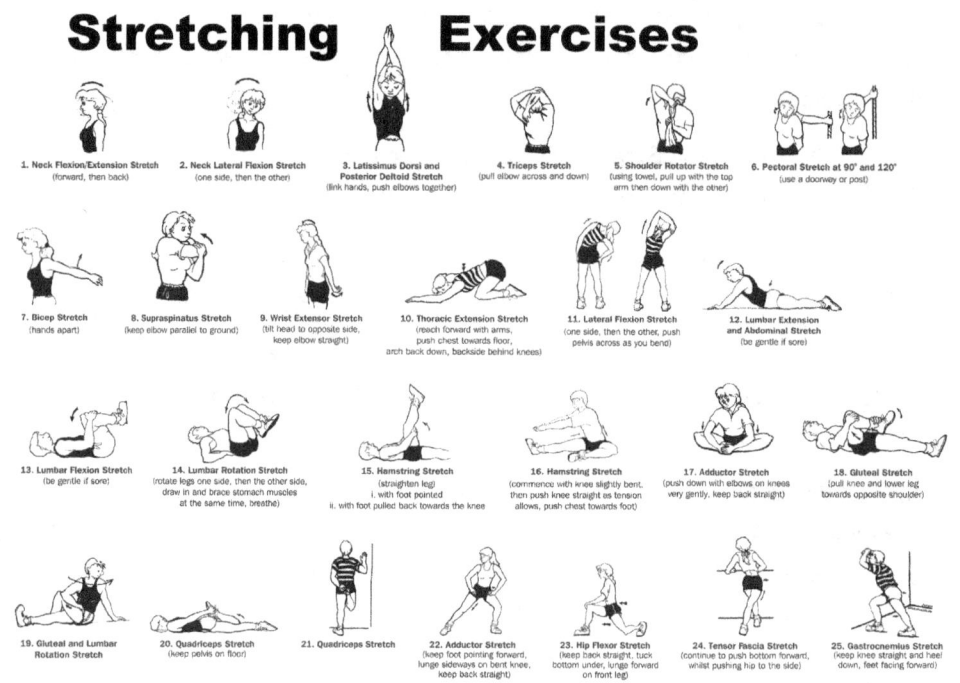

Back and Hip Stretching Routine #1

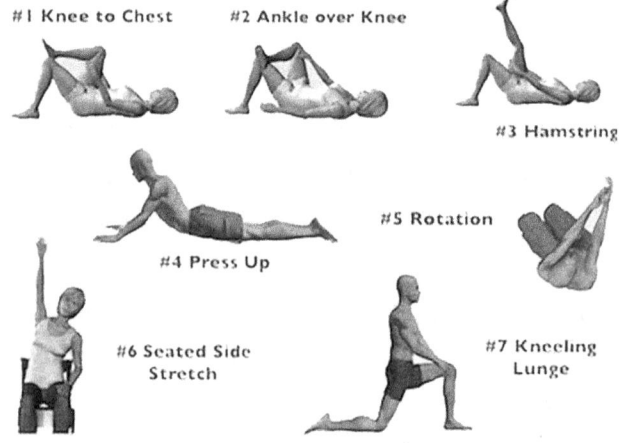

Easy stretches for your back and hips.

Now are these easy, low-no sweat exercises or what? The goal is to move in a new position throughout the day to avoid repetitive stretch injuries. Also consider standing up while you are on the phone or eating lunch. Can you get a flexible standing desk (ergonomic furniture) that you can set on your desk and alternate between typing-writing-reading while

MODULE A6: PROTOCOL EXERCISES

Computer & Desk Stretches
Approximately 4 Minutes

Sitting at a computer for long periods often causes neck and shoulder stiffness and occasionally lower back pain. Do these stretches every hour or so throughout the day, or whenever you feel stiff. Photocopy this and keep it in a drawer. Also, be sure to get up and walk around the office whenever you think of it. You'll feel better!

sitting and then while standing nice and straight? Get up from your chair every hour or so and take a quick, short stroll around the office, your house, or to the lavatory. Going outside to grab a smoke is not part of the process, nor is taking a trip to the pantry or refrigerator or handy cookie-jar. Chug down water throughout the day (*Healthline*, Deskercise March 1, 2017).

No time you say? Try these easy stretches to loosen up your sore spots while at work. Low-impact. No sweat. No equipment needed.

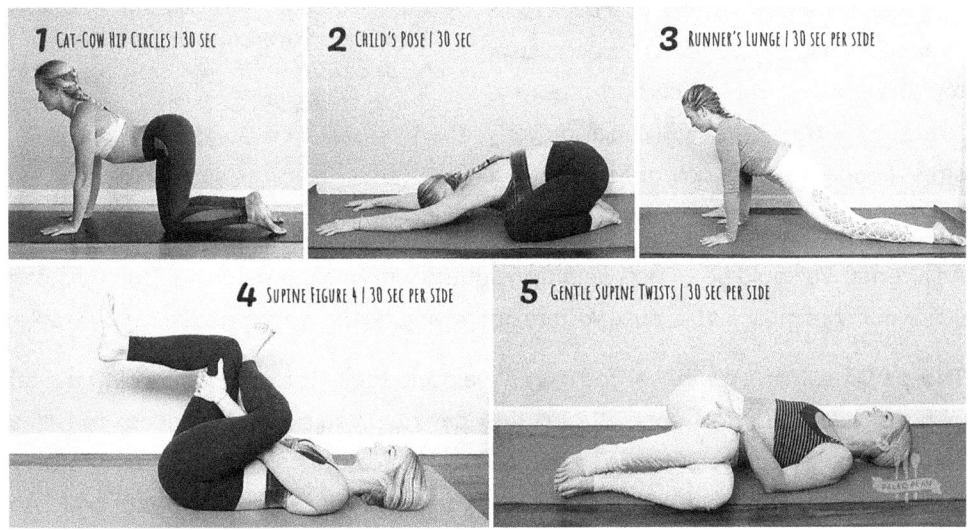

Back and hip stretching exercises.

289

Exercises to Avoid

If you are younger and in great shape and conditioning, you probably could do the following exercises without any short-term problems. No doubt, you will see folks engaging in these exercises. If you continue to do these over the longer-term you may develop some shoulder or upper-body problems. Who can tell? Regardless, you may want to avoid these and certainly check with your physician or therapist about the risk to you, especially if you have shoulder, arm or upper body issues. These three exercises and the illustration are exercises to avoid: Smith Machine, Triceps dips (2)

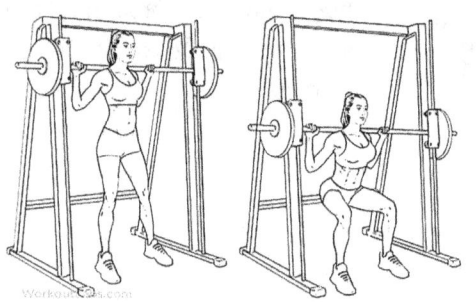

Smith Machine Squats may not be a wise choice for everyone. Check with your physician first.

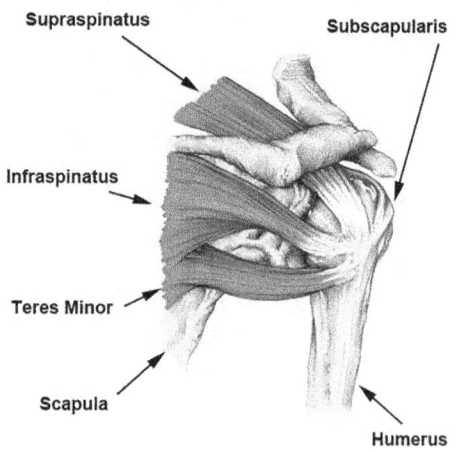

*There are four shoulder rotator cuff muscles- the **subscapularis**, **supraspinatus**, **infraspinatus** and **teres minor** muscles. These small muscles connect the scapula to the **humerus** and provide support for the **glenohumeral joint**. If you are rehabbing a rotator cuff injury, use lighter weights. Check with your therapist about using weights and what stretch exercises to incorporate as well.*

Smith Machine Squats. Maybe not. According to Lou Schuler, co-author of *The New Rules of Lifting Supercharged,* "when you lower into a squat using a Smith machine, your back stays straight and almost perfectly perpendicular top the ground, which compresses and stresses the vertebrae." You can also overly stress your knees; you do not fully contract your glutes or hamstrings; and you don't train your core. So there.

An alternative could be to use weighted squats without the machine. Doing so can build your core muscles because you are not relying on the machine to keep you stable.

Triceps Dips. Don't do these. You may have done these (or seen folks doing these) with a bench to support yourself. Yes, they can help you build your triceps muscles and they could also overload the small muscles that comprise your shoulder's rotator cuff. You could experience some injury when your upper arms are behind your body. An alternative and great way to build your triceps is to use cable pushdowns. Keep your arms in front of your body and bring the bar down to your chest and you should be fine.

MODULE A6: PROTOCOL EXERCISES

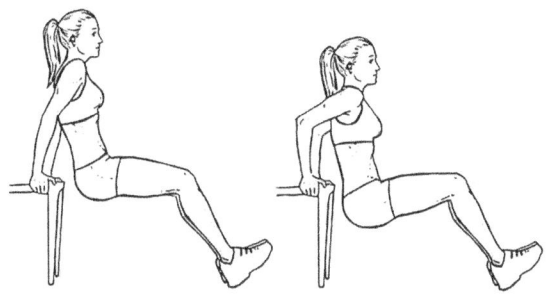

Triceps dips. Your club may have a similar apparatus or benches. You could experience pain and perhaps injury working your triceps in these two ways. Check with your care-team before you decide to do any of these squats or dips.

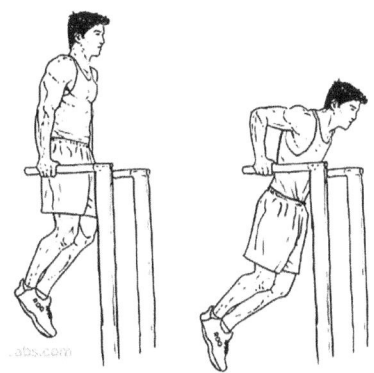

This type of exercise in this position could adversely affect the smaller muscles in your rotator cuff. Use caution.

There are two other triceps dip exercises that you may want to avoid using and are illustrated above.

Non-Food Diet for Weight Loss and Conditioning

Maybe you have tried one of those diet programs. Sometimes the folks you see talking about a weight loss program and how many pounds they lost in a week probably had a zero fat-level and are under thirty-years of age and don't look anything like you or anyone you know. That also applies to folks who chat-up their special exercise program designed to help you lose weight. How about considering a low-impact exercise diet without all the hype? It can work for you so long as you are willing to carry it through, both pre- and post-surgery. And it is free.

You can do any of these low-impact exercises by yourself or with a pal or in a group. Doing so can provide you and the others with positive reinforcement and a social-bond. If you are just starting these exercises, you may not want to join the most advanced group. Find one that seems to fit what you want to do in the most effective way possible. Chat with the instructor. Chat with others who are in the group. What do they like about the group? What progress have they made? You read about some of these suggestions earlier in this book.

- Begin this *diet* by **walking** and keep it in your ADL routine. If you are a bit over- weight or a lot overweight, walking could be difficult for you. Your gait might rock a bit, from side to side because you have pain in your hips or knees or both. But you can do this. Forget about speed walking. You can still burn off some calories by walking slowly, even with a cane or walker. You are burning some calories, even if you carry some extra weight, because your body has to exert more energy to move you. You are up, standing vertically, and walking versus sitting down. Walking is a free exercise and you can easily measure your walks and progress by noting the distance or time that you walk. Are you getting more confident from walking? Consider joining a 3K or 5k race where you do not have to run or jog but can walk the distance or at least as much as you can. Many races include walkers, joggers, folks in wheel-chairs and runners of all shapes and sizes and ages.

- Add **water aerobics** to this *diet*. Bouncing up and down and doing exercises in water, or just walking in water, makes you feel lighter. The water supports your weight and reduces the impact on your joints, which should mean less pain for you, especially in your hips and knees. You could be doing this on your own of course but enroll in a group fitness class at your local club, pool or YMCA. Usually, those classes are free. If the pool has a Vortex system, you can create more resistance for yourself by walking against the flow of the system as opposed to walking with the flow. And you don't have to worry about sweating or glowing while you are in the water.

- Consider adding **aqua-jogging** to the *diet*. As with water aerobics, aqua-jogging could be a great exercise for you if you have joint pain or find it difficult just to move around. I am not talking about lap swimming, which could be a tad intense for folks. What is aqua-jogging? Basically, it is running in water with the help of something that keeps you afloat, e.g., a buoyancy belt. You get the benefits of running, without the stress and impact on your joints. Get your body out to the deep end of the pool or at least where the water is chest-deep. Not to worry if you can't swim. The buoyancy belt keeps you up. Just in case you are a tad nervous about getting into deep water, start where you are comfy, say waist deep, and as you gain confidence move out where the big boys and big girls are splashing. Join in on the splashing.

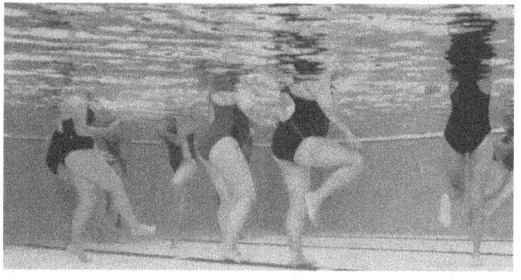

Aqua-jogging is a great way to get in the water, allowing you to get in better condition and lose some weight. You can jog in place or jog as you move forward. If the thought of jogging is not something you are not keen about, consider jogging in place or lifting your legs up to your waist while in the pool.

No pool? Do you live by the ocean? Get into the surf up to your knees or waist and walk parallel to the shore. Be careful not to venture out too far if there is a rip-tide or other posted warnings. As you walk, the resistance of the water and low wave action can provide you with positive benefits.

MODULE A6: PROTOCOL EXERCISES

- A fourth addition to this *diet* would be a **seated, stationary bike**. This is the recumbent bike with a backrest. You may have a problem with a regular stationary bicycle if you are overweight because, usually, you lack a strong abdominal core making sitting upright on that type of bicycle difficult and maybe even painful. And, besides, the seats are not the most comfy. Recumbent bikes are less stressful on your lower spine. You can adjust the tension level and burn more calories. Some have a monitor that allows you to entertain yourself listening to music or watching a news program so you can listen to the latest hollow-promises from politicians.

- A fifth addition could be the **treadmill**. This is a great addition to the *diet* whether walking is easy for you to do or not. Start slowly, very slowly, and keep the elevation or incline angle to zero. Start short and walk for five minutes, ten or fifteen and build up your time when you feel comfy. Use the grab bars for balance. Don't lean on them with your body weight. Stand erect. Treadmills can be a lot safer than walking on a sidewalk or along a street or highway. Treadmills are flat. You can control the speed and watch the monitor for entertainment or to track your progress. They can tell you how many calories you are burning and check your heart rate. Jogging is not necessary. Walk at a pace that allows you to chat with your friend who is using the machine next to you. Don't get out of breath. You can always stop the treadmill and rest a bit. Or, simply lower the speed and walk at a slower pace. Easy. Include a cool down period of several minutes. You can increase your workout by raising the incline to mimic a rolling-hill route or set the machine to interval, which will automatically set a speed and incline by alternating a faster walking speed. Need some guidance? Contact the personal trainers for their suggestions.

- A sixth addition could be **dancing**. Join a class that features the type of dance that you like to do or would like to learn how to do—ballet, ballroom dancing, hip-hop, line dancing, square-dancing or special dances for seniors or overweight folks. And you get to meet some other folks.

- A seventh addition involves **strength** training that can help correct postural issues. Do you have access to a facility that has certified trainers to help you? Often, one or two sessions are all you need to identify what type of strength training would benefit you the most, how to do it, when to increase your duration and how to adjust the machines on your won. Once you understand the what and how, you should be able to do the exercises at home. However, initially it may be wise to buy a package of sessions so you not only learn how to use the machines or weights or exercises but also get feedback throughout the session over time.

- An eighth component is **cardio conditioning**. If you belong to a club or the YMCA, you should have access to a wide range of machines and free weights. Treadmills and rowing machines and elliptical machines and the Stairmaster can also provide you with a good cardio workout. Do any exercise slowly at first until you are comfy with the mechanics, then up your game a bit, pain-free (*www.evelo.com*). Walking faster, rowing with more resistance and lifting heavier weights or doing more sets, for example, can increase the benefits to your heart, lungs and cardio conditioning in general. Make sure the trainer demonstrates how to use each exercise properly. Learn the proper form. Then do it. Consider exercise classes. Some will be low-impact and some will get your heart pumping. Check those out and sign-up for those you feel comfy doing.

If you do belong to a club, you may find that some machines may not accommodate a larger body-frame. Weight benches are usually too narrow to lie on and getting up and down on the floor for mat exercises could be difficult if you are overweight or obese or have arthritic knees or hips. Use a chair for upper and lower body exercises—biceps, triceps, leg-lifts and so on. Don't overdo the exercises. Start slowly. Consistency is the key. If you overdo yourself on those first days, you may get discouraged and give up. If you experience pain or just feel exhausted, stop.

Using the recumbent bike, a cross-trainer machine and light-weight dumbbells are all part of strength training. Yoga and Qigong classes can be included, but sometimes the movements are difficult for overweight folks. Tai Chi could be a better alternative if you are looking for a low-impact class (Frey Malia, *Verywellfit.com*).

In short, there are multiple benefits for lifting weights and dieting with a non-food diet. You can increase your strength and endurance, boost your metabolism, decrease your body fat, boost your confidence and self-image, maintain your bone density, improve your balance and relieve stress.

Obese men and women can benefit from a complete—cardio and strength training—exercise plan. Obese people are prone to diabetes, heart disease, high blood pressure, and several forms of cancer. Check with your primary physician before beginning an exercise program. You may have certain restrictions or requirements, depending on your age, physical condition and health history. The basic and very simple formula for weight loss is to burn more calories than you take in. Exercise can speed up your metabolism, so you typically burn more calories even when you are resting in a comfy chair. Consider including the two main components of a good exercise program—cardio workouts and resistance or strength training.

Cardio workouts elevate your heart rate and can strengthen your heart, lungs, arteries and muscles and burn off calories. Consider walking, cycling, swimming, hiking on trails or pathways that include some easy-incline hills. Resistance training can include free weights and machines. Consider including pull-ups, push-ups, crunches, plank, bench presses, bicep curls, triceps extensions, squats and lunges

Non-Food Diet for Smokers. These exercises are beneficial for smokers who want to graduate to the Ex-Level. Exercises for ex-smokers can begin with a cardio workout, such as **walking** initially for ten-minutes at a time. Breath in deeply with each step. Once you get use to walking, increase your time; shift into second or third-gear by walking more briskly or, possibly, jogging. Do not go any faster or longer than you need to unless and until you can do so in a comfy way.

Stretching will help you loosen up before any exercise. Stretch your hamstrings. Using weights can benefit you as well. If you want to create muscle mass, then lift heavier weights. If you want to create definition, *cuts* or *rips* or *pipes* in your arms for example, then use less weight with more repetitions. Free weights are fine. Most machines target and isolate specific muscle groups, so choose those that you want to develop for, say, your legs or arms or back. Biceps curls build your biceps muscles; squats and lunges will tone up your legs and glutes; the bench press can focus on your chest. Developing specific body parts can be beneficial. Better to develop a whole-body program that includes your shoulders down to your feet.

Crash diets and fad diets all sound easy to do. For any program to succeed you need to change your behavior and how you go about your ADLs. Exercise can help. The key here is to start and make it part of your daily routine. Focus on what you can do at that moment and don't get bogged down and discouraged by focusing on what you cannot yet do. As your fitness improves, you will start to scare yourself about what you have been able to do and what you could now do to make your *diet* more challenging and still be enjoyable and fun to do.

Keep track of what you are doing. Build positive habits. Exercise with a friend. No friends? Join the YMCA, join the senior center, enroll in a class or two and make new friends.

Exercise Machines

Proper use of free weights will get you in shape. The problem, sometimes, is that you can tend to favor one side of your body when pushing, lifting or pulling the machine's bar or plate. You may not even know you are doing this. For example, if you were doing leg presses you may be pushing off on your left leg with more force than the right leg, or vice versa. How can you tell?

One easy way to check that is to set a lower weight and *only* push or pull or lift with one leg or arm for that set, then do it with your other extremity. Does one arm or leg seem stronger than the other? Did you feel a little pain or more resistance in one leg versus the other? If so, working one leg at a time could benefit you overall. You should use a lower weight until your body tells you to increase the tension or weight.

Some machines will allow you to work multiple muscle groups and others target a single group. Generally, machines are a bit safer to use in that the bar of weights, for example, will not fall on your head or other body part and cause an injury, which is a handy feature. Then again, stuff happens. Regardless whether you use free-weights or machines, start easy with lighter weights and build up to whatever it is that makes you work in a safe way.

Here are just a few machines to consider. Look for these machines (and others) at your local YMCA, club or exercise facility.

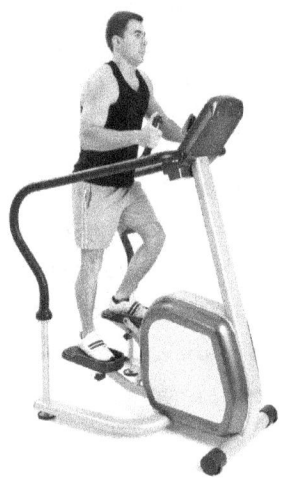
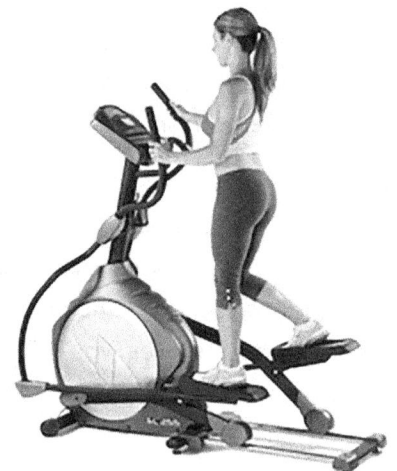
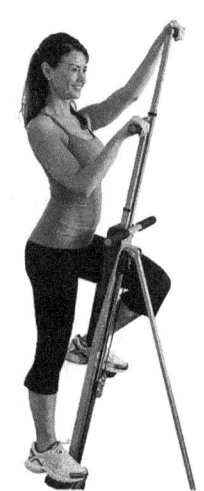

A stepper-type machine for lower-body, cardio and aerobic exercising. You are strengthening your legs, not your arms. This machine involves an up and down movement that you control.

Dual-purpose machines can work your legs and arms and provide you with a cardio workout while you are in a standing position. Some have screens that can monitor your efforts.

Want cardio? Want to strengthen your legs? This rock-climbing stepper could get your heart racing.

MODULE A6: PROTOCOL EXERCISES

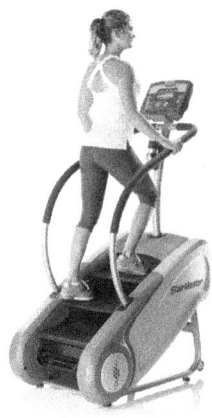
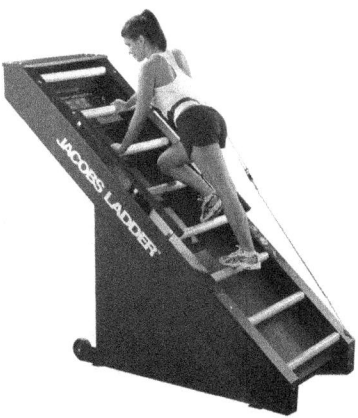
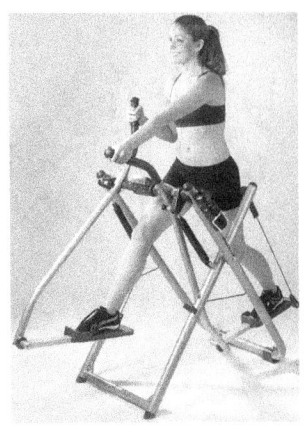

This machine will work your legs and provide you with a cardio-workout. You can control the speed. You set the speed and the steps move, like an escalator, at that speed. Keep your hands on the side-rails for balance and safety.

You may be in the big leagues with this baby. Legs, cardio and your arms could get a good workout with this machine. And, just as a reminder: for any machine check with your physician or (better) with a physical therapist trainer about your current health situation and whether a particular machine would be good for you to use.

The strider or air walker will help you work your upper and lower body and give you a good cardio workout.

There are exercise machines that you can use standing or sitting or lying down on your back and maybe even other body parts. If standing is not high on your wish-list, check out machines that allow you to sit. These are not necessarily either-or machines. That is, you should be able to find a do-it-while-standing machine and a do-it-while-sitting machine. Both types will give you a good exercise based on the energy you expend, sitting or standing.

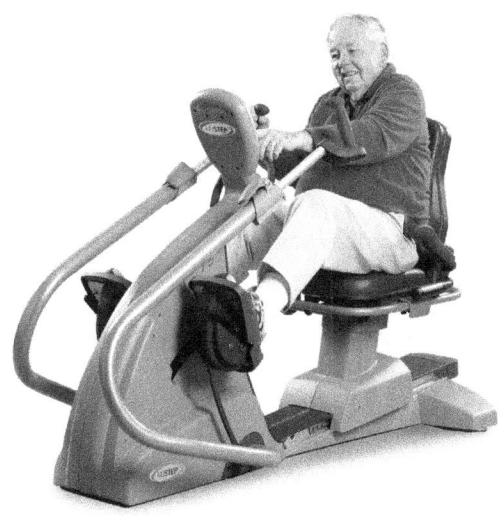

How about resting after you did all that standing? There are a wide range of machines that will give you an excellent workout by sitting versus standing. This machine will work your legs and arms and, depending on your effort, give you a good cardio workout as well.

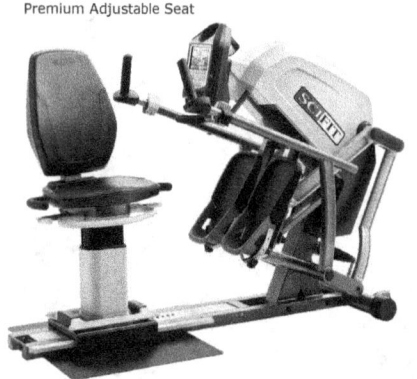

Premium Adjustable Seat

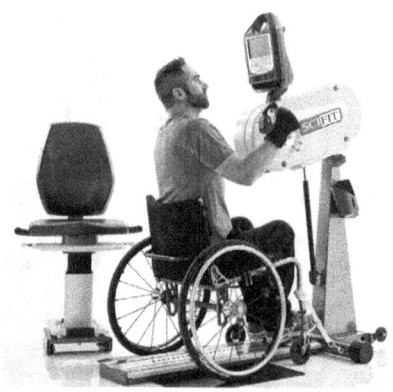

Swivel and sit. If you have trouble getting in and out of the chair, consider machines that have a swivel seat. As illustrated, you would turn the seat, back into it, then swivel it back so you are facing the machine. Some of these machines will only work your legs, while others will give you a good upper and lower body workout.

Some machines may have a removable seat to allow for easy wheel-chair accessibility. Your friendly personal trainer or staff-person will remove the seat for you, so not to worry. This machine can help build upper arm strength and flexibility and allow you to monitor your progress.

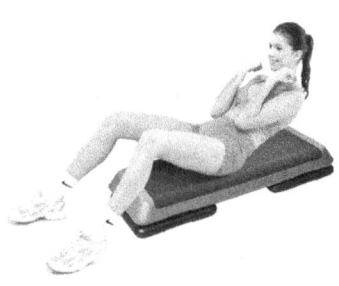

These steppers are not exactly machines, but you can stack them to jump up and down on them, recline on them to do crunches and other exercises. You will probably see these in exercise classes. No moving parts here, except your favorite body.

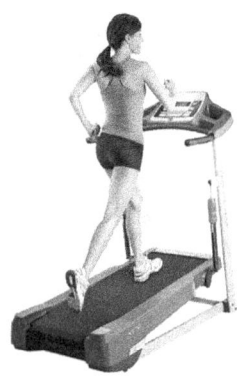

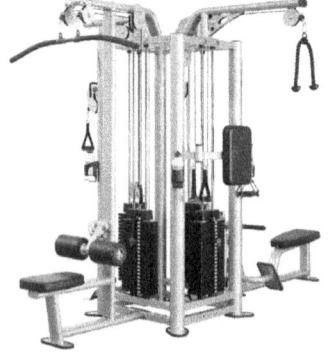

*Do you want to walk but are afraid to walk? Treadmills are great for an indoor walking routine. As mentioned earlier, you can control the incline level, the speed, and whether you want to **walk** on hills or a mountain trail or around an oval track. Treadmills should have an emergency stop button and side handles to help you keep your balance if necessary and to stop suddenly if necessary.*

*If you could only buy or have access to one machine, consider the **universal** machine, which has multiple stations in a relatively small footprint. Lat pull-downs, triceps, biceps, back extensions, squats and rowing are some of the exercises you can do to build strength and general toning. These are **one-stop** machines. You could do a well-rounded strength and conditioning program with this one machine without having to travel all over the club.*

BIBLIOGRAPHY

General References

Artnowandthen.blogspot.com.com/2018/John-Wagner-and-Maxine.

Department of Health and Human Services. "A Guide to Selecting Non-Powered Hand Tools." Cal/OSHA publications at: *http://www.dir.ca.gov/dosh/puborder.asp*

http://sporty7.blogspot.com/2011/05/tai-chi-for-beginners.html

http://www.ast.org/pdf/Professionals/Ortho_CE_Package_Consolidated.pdf?) Retrieved 201312-14.

http://www.dailymail.co.uk/femail/article-2808799/Healthy-No-honey-WORSE-sugar.html

http://www.mayoclinic.org/diseases-conditions/arthritis/in-depth/arthritis/art-20047971

http://www.osha.gov/SLTC/ergonomics/index.html

https://blog.supplysideliberal.com/post/83271629813/so-what-if-we-dont-change-at-all-and-something-magical-happens

https://qi.elft.nhs.uk/wp-content/uploads/2014/09/force-field-analysis.png

https://skinnyms.com/9-proven-health-benefits-of-lifting-weights-2/

https://www.freedom-distributors.com/wp-content/uploads/2015/03/ergonomics_graphic.jpg

https://www.hennepinhealthcare.org/specialty/orthopedics/joint-replacement/

https://www.livestrong.com/article/431042-tai-chi-basic-steps-for-beginners

https://www.mayoclinic.org/diseases-conditions/arthritis/symptoms-causes/syc-20350772).

https://www.nhs.uk/chq/Pages/2615.aspx?CategoryID=69

https://www.psychologytoday.com/us/basics/groupthink

https://www.sportsinjuryclinic.net/images/shoulder/shoulder_rotator_cuff474.jpg

https://www.verywell.com/physical-therapy-abbreviations-2696107

https://www.verywell.com/recovering-from-surgery-what-to-expect-3156826

https://www.verywell.com/what-is-arthroscopic-surgery-2548501

https://www.webmd.com/healthy-aging/features/rehab-mistakes#1

Institute for Quality and Efficiency in Health Care. "What Can Help Relieve Anxiety Before Surgery?" PubMed Health. U.S. National Library of Medicine. Updated May 21, 2014.

Nelson, J. A. (2015). "Fearing fear: Gender and economic discourse." Mind & Society, 14 (1), 129-139. Doi.10-1007/s11299-014-0148-6.

www.youtube.com/watch?V=Pl1u_UCygml. (Mnemonic)

Gardening References

Cipolla, Larry. *Hydroponic Gardening The Very Easy Way. January 2018.* Amazon.com and Okikumapress@gmail.com. *www.gardeningconnections.com*

Cipolla, Larry. "Hydroponic Gardening: webinar." February 2019. Power Point Presentation.

---. "Singapore Community Gardens." January 2011. Power Point Presentation.

---. "Japanese Garden Designs." March 2011. Power Point Presentation.

---. "Water Gardening in Zone 4." February 2012. Power Point Presentation.

---. "Basic Gardening Techniques." March 2012. Power Point Presentation.

---. "Container Gardening." April 2013. Power Point Presentation.

---. "Backyard Composting: The Easy Way." August 2013. Power Point Presentation.

---. "Your First Garden." March 2014. Power Point Presentation.

---. "Totally Tomatoes." March 2016. Power Point Presentation.

---. "Advanced Vegetable Gardening." February 2015. Power Point Presentation.

---. "Growing Garlic in Zone 4." March 2015. Power Point Presentation.

---. "Planting by Artists." June 2015. Power Point Presentation.

---. "HCMG Square Foot Gardening." June 2015. Power Point Presentation.

---. "No Soil, Early Frost, No Problem." March 2016. Power Point Presentation.

---. "Flowerless Flower Gardens." June 2016. Power Point Presentation.

---. "Hydro for Year-Round Gardening: webinar." January 2017. Power Point Presentation.

---. "Gardening After Surgery: Deliverance." August 2018. Power Point Presentation.

---. "Gardening Before Surgery: Proactive Preparation." October 2018. Power Point Presentation.

"Plants Clean Air and Water for Indoor Environments," NASA, *http://spinoff.nasa.gov/Spinoff2007/ps_3.html*.

(*https://lpi.oregonstate.edu/*).

"Benefits Stemming from Space Exploration," NASA, September 2013, *http://www.nasa.gov/sites/default/files/files/Benefits-Stemming-from-Space-Exploration-2013-TAGGED.pdf*.

BIBLIOGRAPHY

Dickson, Ryan and Fisher, Paul. "Edible crop species differ in their pH effect in hydroponics." Producer Grower, August, 2017.

Funkenbusch, Karen, MA and Willard Downs, PhD. "Tips and Techniques for The Senior Gardener. Agricultural Engineering Extension, University of Missouri Extension Center

Heather L. Papinchak, et al., "Effectiveness of Houseplants in Reducing the Indoor Air Pollutant Ozone," Hort Technology, April-June 2009; 19(2): 286-290, *http://horttech.ashspublications.org/content/19/2/286.full*.

Heather. "Best Liquid Fertilizer Nutrients for Hydroponics Plant Growth in 2019." June 2, 2018. Copyright by Origin Hydroponics, 2019.

Hopper, Eric. "Dry Fertilizers vs Liquid Fertilizers." Fertilizer & Plant Nutrition Articles, April, 2016.

http://chiropracticasleytdj.storybookstar.com/some-fundamentals-on-major-issues-in-when-sciatica-is-cancer

http://http://americanhostasociety.org/

http://sporty7.blogspot.com/2011/05/tai-chi-for-beginners.html

http://www.careukgroup.com/news/resume-gardening-after-a-total-hip-or-knee-replacement-professional-advice-from-a-physiotherapist

http://www.dowlingcommunitygarden.org/pages/projects.htm

http://www.motherearthnews.com/organic-gardening/gourmet-garlic-hardneck-vs-softneck-zbcz1404.aspx

http://www.universaldesignstyle.com/terraform-wheelchair-accessible-garden-kit/

http://www.webgrower.com/regional/pdf/Winter-Gardening-OR_pnw548.pdf for charts and information for the Pacific Northwest.

https://bonesmart.org/wp-content/uploads/2010/10/Knee_arthritic-1000-1024x790.jpg

https://extension.umn.edu/yard-and-garden

https://www.bing.com/images/search?q=Handicapped+Raised+Bed+Gardening+Plans&FORM=IDINTS

https://frameimage.org/calend%C3%A1rio-2018-feriados-rj-e-nacionais-para-imprimir/

https://i.pinimg.com/736x/3f/ab/6b/3fab6b38efab470332859a6639dab31f.jpg (Potatoes-Chinese Scientist)

https://live.staticflickr.com/8496/8411942287_8fb43aa849.jpg

https://originhydroponics.com/best-fertilizer-nutrients-for-hydroponics/ <<liquid vs granular; organic vs. synthetic

https://permaculturenews.org/2014/10/04/plants-attract-beneficial-insects/

https://time.com/5105027/indoor-plants-air-quality/

https://www.flora.dempstercountry.org/Flower.Glossary.html

https://www.gardeningknowhow.com/.../containers/plants-in-galvanized-containers.htm

https://www.gardeningknowhow.com/edible/vegetables/vgen/raised-vegetable-gardens.htm

https://www.gardeningknowhow.com/garden-how-to/lifestyle/garden-fitness-more-than-a-hobby-its-good-for-you.htm

https://www.gardeningknowhow.com/garden-how-to/lifestyle/the-love-of-gardening-one-of-americas-most -addictive-hobbies.htm

https://www.gardeningknowhow.com/special/accessible/sensory-garden-ideas.htm

https://www.goodreads.com/author/show/186361.Jeff_Gillman

https://www.healthline.com/health/tetanus.htm

https://www.healthline.com/nutrtion/oxalate-good-or-bad

https://www.mayoclinic.org/diseases-conditions/e-coli/symptoms-causes/syc-20372058

https://www.motherearthnews.com/organic-gardening/pest-control/plants-to-attract-beneficial-insects-zl0z1005zvau

https://www.msn.com/en-us/news/markets/us-vertical-farms-are-racing-against-the-sun/ar-AADTH97?ocid=News

https://www.oercommons.org/authoring/24036-introduction-to-anatomy/view

https://www.seedsnsuch.com/gardener'sgreenroom.html

https://www.shawangunkjournal.com/sj/180614/5162/Jumping-Worms-Will-Eat-Your-Lawn!.html.

https://www.thespruce.com/is-gardening-good-exercise-1401896

https://www.treehugger.com/lawn-garden/terraform-raised-bed-makes-gardening-accessible-mobility-impared.html

https://www.webmd.com/mental-health/news/20041022/pungent-onions-make-potent-cancer-fighters

https://www.wikihow.com/Dress-After-a-Shoulder-Surgery

Luz Claudio, "Planting Healthier Indoor Air," Environmental Health Perspectives, October 2011; 119(10): a426-a427, http://www.ncbi.nlm.nih.gov/pmc/articles/PMC3230460/.

Sustainable Gardening: The Oregon-Washington Master Gardener Handbook, EM 8742 (Oregon State University, Corvallis, published 2000.

www.PartnershiForTick-borneDiseasesEducation.org.

BIBLIOGRAPHY

Arthritis References

https://liem-acupuncture.com/arthritis/ [normal-arthritic joint]

https://www.health.com/health/gallery/020443624,00.html

https://www.ndtv.com/health/rheumatoid-arthritis-lose-weight-and-quit-smoking-for-treatment-1877015

https://www.timesleader.com/features/710910/to-your-health-understanding-arthritis-may-help-with-treatment-for-pain

https://www.webmd.com/osteoarthritis/guide/options-basics?print=true

Startribune.com. "Cutting 300 calories can improve health." (June 28, 2019).

www.Mayo Clinic, diseases, arthritis, symptoms, 20350772

Collaborating with Your Care-Team

Guenard, Rebecca. "The Allergens in Natural Beauty Products", January 21, 2015. https://www.theatlantic.com/archive/2015/01/the-allergens-in-natural-beauty-products/384326

http://holycrossleonecenter.com/blog/top-20-questions-to-ask-your-orthopedic-surgeon-prior-to-surgery/

http://www.chirosportspecialists.com/wp-content/uploads/2017/05/Stretch-5.jpg

http://www.wrha.mb.ca/extranet/nutrition/files/ClientEd-HealthLifestyles-SurgeryAlcohol.pdf

https://365daystoendingheartdisease.files.wordpress.com/2013/01/dr-willett-dood-pyramid.jpg FOOD Pyramid

https://anesthesiology.pubs.asahq.org/data/Journals/JASA/930989/18FF01.png

https://cdn.shopify.com/s/files/1/0705/2895/files/7008_One_Arm_Bent_Over_Back_Rows_Lawn_Mower.png?195

https://cdn1.dailyhealthpost.com/wp-content/uploads/2017/09/9neckexercisesinfographics.jpg (((NECK))

https://exercisesforinjuries.com/wp-content/uploads/2014/11/Wall-Push-Up-Plus.jpg

https://my.clevelandclinic.org/patients/information/questions-to-ask-your-doctor

https://nusantarafood.me/ [desk exercises]

https://pbs.twimg.com/media/Dz5ZD_IXQAA3kWS.jpg

https://qph.fs.quoracdn.net/main-qimg-ec1b7fd77871e742eaeeeb043ad725fe-c [neck exercises]

https://www.bing.com/images/search?q=dr.+willett+food+pyramid&qpvt=Dr.+Willett+food+pyramid&FORM=IQFRML

https://www.bing.com/images/search?q=Plantar+Flexion+Movement&FORM=IDINTS

https://www.bpp2.com/treating-tennis-elbow-tyler-twist/

https://www.fitness19.com/aerobic-and-anaerobic-exercise-what-is-the-difference/

https://www.footlevelers.com/school-resources/876-5-simple-exercises-to-help-keep-your-feet-healthy

https://www.healthline.com/health/fitness-exercise/exercise-for-obese-people#1

https://www.healthline.com/health/pain-in-buttocks

https://www.healthline.com/health/rotator-cuff-injury-stretches

https://www.healthline.com/health/shoulder-pain/stretches-at-work#prevention

https://www.healthydietbase.com/the-best-exercises-for-ex-smokers/

https://www.hopkinsmedicine.org/healthlibrary/conditions/surgical_care/questions_to_ask_before_surgery_85,P01409

https://www.medicinenet.com/surgery_questions/article.htm

https://www.nbcnews.com/better/health/real-reason-going-doctor-gives-you-anxiety-ncna795566

https://www.shape.com/fitness/tips/worst-exercises-equipment

https://www.surgeryencyclopedia.com/

https://www.webmd.com/healthy-aging/features/ask-surgeon?print=true

https://www.webmd.com/pain-management/neck-exercises-dos-donts?print=true

https://www.wfaa.com/article/news/nation/yoga-vs-tai-chi-which-is-better/311901475

https://www.whyiexercise.com/images/illustrated.stretching.exercises.thumbnails.jpg ((stretching X))

https://www.wisegeek.com/what-is-the-difference-between-aerobic-and-anaerobic-exercise.htm

Karen E. Dennis, Andrew P. Goldberg. Women. "Addictive *Behaviors* January – February 1996.

Kelly H. Webber, Deborah F. Tate, J. Michael Bowling. *"A randomized comparison of two motivationally enhanced Internet behavioral weight loss programs." Behaviour Research and Therapy* September 2008.

Kelly H. Webber, Ph.D., MPH, RD., Deborah F. Tate, PhD., Dianne S. Ward, EdD, J. Michael Bowling, Ph.D. *"Motivation and Its Relationship to Adherence to Self-monitoring and Weight Loss in a 16-week Internet Behavioral Weight Loss Intervention." Journal of Nutrition Education and Behavior* May – June 2010.

Lora E. Burke, Ph.D., MPH, Mindi A. Styn, Ph.D., Susan M. Sereika, Ph.D., Molly B. Conroy, MD, MPH, Lei Ye, BMed, Karen Glanz, Ph.D., MPH, Mary Ann Sevick, ScDd, Linda J. Ewing, PhD. *"Using mHealth Technology to Enhance Self-Monitoring for Weight Loss: A Randomized Trial."* American Journal of Preventative Medicine July 2012.

Noreen M. Clark, PhD., Julia A. Dodge, MS *"Exploring Self-Efficacy as a Predictor of Disease Management."* Health Education and Behavior. February 1999.

Victor J. Strecher, Ph.D., MPH., Brenda McEvoy DeVellis, PhD., Marshall H. Becker, Ph.D., MPH, Irwin M. Rosenstock, Ph.D. Change. "Health *Education and Behavior."* March 1986.

www.custompilatesandyoga.com/cat-cow-exercise/

www.dermatologypa.org "Fragrance and Botanical Free Regimen."

www.mckessoncorp.com

www.sepalika.com

Long and Ridiculously Long Urls

You are reading the first paperback printing which includes URLs that are a tad long. A bit difficult to copy and paste them into your browser which could result in errors or a message that indicates that that URL is an outdated website or a website that non longer exists. I have not included the entire URL for your viewing pleasure. Instead, I have relied on https://tinyurl.com/ to shorten the URL. In any event, I trust this will help you find some of the illustrations, photos and cartoons that I used to research the content of this book.

httops://tinyurl.com/sgbjymt [top 5 Alcohol Support Supplements of 2019]

https://tinyurl.com/gk3k54g [Vegtrug planter]

https://tinyurl.com/ru7g4ax [square foot designs]

https://tinyurl.com/s78b7s5 [exercises for losing weight]

https://tinyurl.com/sz9f5or [spiral beds]

https://tinyurl.com/tc2c7ze [triceps]

https://tinyurl.com/tm72wnb [active hydroponic illustration]

https://tinyurl.com/u5mjer9

https://tinyurl.com/u5yjfea

https://tinyurl.com/u6hcobq [range of Motion illustrations]

https://tinyurl.com/ufffvf5 [stretching exercises]

https://tinyurl.com/ugwz5h8

https://tinyurl.com/uw3thrk [straw bale gardening]

https://tinyurl.com/vcpnp46 [tai chi symbol]

https://tinyurl.com/w2z96sv [Seppo cartoon and insecticide sprays}

https://tinyurl.com/w7qdlp2 [elective surgery]

https://tinyurl.com/wmegxyv [neck exercises illustrations]

https://tinyurl.com/yxy3oeqp [raised bed designs]

https://www.researchgate.net/profile [Comparison-between-a-normal-and-diseased-joint.png]

INDEX

Action Planning
    Force-Field Analysis, 277-278
    Self-Directed Action Plan, 180-181
Arthritis, 4-6
    Cancer, Alzheimer's, 231-233
    Cartilage, 6-8
    Natural Remedies, 229-230
Balance, Increasing, 18-19
    Preventing Falls, 236-237
Behavior Change, 26-29; See also Non-Food Diet
    Denial, 29-32
    Fear of, 32-34
    Resolutions, making, 279-280
    Soil to water, 118-120
Botanicals, Lavender, Allergies, 241-246
Critter Control, 246-248; See also Yard and Garden
    Integrated Pest Management, 89-90
    Jumping Earthworms, 248-249
    Ticks, 249-250
Elective Surgery, 2-3; 273; See also Medical Team
Ergonomic Toys, Tools, 100-104
    Checklist, buying, 102
Exercise, 188; 279-280; See also Pain Management; Tai Chi; Yoga
    Chart, Aerobic, Anaerobic, 284-285
    Classes, 19-21
    Non-Food Diet, 291-295
    Resolutions, making, 279-280
Exercising Body Parts; See also Non-Food Diet
    Assistive Devices, for, 189-190
    Core, 204-206
    Cross-Training, 222-224
    Elbows to Hands, 200-205

    Hips to Feet, 210-222
    Machines, 295-298
    Neck to Shoulders, 190-200
    Range of Motion, 185-188
    Spine-Thoracic, 206-210
    Standing or Sitting, 285-289
Food Ailments
    E. coli, 259
    Oxalic Acid, stones, 259-260
    Pesticides, 256-258
Foodies, food for
    Diet Pyramids, 265-272
    Dining out, 233
    Eat the Rainbow, 144-145
    Garlic, 254-256
    Super foods, 232-233
    Surgery, pre-post, 174
    Veggies, sugar in, 253-254
Hydroponics, 112-115; 150; See also Strawberries
    Advantages, 116-117
    Aquaponics, 141-142
    Basic Materials, 121-123
    Buckets, tool-free start, 123-124
    Containers, Food Safe, 123; 129
    Deep-Water Passive System, 120-121
    Disadvantages, 117-118
    Earth and Space, In, 260-263
    Fertilizers, 136-138
    Floating Gardens, 140-141
    LECA, 135-136
    Lighting, 130-131
    Net pots, 126-127
    Plant Options, 142-148
    Plants, store bought, 124-126
    PVC Pipe, Tubes, 127-129
    Starting Seeds, 132-133

Substrates, 131-132; 134 136
Sustainability, 262-263
Taste, 263-264
Totes, 127
Water Changes, 139-140
Watering Options, 138-139
Lifestyle Changes; *See also* Non-Food Diet
   Alcohol, 158-160
   Losing Weight, 157-158
   Smoking, 154-157
Medical Team, trust your, 160-162
   Anesthesia, 165
   Post-Surgery Checklist, 274-277
   Pre-Surgery Checklist, 171-174
   Questions, asking, 5Ws, 166-167
   Questions, answering, 168
   Surgery day, expectations, 175-177
   Surgery, Go, no go, 170-171
   Procedures, 163-165
Navigating After Surgery, 53; See also
   Planning, yard, garden
   Assistive Aids, Transferring from, 54-56
   Bum Bumping, 60-61
   Crutches 57-60
   Dressing, Undressing, 61-63
   Wheel-chairs, 56-57
Non-Food Diet, 291-295
NPK: Mnemonic, 264-265
Organizing, indoors
   Checklist, 44-53
Pain Management, 9
   Classes, 19-21
   Exercise, barriers, 14-15
   Exercising, 13-14

Lifting Weights, 21-23
Meditation, 23-26
Non-Surgical Options, 11-13
Pain Meds, 9-11
Walking, 15-19
Planning, Yard and Garden, 69; *See also*
   Critter control; Ergonomic toys, tools
   Accessibility Options, 90-100
   Animal Manures, 77; 259
   Benefits, 240-241
   Coconut coir, 73;132
   Companion Planting, 87-88
   Compost-Mulching, 74-76
   Container Options, 82-86
   Elevated Beds, 97-98
   Gardening, square foot, 92-94
   Green Manures, 72
   Integrated Pest Management, 89-90
   No-Till, 73
   Pathways, 76-77
   Pruning, 71-72
   Raised Beds, 94-97
   Season Extenders, 77-81
   Soil, pH, 104-106
   Watering Options, 106-107
   Wheel-chair Gardening, 98-100
   Winterizing and Springerizing, 69-77
Sports Envy, 38-44
Strawberries, growing, 146-149
   Checklist, 146-147
   Vernalization, 146
Tai Chi, 280-283
Yoga, 283-284

A LAST WORD OR TWO

My intent was to provide you with a wide range of practical suggestions and ideas. Some may not be practical for you. Some may not be compatible with what you believe you may or may not need to do to prepare for your upcoming elective procedure. And some of my suggestions may seem to infringe on your right to be, well, to be you. I understand that. You are responsible for the decisions you make. Whether those decisions result in a positive outcome for you rests with you. Yes, there can always be unforeseen consequences for decisions you make to do something or not to do something. All of that said, here is a bit of philosophical wisdom that may apply to you.

Change what you do because you believe that will be in your best interests. Live your life as you want. Do not change your life for others so that you will be accepted by them. Enjoy your life and time and dreams. It is your life and it will be the only one you have while on this planet. Embrace your circle of life. And, accept the consequences (whether they are positive or negative). Where are you now? Where would you like to be? It is your choice.

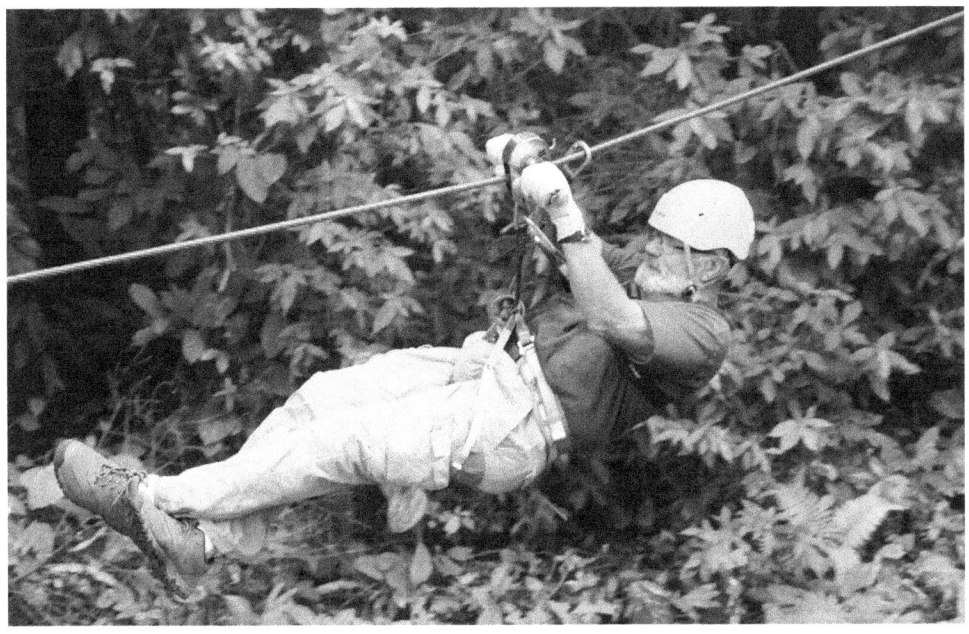

Zip-lining 1000 feet above a river gorge in Costa Rica after hip and knee surgery. Close to a real rush, 2019 (the zip-lining part).

BIOGRAPHY OF AUTHOR

Larry Cipolla was born and raised in Connecticut and has lived in Minnesota since 1970. He attended Manchester Community College, the University of Connecticut and the University of Minnesota, Graduate School and Spencer Foundation Research Fellow. He has been published since 1966 with more than 300 articles on leadership and management topics. He is an internationally recognized performance management and organizational development consultant and executive coach. He founded his company in 1976 and has traveled extensively, visiting more than forty countries to serve his client base. He is a US Air Force veteran and served in Europe and Asia from 1961-1965. Larry is a master gardener and life-long learner and frequent speaker to other master gardeners and garden clubs.

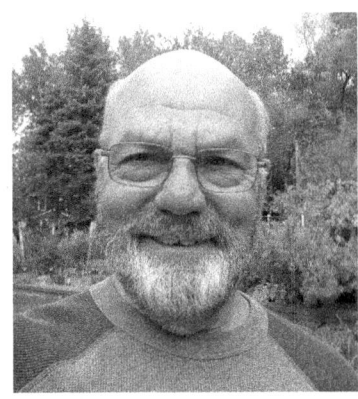

Thank you for buying my book.

Other books by the author

Hydroponic Gardening The Very Easy Way is the first comprehensive, step-by-step guide on how to grow fresh vegetables and herbs year-round, without pesticides, using the deep-water culture system. No gardening experience required. Through fifteen modules and dozens of photos, case studies and DIY projects, Larry Cipolla shows you how to build and use simple Deep-Water Culture systems to grow everything your taste buds crave, from sweet basil to salad greens to luscious tomatoes. You will learn how to build your own system with inexpensive food-safe buckets, totes and PVC tubes; what types of fertilizer and growing medium to use; what

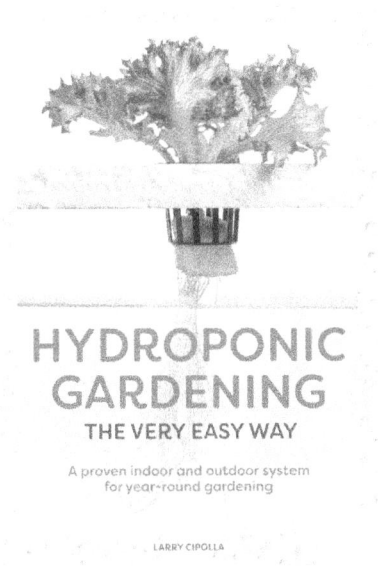

types of lighting units to buy and how to build your own portable light frames, and more. This book is for anyone who wants to grow and enjoy healthful, pesticide-free produce quickly, easily and inexpensively, both indoors and out. This type of hydroponic gardening works especially well for those who live in apartments, condos, and assisted-living and healthcare facilities.

© 2018, CCi Gardening Connections, ISBN: 978-1-975919-37-5. BISAC: Gardening/Techniques.

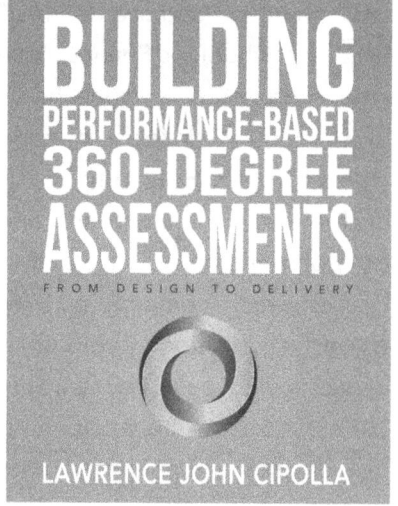

Building Performance-Based 360-Feedback Assessments: from design to delivery is the first book to focus on developing and delivering more effective 360-degree feedback assessment tools through web-based software. The book is substantive versus anecdotal. Larry Cipolla provides you with a step-by-step format that guides you through the essential process for creating dynamic assessments for any target population. It helps you assess the behaviors and practices that must be measured and optimized in our age of national and global competition. Internal and external HR trainers and OD consultants will be able to build powerful performance-based assessments that work for any target population in business, industry, government and educational organizations for the purpose of helping employees at all levels reach their performance potential.

© 2006-2008, Cipolla Companies, Inc, ISBN: 10-1-97924-558-4. BISAC: Reference.

Both books are available through the author and *www.Amazon.com*.

www.ingramcontent.com/pod-product-compliance
Lightning Source LLC
Chambersburg PA
CBHW080538220526
45466CB00010B/2963